Low-Calorie Dieti
For Dummies®

D1549029

What's in a Serving?

One way to keep track of how much food you're eating is to focus on portion sizes, rather than on individual calorie counts. Here's a quick-reference guide to standard portion sizes of different foods within each food group that provide approximately the same number of calories. Keep in mind that these guidelines are general; calories actually vary within each food group, depending not only on the food itself, but also how it's prepared. Use this chart to substitute one food for another and stay within your calorie range. See Appendixes A and B for additional calorie counts on a variety of foods.

Vegetables

One serving from this group, in the amount shown, provides about 25 to 45 calories.

- 1 cup spinach, lettuce, kale, collards, or other raw leafy green or uncut vegetables such as green beans, mini carrots, or snow peas
- ½ cup any other nonstarchy vegetables, cooked or finely chopped raw
- ½ to ¾ cup vegetable juice

Grains and starchy vegetables

One serving from this group, in the amount shown, provides about 80 calories.

- 1 slice bread
- 1 small (6-inch) tortilla
- ½ English muffin
- ½ small bagel
- ½ small (6-inch) pita
- ½ cup hot cereal
- ½ to ¾ cup cold cereal (1½ cups puffed cereal with no milk)
- ½ cup cooked pasta or rice
- ½ cup starchy vegetables such as peas or corn

Proteins

One serving, in the amount shown, provides between 150 and 250 calories.

- 3 ounces cooked lean meat, poultry, or fish
- 1 cup cooked dry beans, lentils, or split peas
- 1 to 1½ cups (2 to 3 ounces) tofu cubes
- 2 to 3 eggs
- 2 tablespoons peanut butter

Fruit

One serving from this group, in the amount shown, provides about 60 to 80 calories.

- 1 small to medium apple, banana, orange, peach, or other whole fruit
- ½ grapefruit or mango
- ½ cup chopped fruit
- 15 grapes or 12 cherries
- 7 dried apricot halves, 3 prunes, or 2 tablespoons raisins
- ½ cup fruit juice

Fats

One serving, in the amount listed, provides about 35 to 40 calories. Reduced-fat spreads often contain fewer calories.

- 1 teaspoon butter, margarine, regular salad dressing, regular mayonnaise, or vegetable oil

Milk and dairy products

One serving, in the amount listed, provides 150 to 200 calories. Lower-fat and fat-free dairy products often contain fewer calories. For instance, whole milk contains about 150 calories per cup while 2 percent lowfat milk contains 120 calories per cup, and skim milk contains only 90 calories per cup. When considering flavored yogurts and other dairy products, however, be sure to check the nutrition labels for actual calorie counts because lower fat doesn't always mean fewer calories.

- 1 cup whole milk or yogurt
- 1½ ounces cheese such as cheddar, muenster, brie, blue, Swiss, or mozzarella
- ½ cup ricotta cheese
- ⅓ cup grated Parmesan or Romano
- 2 ounces American cheese

Low-Calorie Dieting For Dummies®

Cheat Sheet

Surveying Sample Low-Calorie Menus

You can take the following calorie-controlled menus with you wherever you go to use as guidelines for how much food you can eat throughout the day while sticking to a 1,500-, 1,200-, or 1,000-calorie diet plan. Use the portion size chart on this Cheat Sheet to make smart substitutions within each food group.

Sample menu: 1,500 calories

Breakfast

½ cup orange juice

1 cup mini shredded wheat cereal (add up to 2 tea-spoons sugar, if desired)

1 cup blueberries

1 cup skim milk (for cereal and coffee or tea)

Lunch

1 cup black bean soup

12 baked (6 regular) tortilla chips or 1 small soft roll

2 cups mixed green salad with 4 thin slices avocado (¼ of an avocado) and 1 tablespoon light dressing

1 fresh pear

Dinner

3 ounces skinless chicken breast

½ cup cooked rice (any variety)

½ cup roasted red peppers tossed with ¼ cup moz-zarella cheese cubes

Snacks

1 cup cantaloupe cubes

2 graham cracker squares

1 cup soft-serve or ½ cup regular frozen yogurt

Sample menu: 1,200 calories

Breakfast

1 small muffin (any flavor)

6 ounces flavored lowfat yogurt

¼ cup skim milk for coffee or tea

Lunch

1 cheese and tomato sand-wich made with 2 slices light bread, 2 ounces cheese (any variety), and 4 thin tomato slices

½ cup mixed fresh fruit salad

Dinner

3 ounces broiled salmon

½ cup mashed potatoes

1 cup steamed green beans

½ cup baby carrots

Snacks

2 rice cakes topped with 2 tablespoons apple butter

Sample menu: 1,000 calories

Breakfast

½ grapefruit (with up to 1 teaspoon sugar, if desired)

1 scrambled egg

1 slice light bread with 1 tablespoon jam

¼ cup skim milk for coffee or tea

Lunch

6 ounces (¾ cup) lowfat vanilla yogurt topped with 2 tablespoons lowfat granola

1 small banana

Dinner

½ cup cooked rotelle pasta or other small shaped pasta

¼ cup marinara sauce

2 teaspoons grated Parmesan cheese

1 lean turkey sausage (about 2 ounces)

1 cup steamed broccoli or ½ cup steamed spinach

Snacks

12 grapes

½ ounce cheese (any variety)

For Dummies: Bestselling Book Series for Beginners

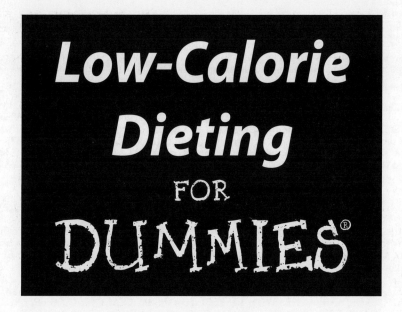

Low-Calorie Dieting FOR DUMMIES®

by Susan McQuillan, MS, RD

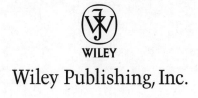

WILEY

Wiley Publishing, Inc.

Low-Calorie Dieting For Dummies®

Published by
Wiley Publishing, Inc.
111 River St.
Hoboken, NJ 07030-5774
www.wiley.com

WILEY

About the Author

Susan McQuillan, a registered dietitian, writes about food, nutrition, and weight control from her home in New York City. She received her bachelor's degree in dietetics management from New York University and her master's degree in human nutrition from Hunter College, both in Manhattan. She was formerly a food and nutrition editor at *American Health* magazine and *Reader's Digest* general books division. Susan is the author of *Breaking the Bonds of Food Addiction* (Alpha/Penguin) and a contributor to many health and nutrition-related books and cookbooks. Her articles and recipes have appeared in *Woman's Day, Family Circle, Cooking Light, Prevention, Fitness, Women's Sports and Fitness, McCall's,* and *Fit Pregnancy* magazines.

Dedication

To Molly, who never misses a meal, but who often has to wait for dinner while her mom is helping other people find better ways to eat.

Author's Acknowledgments

First, I must thank my acquisitions editor, Mikal Belicove, who recommended that I write this book and then worked very hard to get it off the ground. My project editor, Georgette Beatty, was my best motivator throughout this project, showering me with words of praise and encouragement at every turn. Thank you, Georgette! Many thanks also to Chad Sievers, copy editor extraordinaire, for ensuring clarity and adding a touch of humor, and to Emily Nolan and Patty Santelli, for double-checking the accuracy and taste of the recipes and making sure my calorie counts were correct.

I'm in great debt to every dieter who has ever shared his or her weight-loss story with me and every weight-control expert who understands that it's not just about the food. Your contributions are invaluable.

Much gratitude goes, as always, to the ever-growing list of people who provide me with such generous amounts of friendship and support. Special thanks to David Ricketts, Dui Seid, Ray Robbenolt, Lorraine Kenny, Sally Xuereb, Juliette Knight, Andrea Sperling, Esther and Jaimie Meyers, and last, but never least, my mother, Irene McQuillan.

Publisher's Acknowledgments

We're proud of this book; please send us your comments through our Dummies online registration form located at www.dummies.com/register/.

Some of the people who helped bring this book to market include the following:

Acquisitions, Editorial, and Media Development

Project Editor: Georgette Beatty

Acquisitions Editor: Mikal Belicove

Copy Editor: Chad R. Sievers

Technical Editor: Stacey Lyn Faryna, RD, ACSM Health/Fitness Instructor

Recipe Tester: Emily Nolan

Nutritional Analyst: Patty Santelli

Editorial Manager: Michelle Hacker

Editorial Assistants: Hanna Scott, Nadine Bell

Cover Photo: © Wiley Publishing, Inc.

Cartoons: Rich Tennant (www.the5thwave.com)

Composition Services

Project Coordinator: Kathryn Shanks

Layout and Graphics: Mary Gillot, Lauren Goddard, Stephanie D. Jumper, Barbara Moore, Julie Trippetti

Special Art: Elizabeth Kurtzman

Proofreaders: Laura Albert, Leeann Harney, TECHBOOKS Production Services

Indexer: TECHBOOKS Production Services

Publishing and Editorial for Consumer Dummies

Diane Graves Steele, Vice President and Publisher, Consumer Dummies

Joyce Pepple, Acquisitions Director, Consumer Dummies

Kristin A. Cocks, Product Development Director, Consumer Dummies

Michael Spring, Vice President and Publisher, Travel

Kelly Regan, Editorial Director, Travel

Publishing for Technology Dummies

Andy Cummings, Vice President and Publisher, Dummies Technology/General User

Composition Services

Gerry Fahey, Vice President of Production Services

Debbie Stailey, Director of Composition Services

Contents at a Glance

Recipes at a Glance

Dinner

Snacks and Desserts

Table of Contents

Introduction

*I*f your love affair with food is out of hand or if you've developed a love-hate relationship with food that makes eating an unpleasant experience, you have the right book in your hands. I've been a dietitian, and a food and nutrition writer and editor, for almost 20 years. I've seen it all when it comes to weight control — every diet, every gimmick, every scheme devised to trick people into thinking that weight loss will come easy if you just buy the right product or read the right book. I'm here to convince you that the only real solution to weight control is to eat right, exercise regularly, and stay away from fad diets. I offer no gimmicks, but I can make this promise: If you're ready to give up on quick-fix diets and commit to a low-calorie lifestyle, you'll shed pounds and maintain a healthier weight for good.

Whether you're trying to lose 15 pounds or 150 (or some number of pounds in between), there's only one sure way to do it. You must eat less and exercise more. If that's all you need to know, then you can close this book and start losing weight. If you need a little more guidance, read on.

About This Book

In this book you can find a low-calorie diet plan, complete with weeks and weeks of calorie-controlled menus and more than 60 optional recipes. (Optional means that the recipes fit right into menu plans, but you don't have to use them if you don't feel like cooking.) You can skip the first five chapters of this book, if you prefer, and go straight to the plan. Or, if you need some time to prepare yourself, you can start reading anywhere in this book and pick up plenty of weight-loss advice and inspiration.

I like to think that as soon as you start reading, you won't be able to put this book down; you'll want to consume every word (so to speak) from cover to cover. Every chapter is an independent, self-contained unit. If one chapter has something that needs explanation or information found in another chapter, you find a reference. You know where to go for more information.

Much of what's in this book may not apply to you right now. Weight loss happens in stages, and this book covers all those stages, so you probably want to find out what you need to know to get through the stage you're in right now. Then, when you're ready to move on to the next stage, you can flip to the appropriate chapter and read more.

That's the great thing about *For Dummies* books. You can open them up to any chapter and start reading; you don't have to start at the beginning and end at the end. In fact, *For Dummies* books never really end. They're reference books that you can keep on your bookshelf to refer to again and again.

Conventions Used in This Book

This book contains more than 60 recipes and several conventions hold for them. The best way to prepare any dish from a recipe, by the way, is to read the recipe through before you begin, gather all the required equipment and ingredients, and measure and prepare any ingredients as indicated in the ingredient list before moving on to the general directions.

For successful cooking, follow the recipe directions in step-by-step order and be aware of the following conventions:

- ✔ Ingredients are listed in the order in which they're used. Arranging them in this order on your work surface can be helpful.

- ✔ All measurements are level. Flour, sugar, and other dry ingredients are measured in graduated metal or plastic cups that can be filled to the top and leveled off with a metal spatula or the dull side of a knife. Liquid ingredients are measured in a spouted glass or plastic measuring cup with extra room at the top to prevent spilling. Place the measuring cup on a flat surface and fill with liquid, bending to read the measure at eye level, if necessary.

- ✔ Dairy products are usually reduced-fat or fat-free varieties unless otherwise specified.

- ✔ Eggs are large.

- ✔ Onions are yellow unless otherwise specified.

- ✔ Salt is table salt.

- ✔ Pepper is freshly ground black pepper unless otherwise specified.

- ✔ Preheating directions are included in all recipes that call for the use of an oven, grill, or broiler. Allow at least 15 minutes for the oven to come to the correct temperature.

- ✔ All temperatures are Fahrenheit. (Check out Appendix C for information about converting temperatures to Celsius.)

- ✔ A recipe that yields 4 servings may serve four people or it may serve only two or three, depending on the eating habits of your fellow diners. For you and anyone else who is following a low-calorie diet plan, a single serving fits the parameters of this diet.

✔ The nutrition information at the end of each recipe is based on the ingredients called for in that recipe. If you change the ingredients, the nutrition information will change too.

↻ If you need or want vegetarian recipes, scan the list of "Recipes in This Chapter" on the first page of each chapter in Part IV. A little tomato in front of the name of a recipe marks that recipe as vegetarian. (See the tomato to the left of this paragraph.)

Here are some other nonrecipe conventions you find in this book:

✔ *Italic* emphasizes and highlights new words or terms that are defined in the text.

✔ **Boldfaced** text indicates the action part of numbered steps.

✔ Monofont identifies Web addresses.

When this book was printed, some Web site addresses may have been broken across two lines of text. If you come across one like that, rest assured that I didn't put in any extra characters (such as a hyphen) to indicate the break. When you go to find the site, you can type in exactly what you see in this book, as if the line break doesn't exist.

What You're Not to Read

In a handful of instances in this book, you may find text preceded by a Technical Stuff icon. You can ignore this information if you're not interested in knowing more about the topic at hand. If you're in a hurry, you can also ignore the few sidebars (those shaded gray boxes) you see throughout the book. Although the information in these sidebars is topical and interesting, it's not essential to understanding the subject. Sidebar material and anything marked Technical Stuff both fall into the category of information that is merely nice to know.

Foolish Assumptions

I make very few assumptions about my readers, but I do know that some of you have been down this road before. Using this book may not be your first attempt at losing weight. If that's true, I can assume that you already know a lot about the basics of low-calorie dieting, so I try to keep everything as interesting and eye-opening for you as it is for first-timers.

Regardless of how many diets you've been on in your life, I can assume that right now you're looking for motivation and a good weight-loss plan because you're holding on to a strong vision of a leaner, healthier, you. Rest assured; this plan can help turn your dream into a reality.

How This Book Is Organized

This book contains 17 riveting chapters that have been organized into six parts, including the three appendixes. What follows is a summary of what you can find in each part.

Part I: Understanding the Basics of Low-Calorie Dieting

This part of the book helps you start a low-calorie diet plan by introducing you to easy-to-read weight charts and simple formulas so you can figure out how much weight you can realistically expect to lose and how many calories you need to cut from your diet in order to lose them. This part assists you to evaluate your weight-loss history, understand your metabolism, and see why eating well is so important on a low-calorie diet.

Part II: Getting Started: The Four-Week Plan and Beyond

In this part of the book, you establish your diet and fitness goals and discover how to prepare yourself (and your kitchen) for living a low-cal lifestyle. This part provides the actual diet plan, including four weeks of calorie-controlled daily menus you can follow strictly or use as guides to low-calorie eating. You can find food shopping tips and "alternative" menu plans to help keep your diet interesting. One of the most important chapters in this part helps you examine your attitude and see how it affects both your behavior and your ability to lose weight and maintain a healthier weight. You also find tools to help you improve your eating habits, increase your physical activity to burn more calories, find the motivation you need to stick to your plan, and track your progress.

Part III: Overcoming Obstacles and Moving On

Even though food is a central theme for dieters, it's really only one piece of the weight-loss puzzle. Losing weight and living a low-calorie lifestyle is also about facing the issues that drive you to overeating and finding nonfood ways to cope with stress, boredom, and other day-to-day frustrations that may or may not have something to do with your diet. In this part, you discover how to deal with situations that trigger overeating in and away from home. You figure out how to stick to your low-calorie lifestyle, prevent weight gain, and maintain your new, healthier weight after you've reached your goals. You also find resources for helping yourself and getting outside help when self-help isn't enough to keep you on your diet.

Part IV: Trying Time-Tested Low-Calorie Recipes

This part of the book is what my friends like best because here is where the food is, and my friends are the ones who get to taste most of the recipes before the book goes to print. Besides recipes and good ideas for low-cal breakfasts, lunches, and dinners, you also find plenty of treats and sweets. Along the way, this part helps you figure out just how to fit all this fabulous food into your low-cal diet plan.

Part V: The Part of Tens

Every *For Dummies* book has this part, which gives the author an opportunity to highlight important information. My favorite chapter in this part is the one that contains weight-loss inspirational stories from men and women who shared their own success stories. In this part you also find the "best of the best" reasons for losing weight and living a low-calorie lifestyle.

Part VI: Appendixes

Here you find two ways of counting calories — by individual foods and by food groups — plus a useful metric conversion guide.

Icons Used in This Book

Throughout this book, in the left margins, you find icons, or symbols, that serve as a guide to the type of material you're about to read. Here's what those icons mean:

The Remember icon points out information that has been summarized to make an important point. All information marked with a Remember icon is worth remembering!

The Tip icon marks helpful or practical information. It's not just reading material, it's news you can use. Wherever you see this icon, you can find advice, tips, and shortcuts for eating leaner, thinking smarter, moving more, and feeling better about yourself and your weight-loss plan.

When you see a Warning icon, it doesn't mean you're about to hear bad news or that anything scary is about to happen or that you need to avoid that particular paragraph. Au contraire! Warning icons point out information that can help prevent bad and scary things from happening, so don't step around that paragraph; read it just in case it applies to you.

Any information marked with the Technical Stuff icon is material that is a bit more academic than the rest. You can read it or skip it. It's not essential information, but if you do read it, you may find out something new.

Where to Go from Here

Every dieter is different, so a book like this one has to include a wide breadth of information and a variety of suggestions to help satisfy many needs. Many of the tips and advice in this book can help you. Depending on how long you've been trying to lose weight, you may have heard some of them before.

Your task, if you choose to accept it, is to decide, while you're losing weight, what will and won't work for you in the long run. Start wherever you want and work your way through this book to see what's in it for you. Regardless of where you begin, you'll end up knowing just what it takes to stay at a healthier weight.

Part I
Understanding the Basics of Low-Calorie Dieting

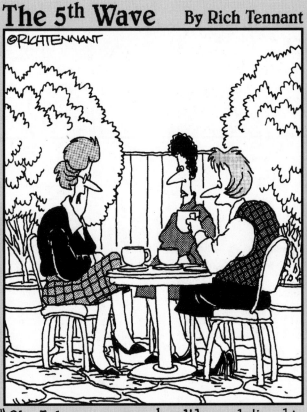

The 5th Wave   By Rich Tennant

@RICHTENNANT

"Oh, I have a very healthy relationship with food. It's the relationship I have with my scale that's not so good."

In this part . . .

Reading this part can help you ease into your low-calorie diet plan. In this part, you find help figuring out how overweight you are, how much weight you need to lose, and how best to approach a low-calorie plan. I hope you come away with a better understanding of how your metabolism works, the role of calories in weight control, and how important planning a nutritious diet at any calorie level is.

Chapter 1

Living a Low-Calorie Lifestyle

On any given day, one out of four Americans is doing something to try to lose weight. They change their diets, join gyms, swallow pills, and even undergo elective surgery in a never-ending attempt to shed those excess pounds. In spite of all these efforts, relatively few people are successful at losing weight and keeping it off. Most diets and weight-loss gimmicks are, at best, short-term solutions for weight control, and short-term means it's only for now, not forever.

By definition, your diet is simply the food you eat from day to day. With or without a plan, you could be following a vegetarian diet, a low-fat diet, a high-fiber diet, or a low-carbohydrate diet. Whatever it is, your current diet is how you choose to eat. A low-calorie diet is another story, though, with an altogether different meaning. To some people, it implies deprivation, suffering, and hunger. I'm here to change that point of view.

To say you're going on a diet implies that, at some point, you'll come off that diet and eat differently. It's temporary, and a temporary way of eating only has temporary effects. Look at it this way: If you have heart disease, your doctor or dietitian will probably recommend a low-fat diet. You can't follow that diet for just six months and expect it to keep your arteries clear forever. You must cut calories to lose weight and, at the same time, develop healthier eating habits. You can't turn back to your old habits if you expect to maintain a healthier weight for the rest of your life.

This chapter introduces the idea that the key to successful weight control is developing a low-calorie lifestyle plan. This chapter also explores the many facets of living a life devoted to lighter eating and better health. In this chapter you can find an overview of the tools you need, the plan's details, and the resources available to help you lose weight without fear of gaining it back. I discuss everything in greater detail throughout the book.

Deciding How Much Weight to Lose

Think about a time when you were at a comfortable weight. Now, think about how much you weigh right now. The difference between the two is probably the number of pounds you're aiming to lose. That's probably your long-term goal (which means you don't expect it to happen tomorrow, this week, or even this month, but you do expect it to happen eventually). Of course, you can rely on much more scientific ways to determine how much weight you can or need to lose. In fact, government health experts have established standards for healthy weights that you can use to gauge your own weight.

Check with your doctor before you start any weight-loss program to be sure that your weight-loss goals and strategies are appropriate for your age and state of health.

In this book, you can find six easy steps to help you figure out how much weight you need to lose, whether or not your weight is putting you at risk for serious health problems, and how to calculate a safe and effective calorie range within which you can lose excess weight. You can find more info on the first three steps in Chapter 2 and the last three steps in Chapter 3.

1. **Consult the healthy weight range chart in Chapter 2 to figure out how far you are from a healthy weight for your height.**

   Using charts and formulas for figuring out how much weight you need to lose, or how much you need to weigh after you lose the weight, helps keep your expectations within realistic limits. Your healthiest weight isn't necessarily the same as someone else's, even if that person is the same height. You may be built differently. That's why, when you look at a healthy weight range chart, you can see a range of acceptable weights for each height listed.

2. **Figure out your Body Mass Index (BMI) from the chart and formula.**

   This step helps you figure out whether or not your weight puts you at risk of developing or worsening chronic medical conditions such as high blood pressure, diabetes, and heart disease.

3. **Determine your waist-to-hip ratio.**

   This ratio tells you if the way your weight is distributed on your body puts you at higher risk of developing chronic medical conditions.

4. **Figure out your basic calorie needs.**

   Knowing this information can help you figure out the minimum number of calories you need in your diet every day.

5. **Calculate the number of calories you can eat and still lose weight.**

   This information is vital because it tells you the maximum number of calories you can allow in your diet every day.

If you've overweight, blame your fat

When you're overweight, you're also overfat. Otherwise, being overweight would mean that your excess weight is coming from muscles, bones, skin, and water. That's not likely unless you've built up so much muscle from strength training that you've gained weight from it, or you're retaining fluids for some reason, or you have impossibly dense bones that are adding to your normal weight. At most, you may be a few pounds over your usual weight if your extra weight is muscle from working out or water retention from hormone fluctuations. But neither of these are weight concerns.

Being overweight from extra fat, however, means that losing weight will probably be beneficial to your health. If you have a family history of high blood pressure, heart disease, diabetes, high cholesterol, or certain types of cancer, losing weight by cutting calories and getting more exercise can lower your risk of developing these conditions. If you already have these conditions, losing weight may improve them. (You can find more information about weight-related medical conditions in Chapter 16.)

6. **Give yourself a range of calories within which you can eat and still lose weight.**

   If you know this information, you can try to stick to the bottom of the calorie range and on days when you feel you need to eat more food, you can go as high as the top of the calorie range.

Many dieters aim for an unrealistic weight. If you have a tendency to compare your weight and shape to other people, you may find yourself wanting to lose more weight than is reasonable. Don't compare your size and shape to others. The combined effect of your age, rate of metabolism, body type, genetic predispositions, exercise habits, dieting habits, and the number of fat cells you carry in your body ultimately determine how much weight you can lose and what your body will look like at any weight. That package of factors belongs to you and nobody else and that's what makes everyone's body different. You can't stretch yourself any taller, change your bone structure, or borrow someone else's genes. Be realistic in your expectations and goal setting and spend your time planning to get into your own best possible shape.

If you're a control freak, you're not going to like the fact that even though you can control the amount of food you eat, and the amount of exercise you do, and even the way your mind works when it comes to losing weight, you may not have as much control as you want over how much you actually weigh. You can make every effort in the world to get down below, say, 120 pounds, but nothing short of starvation will get you there or keep your there if it's not a reasonable weight for you.

Understanding How to Live a Healthy Low-Calorie Lifestyle

Living a low-calorie lifestyle means adopting healthier eating and exercise habits for the rest of your life. It starts with a diet plan that cuts back on the number of calories you've been consuming so that you can achieve a healthier weight. Your new diet plan is designed to help you lose weight safely and effectively, and to grow into a lifelong plan for weight maintenance.

A safe low-calorie diet not only supplies enough energy to get you through each day, but it also provides the essential nutrients you need to get from food to stay healthy. The fewer calories you consume, the harder it is to get enough of those essential nutrients. The way to get the most nutritional value from your diet at any calorie level is to eat a well-balanced diet that contains a wide variety of foods. In Chapter 3, you find more information about the nuts and bolts of a nutritionally sound low-calorie diet.

Knowing exactly how many calories actually go into a low-calorie diet is also crucial. Chapter 6 contains four weeks of daily menu plans that contain from 1,000 to 1,500 calories a day. You may be thinking these menus contain the maximum number of calories you need to consume on a low-calorie diet, but in fact, I call them minimum-calorie menus. Yes, you need to put a top limit on your daily calories when you're on a low-cal diet to lose weight. But you need to put a bottom limit on your calorie count too, because if you go too low, you'll just trip yourself up. You'll find yourself caught in the type of starve/binge cycle that sabotages many a dieter's best intentions. When you start cutting calories, you can work within this range of 1,000 to 1,500 calories because most people can lose weight in this range. The top of this range (1,500 calories) may even be too low for you. If that's the case, you can add calories back in until you get to a point where you're more satisfied with the amount of food you're eating and still able to lose weight. You can always cut back again if you stop losing weight before you reach your goal.

You *never* want to go lower than 1,000 calories on a self-help diet plan. Just about anyone who needs to lose weight can lose it on a diet that allows between 1,000 and 1,500 calories, so you don't need to deprive yourself and eat less. Keep in mind that the closer you get to your goal weight, the more you may have to cut calories in order to keep losing. So first start your diet at the highest calorie count that, combined with enough physical exercise, allows you to lose about a pound or two a week.

Two things happen when you don't consume enough calories.

✔ Your body puts the brakes on your metabolism and you start burning calories less efficiently. That's your body's way of saving itself when it's afraid you're going to starve. If you don't give your body enough food, it has no way of knowing whether or not you'll be giving it more and so it prepares itself for living on less by slowing down the rate at which it uses food to produce energy.

✔ The other thing that happens when you don't eat enough is more immediate and more obvious: You get very hungry. If you allow yourself to get too hungry, guess what happens? You overeat. And there goes your diet.

Getting Started on Your Low-Calorie Plan

Living a low-cal lifestyle means putting your all into it — setting your life up in ways that accommodate your diet, such as stocking your kitchen with low-calorie cooking equipment, discovering new cooking techniques, if necessary, committing to an exercise program, and taking the time to find out as much as you can about food, nutrition, and fitness.

The very first step in a self-help weight-loss plan, though, is to look inward and figure out everything you can about yourself and about your eating and exercise habits. Then you can begin to change your bad habits and practice healthier new ones. Awareness is the first step because you have to know what you're doing wrong before you can make it right. (See Chapter 4 for more about looking inward.)

Psyching up with goals, tools, and more

Planning and record keeping are essential tools for weight loss because they provide both structure and a way of monitoring whether your program is working for you. I treat the following tools of the trade separately in this book, but you can keep these records in one journal. That way, you always know exactly where to find each one when you need it.

✔ Establishing short-term, intermediate, and long-term goals (Chapter 4)

✔ Keeping a food diary (Chapter 4)

✔ Filling in a weight change chart (Chapter 4)

✔ Maintaining an exercise log (Chapter 8)

You can also use this same journal to write down all your thoughts and feelings while you're trying to commit to a low-calorie lifestyle. If your journal is large enough, you can write down any interesting tips or advice you pick up along the way or even store a special low-calorie recipe that you don't have time to prepare right now but hope to use in the future. If you want to be ultraserious with your notebook, a three-ring binder with pocket inserts and tabbed dividers may not be a bad investment.

Setting up a low-calorie kitchen

People who are successful at weight loss often cook many of their own meals as a way of controlling the types and amounts of food they eat. You can find everything you need to know to get cooking in Chapter 5, which discusses healthy eating guidelines and shows you how to use those guidelines to create a nutritionally balanced low-calorie diet plan.

Chapter 5 also contains plenty of aisle-to-aisle advice on the best foods to buy in the supermarket to create healthful, low-calorie meals, how to stock your cupboards with the most healthful convenience foods, and how to equip your kitchen with a good selection of cookware and tools for steaming, poaching, and other great low-cal cooking methods.

Planning marvelous meals

The daily menu plans in Chapter 6, and the alternative "theme" menu plans in Chapter 7, are all designed to keep your diet life interesting by including different types of foods at every meal. If you're a creature of habit, you'll probably pick two or three menu plans at first and repeat them day after day. That's perfectly okay, as long as you don't get bored. And if you do eventually get bored, you have plenty of other menu plans to choose.

I developed the recipes in Chapters 12, 13, 14, and 15, covering breakfast, lunch, dinner, snacks, and desserts, to fit right into the menu plans in Chapter 6. I also designed them to be appealing to friends and family who aren't watching their weight. In other words, they taste good. They don't taste like "diet food," which is the beauty of preparing your own low-calorie meals from scratch, rather than relying entirely on calorie-controlled frozen dinners or liquid meal substitutes from the supermarket. After you've lost weight, you won't have to make a huge transition from "diet" food to "real" food because you're already eating real food every day.

When you cook, pay attention to the serving sizes of the dishes you prepare. If a recipe yields 4 servings, then one-fourth of the dish is the amount of food you can eat. By taking a good look at the portioned-out foods you prepare at home, you can figure out how to eyeball portion sizes when you eat out, and you can develop a good sense of approximately how many calories are on your plate, regardless of where you eat.

Exercising to burn calories and improve your health

As a dietitian, I focus mainly on food and nutrition, so to tell you the truth, it was years before I really understood just how important physical activity is to losing weight, maintaining weight, and staying as physically and mentally fit as possible. In fact, many people focus on food more than anything else when it comes to healthier living. You can only make so many changes at once and when the issue is weight control, it's natural to look at your diet first. But I'm here to tell you now that food is one half of the calorie equation and exercise is the other half. They carry equal weight, so to speak.

In Chapter 8, you find out that strength training is just as important as aerobic exercise. This chapter also discusses the many benefits of mind-body exercises, such as yoga, pilates, and t'ai chi. Make sure you check out the long list of ailments that exercise can help prevent and cure, because it's good motivational material for sticking to an exercise program for life.

Even if you already recognize the benefits of exercise in a low-calorie lifestyle, you may have trouble actually fitting it into your daily routine. Fear not; in Chapter 8, there are plenty of tips for finding your motivation to exercise, choosing the type of exercise that's right for you, and fitting exercise into your already crowded schedule.

As you age, staying the same shape and weight you were when you were younger becomes more difficult. For many, it's a never-ending battle trying to stop your various body parts from getting thick and baggy. Although some health experts say gaining some weight in midlife is normal, you may not like the direction in which your body is moving. I'm with you on that one! Eating light is important for both your weight and health as you get older, but exercise is the real weapon against the stalling metabolism and thinning muscle tissue that causes your weight to creep up with age.

Staying on the Low-Calorie Track

Food isn't everything when it comes to weight control. Sure, excess food packs on the pounds, and a lack of food helps you shed them, so food plays an extremely important role. And you absolutely have to know how to eat better in order to lose weight and maintain a healthier weight for life.

But consider this point: Everyone eats, but not everyone becomes overweight from eating. Some people seem to live on junk food but never gain weight. So there must be something else to this weight stuff, right? Right. And that something else may have more to do with what's happening in your mind than what's happening on your plate.

If you've been on weight-loss diets before, one of your first steps at this point is to look back over your previous diets and see what worked and what didn't. Focus on the time period when you started gaining back the weight you'd lost. What was going on? Why did you start overeating again? Or did you just stop going to the gym? Remembering what went wrong with your past diet plans helps prevent the same thing from happening again.

Even if this time is your first attempt at weight loss, read on, because it pays to be prepared for the challenges faced by most dieters. In the following sections, I discuss the roadblocks you may face, explain when and how to reassess your plan to be sure it continues to work for you, and give you tips for seeking extra help.

Working through challenges

What happens when you're trying to stick to a low-cal diet and you find yourself in the midst of an office party or your parents' 25th wedding anniversary celebration? One thing is for sure: You need a plan. For instance, you can bring a very light lunch the day of the office party and plan in advance to have a light dinner waiting at home. You can spend an extra 20 minutes at the gym the morning of the event.

You can find more ideas for dealing with special circumstances in Chapter 9, but remember that you're not going to blow your diet with one evening of celebratory overeating. The best advice anyone can give you is simply to enjoy yourself, try not to go overboard, and get back on your plan the next day. Every day can't be a party when you're on a low-calorie plan to lose weight, but when you're watching what you eat on a regular basis, you do have room in your calorie budget for occasional excess.

The challenges you face when you're trying to lose weight also include the daily events in your life that trigger you to eat in response to your emotions or to eat when you're not really hungry. The "cure" is to recognize and address these situations so you can eliminate eating triggers that have nothing to do with real hunger. Some of these triggers, such as boredom, loneliness, and anxiety, come from within you; others, such as dealing with an unpleasant work situation or an angry spouse, come from outside.

Regardless of where your overeating triggers come from, you have to figure out how to resist them before you can move on to a healthy weight. Otherwise, you'll continue to turn to food whenever you're coping with emotional situations. Chapter 9 discusses the many forms of emotional eating and offers solutions for dealing with trigger situations head on.

Assessing your progress from time to time

When you take the self-help approach to weight loss, you have to monitor yourself because you're the only one who can do it. (If you have a diet buddy, then you can monitor each other; see Chapter 11 about finding a diet buddy.) Even with a diet buddy, self-monitoring is important. Basically, you're both the dieter and the diet counselor. After you set up the diet plan, the dieter has to check in periodically with the diet counselor to make sure it's working. To self-monitor, stop occasionally and ask yourself the following questions:

- Are you happy with your program?
- Are you losing weight at a steady pace?
- Are you reaching your short-term goals?
- Is your support system working for you?
- What can you do to improve your low-calorie lifestyle?
- Does your food plan need revision?
- What's your next step?

Some of the tools you use to assess your diet include your scale (for weekly weigh-ins), your weight change chart (from Chapter 4), and any other logs and journals you use for keeping track of the food you eat, the calories you consume, the exercise you do, and any other information that may change as you progress from a low-calorie diet into a low-calorie lifestyle.

After you start your low-calorie plan, you can check out Chapter 7 for tips on reviewing your initial progress to make sure you're taking your plan in the right direction to ultimately reach your goals. When you've reached your goal weight and begin a weight-maintenance phase, Chapter 10 is a great resource for advice on adjusting your food and exercise plans and making a lifelong habit of using the weight-control techniques that have worked for you.

Looking for help

Presumably, you bought (or borrowed) this book because you're looking for help losing weight. Good idea! This book can help you figure out everything you need to know about losing weight and keeping the weight off. But that doesn't mean you won't, at some point, need additional help. Don't worry; help is everywhere!

If you're doing everything you know how to do to lose weight but you're just not losing anything, then seek help. Your network of family and friends is the first place to start. Successful dieters have a solid support system in place to cheer them on and help them build and maintain a healthier lifestyle. Most people can't do it alone.

At some point, you may want to look outside your immediate circle of family and friends for additional support and advice. Depending on what type of help you need, you can look in the following places:

- ✔ You can find local branches of commercial weight-loss centers in cities and towns throughout the United States and Canada.

- ✔ Many hospitals have their own in-house weight-loss programs.

- ✔ Some physicians specialize in weight control. Be sure to get a referral from someone you trust.

- ✔ Peer-led groups such as Overeaters Anonymous meet in churches, clinics, and other community centers in most cities and towns.

- ✔ A registered dietitian or state-certified nutritionist is qualified to help you formulate a weight-loss plan.

- ✔ Psychologists who practice cognitive-behavioral therapy sometimes specialize in weight issues.

Chapter 11 provides more information about how to know when you need outside help and how to go about finding it. Chapter 17, which contains ten stories from men and women who've battled their own bulges in a variety of ways, may also be helpful.

If your eating behavior is out of control and you suspect you have a full-fledged eating disorder, you can find a list of eating disorder treatment programs at www.addictionresourceguide.com.

Chapter 2

Figuring Out the State of Your Weight

The health and fitness business is booming, and more information about diet and nutrition is available than ever before. However, government statistics show that at least 30 percent, or almost one-third, of American adults are overweight. Translated to real numbers, approximately 60 million people in this country may improve their health prospects if they lose some of their excess weight. And that figure doesn't include the one out of five American children who are also carrying around more fat than medical experts believe is healthy.

Assessing your current weight situation and figuring out how you arrived in this state of being overweight are important first steps toward permanent weight control. This chapter can help you uncover this information as well as provide many helpful charts and formulas for figuring out just how far you are from your healthiest weight.

This chapter also contains plenty of food for thought to help you examine your weight history and understand its relevance to your current weight-loss goals. This information is necessary for success because you have to know where you are now before you can figure out where you're going next. And you also need to know how you arrived at the weight you are now, so that it doesn't happen again!

Ups and Downs: Discovering How People Gain and Lose Weight

Everyone who struggles with weight control knows at least one person who appears to eat truckloads of food but never gains a pound. It's maddening, isn't it — especially when that other person eats so much of your favorite junk food! Pinpointing the exact reasons why one person gains weight at the mere sight of a doughnut while another person can freely indulge is difficult, but the personal food choices you make and exercise habits you practice on a regular basis greatly impact it. Furthermore, you may not know enough about someone else's habits to judge. But differences in the less obvious, and less controllable, *metabolism,* basically how the body uses food to create energy, also greatly affect how a person loses or gains weight.

In the following sections, I define metabolism, describe its relationship to calories, and explain why some people gain (and lose) weight more easily than others.

Understanding the basics: Metabolism 101

Your *metabolism* is the sum total of all the chemical reactions and changes that are constantly going on in your body. These processes include fat production, protein breakdown, toxin removal, and the general growth, replacement, and repair of body cells that's necessary for overall good health. Concerning weight control, however, the focus is on *energy* metabolism, the process by which your body breaks down nutrients from food and converts them into energy.

Energy metabolism begins as soon as your body digests food and breaks it down into its respective nutrients. Your body can use three different nutrients for energy: carbohydrates, fats, and protein. (Alcohol also supplies energy, but because it contains no nutrients and can potentially damage your health, it's not considered a good source.) Together, carbohydrates, fats, and protein are known as *macronutrients.* (Check out Chapter 3 for more about these and other nutrients.) Your body metabolizes each of these macronutrients differently from the rest.

- ✔ Carbohydrates make energy.
- ✔ Proteins renew body cells in muscle, skin, and other organs, and produce energy if no carbohydrates are available.
- ✔ Fats make energy, or if not used, your body stores them directly as body fat.

In general, your metabolism works the same way as everyone else's, but the rate at which you metabolize nutrients is unique to you. How your body uses the food you eat to create energy, and how the different foods you eat affect your weight and your overall health, is a very individual matter. If you have a fast metabolic rate, you're able to burn calories more efficiently than someone with a slower metabolic rate. Many factors — age, gender, hormones, body composition, body temperature, and your current state of health — affect energy metabolism and help determine how effectively your body uses food to generate energy.

Identifying calories and why they matter

You can't see calories. You can't hear them. You can't even taste them. Even if you had a high-power microscope, you couldn't identify the calories in a sample of food. That's because a calorie isn't a "thing." It's a measurement, like an inch or an ounce or a mile. A *calorie* measures the amount of energy produced when your body metabolizes foods — or more accurately, the macronutrients in foods.

When a certain type of food contains a certain amount of calories, what that really means is that as soon as your body metabolizes a certain amount of food, that food can provide a certain amount of energy. How many calories are in a particular food depends on how much carbohydrate, fat, or protein the food contains. (You can find the calorie content of these individual macronutrients in Chapter 3.)

If the number of calories you consume equals the number of calories you burn, you'll maintain your current weight. If you consume more calories than your body uses on a regular basis, you gain weight and store those extra calories as fat. I'm sorry, but you can't avoid it. If you consume fewer calories than your body burns on a regular basis, you lose weight. There's no other way.

To lose weight and keep it off, you have to find your own individual balance between the calories you consume and the calories you burn. Exercise does boost your metabolism so that you burn calories more efficiently. The more you exercise, the more calories you'll burn. Even when you increase your exercise, however, you only lose weight if you're consuming fewer calories than your body needs to fuel all that additional activity. It's that simple. If your exercise routine is very intense, you may find yourself ravenous after your workouts and, as a result, consuming too many extra calories to lose weight. The solution is to keep an eye on your total daily calorie intake and be sure to factor in some snack calories every day. That way, if your exercise routine leaves you hungry, you can use your snack calories to tide you over until it's time to eat a regular meal.

As you age, your metabolism starts slowing down and the rate at which you burn calories drops by about 2 percent every ten years. If you're still consuming the same number of calories at age 40 that you did at age 20, and you're not exercising more, you can easily start putting on 10 or more pounds a year.

Figuring out why gaining weight is so easy for some people

Gaining weight is easy — many people do it! All you have to do is get into the habit of eating the types and amounts of food that contribute more calories than you can possibly metabolize as energy. That's all it takes. The years go by, and your eating habits catch up with you. Just 100 excess calories a day (the number of calories in a handful of pretzels or a couple of mini muffins) adds up to 36,500 excess calories at the end of a year and those calories result in a 10½ pound weight gain. After just a few years, you have a big weight problem.

You may be the type of person who gains weight just looking at a cheese platter, while your coworker can devour second and third helpings without putting on an ounce. Her metabolism is different from yours. It's probably faster. Chances are, though, her attitude toward food and exercise is different too. She may dislike exercise as much as you do, but she may have figured out what she needs to do in terms of exercise because she feels the payoff is worth it.

Some people simply move more than others throughout the natural course of their day, which helps them maintain a healthier weight. Thanks to a documented phenomenon known as the "fidget factor," these people burn several hundred calories a day just by their use of body language. They often walk fast and talk fast, and they can't sit still for long. Even if their jobs keep them in front of a computer all day, they have to get up frequently and move around. If you know someone who frequently fidgets, you've probably noticed that he or she can get away with eating more food than someone with a calm demeanor.

Everyone who has ever tried to lose weight knows that losing weight isn't always as simple as balancing eating and exercise. Other factors are involved in weight gain. For instance, if being overweight or obesity runs in your family, then you may have a genetic predisposition to easy weight gain. On the other hand, even if your parents, siblings, grandparents, aunts, and uncles are mostly overweight, it may not be in your genes. It may just be that you picked up bad eating habits.

Many of your diet routines — the times of day you eat, the types of food you choose, the reasons why you eat, and even your habits of eating slowly or quickly, reading the newspaper, or watching television while you eat — probably came from your parents, who "inherited" them from their parents, and so on. See "Examining your family history" later in this chapter for more about taking your family history into account.

Recognizing why losing weight is so hard for some people

Unlike gaining weight, losing weight when you're healthy is rarely easy. Why? Losing weight just isn't as simple as gaining weight. To gain weight, you don't have to understand all the different reasons why you're doing it. You just have to overeat or underexercise. To lose weight, and lose it for good, however, you need to have a better understanding of how and why you gained weight so you don't just keep on repeating the behavior. (See the next section to figure out how you reached your current weight.)

For some people, being overweight becomes a chronic condition, just like heart disease or osteoporosis. It won't go away by itself and no quick-fix diet can resolve it. You need a lifetime plan that includes a calorie-controlled diet and exercise program you can comfortably stick with.

Hundreds of strategies for losing weight are available, but not every plan works for every person. Everyone has a different build, metabolism, genetic makeup, and tolerances and preferences for diet and exercise plans. That's why no one-size-fits-all diet exists. You have to participate in the development of your own personal weight-control plan to be successful. Your plan must be flexible, and it has to keep you feeling happy and satisfied or you won't feel motivated to stick to it.

Gaining weight is something you can do by yourself, but to lose weight, most people need the support of family, friends, and, often, strangers in the form of professionals and members of support groups. In the past, if diets have failed you, your support system may have been weak. If so, you may have given up and gone back to your old habits.

Although asking others for help may be difficult, now is most certainly the time to do it! If you don't have much of a built-in support system by way of family and friends, search for a weight-loss support group that you feel comfortable with. Flip to Chapter 11 for more handy tips on asking for help and using outside resources.

A Trip through Time: Taking Stock of How You Arrived Here

What's your weight story? Have you lost and gained weight over the years or is reading this book your first attempt at losing weight? Have you been overweight most of your life or did you put on the "freshman 15" in college and watch your weight story go downhill from there? Maybe you gained weight when you settled down and got married or after you had a baby. Or, maybe you've been watching your weight for quite a while but just can't knock off those last 10 pounds.

Whatever your story is, you need to examine your own weight history to see how you reached your present weight. At the same time, take a look at your family history — your parents, grandparents, aunts, uncles, cousins, and siblings — to identify any pattern you may be following.

Reviewing your weight history

Looking back can be good when you're trying to lose weight. I don't mean looking back and regretting every cookie you ever put in your mouth or remembering all the times you tried to lose weight and failed. Rather, take the time to look back for clues that can help you figure out when and how you became overweight so you can move forward without making the same mistakes you've made in the past. (For ideas about how to deal with old challenges in new ways, see Chapter 9.) If you've tried to lose weight in the past, figure out what worked and what didn't work for you so you can focus on any tips and advice that helped you stay on track (see "Evaluating your diet history" later in this chapter to get started).

The skinny on fat cells

You may be overweight because you have extra fat cells in your body, or because the fat cells you have are jumbo size. When you overeat, you're essentially feeding your fat cells. When you gain weight, each individual fat cell gains weight. When fat cells get to be around three times their normal size, they can split and you end up with more fat cells than you had before. (The point at which a fat cell actually divides varies from person to person.) This process of cell division wouldn't be so terrible if fat cells died the way other old body cells do, but no. Your fat cells live as long as you do.

Researchers once thought that people could only grow new fat cells during specific stages of growth, such as the first year of life and puberty. But it turns out, people can grow them as adults, too. If you've gained a lot of weight as an adult, you may be carrying around many more fat cells than you did when you were younger.

When you lose weight, your fat cells shrink and lose weight, too, but they don't go away. Fat cells are evil. They hang around in your body, just waiting to fill up on more fat. They want nothing more than to sabotage your attempt to lose weight. Don't give in! Don't let them win! The only way to come out on top is to stop overeating and get enough exercise to burn away spare calories from excess food that may find its way into your fat cells.

Overweight babies often turn into overweight adults. If you were a chubby baby who turned into a chubby kid and grew to be an overweight teenager, then you're probably an overweight or obese adult. If you were an overweight child, odds are that you may struggle with your weight as an adult. Don't fret though. You have hope. The best thing you can do is be realistic. Accept the challenge you've been given and move on. (Check out the next section about how your family history can affect your weight.)

If you didn't have weight problems growing up, losing any excess weight you've accumulated in your adult years may be easier, because your weight gain is probably circumstantial. You may have gained weight because you left home and freed yourself from your parents' strict rules about what you could and couldn't eat and started eating more junk food. Now you need to get back on track and make healthier choices. Or you may just need to discover a little more about how your metabolism naturally slows down as you get older and what you can do about it.

Examining your family history

If being overweight is a part of your family history, the bad news is that you may have inherited a genetic tendency to become overweight yourself. That's the sad truth. When you inherit a tendency toward being overweight, it's the same as having a family history of any medical problem. Although you may or may not be affected, you have to be careful and do what you can to prevent the same thing from happening to you. The good news: If you see that you're starting to resemble the heavyweights in your family, you can do something about it. You didn't inherit any actual fat, you only inherited a tendency to collect it. To a certain degree, you can control your tendencies and change your destiny.

If being overweight runs in your family, losing weight is probably going to be harder for you than for someone with leaner relatives. If you inherited bad eating habits along with a genetic tendency to gain weight, losing weight is even more of a challenge. You'll be fighting your genes *and* trying to break a lifetime of bad habits at the same time. You can do it! (Check out Chapter 4 for info and tips on breaking bad habits.)

If you're not the only overweight family member, you may be able to enlist the help and support of other relatives who are struggling with similar issues. If you live with family members who are overweight, you can follow these suggestions and make it a family effort:

✔ **Figure out how your immediate family members can help you and per-haps help themselves at the same time.** The best thing you can do is employ practical solutions. Reading this book is a good start. No lectures, please!

✔ **Cook together or share what you know about low-calorie cooking.** If your mother or significant other does the cooking in the house and you want it done differently, share a few low-calorie cooking tips. You can also spend time and discover tips together. (Chapter 5 is a great place to start.)

✔ **Go food shopping together.** Make grocery shopping a family affair. While shopping, monitor each other's choices as you walk up and down the aisles.

✔ **Exercise together.** Get the family together for group exercises or at the very least, a family walk after dinner (instead of dessert).

A New Beginning: Altering Your Diet Plan

Getting yourself into better shape can start today. It isn't too late. You're never too fat or too old to start eating better, and only certain people with certain medical restrictions have valid excuses for not eating better or get-ting more exercise. Even people with medical problems usually have alterna-tive solutions.

If you're older, or even if you're young but you've been dieting unsuccessfully for many years, you first may need to undo some extra damage. The longer you indulge in unhealthy eating habits, the more ingrained they become and the harder they are to change. The more times you go on a temporary diet, lose weight, and then gain it back again, the more total weight you're likely to gain. After a number of years, you may be heavier than if you hadn't gone on any diets at all.

The trick now is to never give up hope and play an active role in developing a healthful, lower-calorie eating plan you can stick to for your lifetime. The fol-lowing sections provide advice for folks who are new to healthy eating and for those of you who are weight-management veterans. You have the benefit of diet wisdom now. Use it!

For beginners only

You may encounter more weight-loss misinformation floating around than reliable advice. If you're new to the weight-loss game — and it *is* something of a game — you're going to hear and read all types of tips and advice on how to do it, what foods to eat and not eat, and what works and what doesn't. Listen selectively! Listen only to true experts, including seasoned dieters who've been there, tried that, and can tell you the truth about fad diets and other weight-loss gimmicks. Remember that in the diet industry, everyone has something to sell, so spend your money wisely!

The following sections separate dieting myths from truths and give you tips on how to start living your low-calorie lifestyle.

Deciphering weight-loss fact and fiction

Weight-loss myths abound and this section for "newbies" is a good place to dispel as many of them as possible. Experienced dieters have heard these myths before, though some of you old-timers who are reading this info may appreciate the reminders.

Here are six popular diet myths, debunked:

- **Eating in between meals makes you fat.** The truth is, snacking can actually help you lose weight. The purpose of a snack is to prevent you from getting so hungry that you overeat at your next meal. (For more about healthy snacking, see Chapter 15.)

- **You must stick to a strict number of calories to lose weight.** In fact, you can lose weight with a range of calories (for more info, check out Chapter 3). Also, you'll be more successful at weight loss if you give in and cheat a little (with an emphasis on "little") once in while, especially if you feel hungry, than if you allow yourself to get too hungry and end up binge eating.

- **Eating certain specific foods helps you burn calories.** Have you ever heard that you can lose weight by eating only cabbage soup? How about the grapefruit diet? Has anyone ever told you that it takes more calories to digest an apple than the apple itself contains? If you haven't heard any of these stories yet, you will. Unfortunately, none of them are true. Sure, digesting your food does take some energy, and it involves burning calories, but there's no such thing as a "digestion diet." No matter what type of food you eat, the digestion process could never use up enough calories to make any difference in your weight.

✔ **Eating late at night causes you to gain more weight than eating during the day.** Not true. The total amount and type of food you eat is what matters, not when you eat it. Many people often eat after dinner as a form of entertainment or a way to alleviate boredom, not to satisfy hunger, so the food choices tend to be higher calorie snack foods. If food is a form of entertainment for you, the more you feel bored, the more you'll eat. (Chapter 9 talks more about why people eat when they're not really hungry and how to battle this problem.)

✔ **Reduced-fat and fat-free foods can help you lose weight.** Certain naturally fat-free foods, such as vegetables and fruits, can help you lose weight because you can fill up on larger quantities of these foods for fewer calories than if you were to choose food higher in fat. Fat-free convenience food products, however, are another story. Many of these foods contain so much added sugar or other ingredients that they contribute just as many, if not more, calories to your diet.

✔ **Using sugar substitutes helps you lose weight.** As I write, a new wave of diet products is pushing its way onto supermarket shelves. These products all contain the most recently approved sugar substitute that slashes their calories in half. The sudden appearance of these products coincides with a rising trend of eliminating sugar from the diet to lose weight and the release of new dietary guidelines from government health experts, advising overweight people to cut calories to lose weight. How convenient for food manufacturers!

Over the years, I've seen just about every weight-loss trend and gimmick come and go and come back again. You may not have seen it all yet, but you have access to the same facts I do and you can probably put two and two together as well as I can. Check out these two facts:

- On the whole, Americans have gotten fatter and fatter over the past 100 years.

- Sugar substitutes, also known as artificial sweeteners and low-calorie sweeteners, have been around for more than 125 years.

Put two and two together and the answer is that sugar substitutes are *not* the answer to weight control! (Check out Chapter 5 for more information on sugar substitutes.)

Using sugar substitutes is a matter of personal choice. If you're comfortable with the products and you want to use them in your low-calorie plan, it's entirely up to you. The problem with sugar substitutes is that they may lead you to believe you can eat more food because you're not getting as many calories from sugar. Sugar substitutes don't teach you how to eat less food overall, and that's why, in the bigger picture, they don't work as a weight-loss tool.

Starting from scratch

If this diet is your first attempt at losing weight, then you're in luck. Although it's never too late to shape up, doing so is much easier if you aren't already frustrated by years of failed attempts.

Keep an open mind when you set out to lose weight. Initially, you have a big job ahead of you. Sure, you can skip all the reading, journaling, calculating, and planning suggested in Chapters 3, 4, and 5 and just head straight for the actual diet plans in Chapter 6. But chances are, if you do that, you'll be back to this chapter in no time, trying to figure out what went wrong.

The more research you do upfront to understand how you arrived in your state of being overweight and to develop a personal plan for yourself to lose weight, the more successful you'll be in the long run. This first diet may be your last if you approach it somewhat cautiously, rather than diving in head-first. Yes, you want to feel confident, but you also need to know what you're doing in advance. Almost every success story starts with a well thought-out plan, and every chapter in this book counts as part of a bigger plan to help you lose weight once and for all.

For pros

Expectations have a lot to do with success. Your expectations also have every-thing to do with how confident you feel about yourself and about your ability to lose weight. Your expectations must be realistic, of course, or you'll be dis-appointed early on. This book isn't designed to help you lose 10 pounds by the end of next week. This book's intention is simple: to show you the only surefire way to lose weight and help make the path to permanent weight loss a little easier to follow.

If you have plenty of experience with dieting, you're probably more receptive to ideas that worked for you in the past, and skeptical about advice that didn't work or that you didn't enjoy following. That's okay; just remember to be open-minded concerning weight-loss ideas. This book helps you get as much pleasure as possible out of food while you're discovering how to live a low-cal lifestyle. I hope you can find some new ideas in this book that work for you, that make low-calorie dieting as satisfying as possible, and that hold your interest long enough that you can follow through on your goal to main-tain a low-cal lifestyle and feel good about the way you look and feel.

In the following sections, I ask you to look at the diets you've tried, and I explain how to move on to a new low-calorie lifestyle.

Evaluating your diet history

Are you a weight cycler? If you've gained and lost weight repeatedly through-out your life, then you probably fit the bill. If you're a weight cycler, you've probably been on numerous diets. You lose weight while you're on the diet, and then gain it back soon after you stop dieting. So you go on another diet, lose some of the weight you gained last time around, and then gain it all back again. Sometimes you even gain back more than you originally lost. Sound familiar?

This up-again, down-again weight cycling is called *yo-yo dieting*. Some medical experts say that yo-yo dieting is more dangerous to your health than being overweight. They say that you're better off staying at the same weight, even if it's higher than your ideal weight, than you are to repeatedly lose weight and gain it back again. Not all experts agree, however, because plenty of scientific evidence shows clear associations between being overweight and a number of medical conditions, such as diabetes, heart disease, and high blood pressure. So finding a diet plan that helps you stay as close to your ideal weight as possible still makes good health sense. The clue to success is to stick with that plan for the rest of your life. That's why choosing the right plan is essential.

Moving on

If you've been on more diets than you can count and never managed to maintain a healthy or comfortable weight, then the thought of dieting probably aggravates you. You're probably frustrated because every diet you ever went on was somehow about deprivation. Don't eat this food. Don't eat that food. After a while you felt deprived and never satisfied about what you were eating. Are you really surprised that you became discouraged along the way and gave up? No diet will ever work if the focus is on deprivation.

Think realistically about the different diets you've followed in your lifetime and why they didn't work in the long run. Make a list of what you liked and didn't like about all the diets in your life. Reject anything you didn't like because it's probably not going to work any better for you the second time around. Incorporate what you liked and what you found helpful into this plan. You can probably live comfortably on fewer calories than you're now eating, but what's most important for long-term success is that the calories you do eat come from foods you enjoy and that you don't feel unnecessarily deprived.

Low-calorie dieting to lose weight means eating fewer calories than you're currently eating, but you don't have to deprive yourself. You can cut calories and still fill yourself up with plenty of good food. A low-calorie diet that works is one that is flexible enough to allow you to eat any food you want and still stay within your calorie allowance. On this type of diet, you have the choice of eating larger quantities of low-calorie foods or smaller quantities of higher calorie foods, or a combination of both. You have choices and you can change your mind from day to day about how you want to eat to stay motivated and stick to your plan.

Tools of the Trade: Figuring Out How Overweight You Are

When you're overweight, you usually know it. Your clothes feel tight and your body bulges where it didn't before. You feel like you're jiggling when you walk down the street. You look in the mirror and your excess weight is staring right back at you. Ignoring it is difficult because half of your total body fat lies just beneath your skin.

Being overweight means different things to different people. The following definitions clarify it so you clearly understand when health experts use the terms *overweight* and *obese*.

✔ *Overweight* means you're 10 to 20 percent higher than your normal, healthy weight. (You can determine your healthy weight in the next section.) For instance, if a healthy weight for you is 125 pounds, you're overweight if you weigh 13 to 26 pounds more than that, or between 138 and 151 pounds.

✔ *Obese* means you weigh 20 percent or more than your normal, healthy weight *and* your excess weight comes from body fat.

If your extra weight is from muscle you've developed by lifting weights or doing other exercises, you may be several pounds overweight by any of the usual standards. This type of overweight is different from the type of overweight that results from excess fat, and the usual standards don't apply to you. The standards only apply if you're "overfat," which means your excess weight is coming from excess fat and may be a threat to your health.

✔ *Morbidly obese* means you're 50 to 100 percent above your healthy weight or you're sufficiently overweight to have serious health problems.

The following sections are devoted to different ways you can measure yourself and compare yourself to standard weight charts to see just how far you are from your healthy weight. This information can help you establish your long-term weight-loss goal in Chapter 4.

Interpreting a healthy weight range chart

Nutrition experts developed the weight range chart in Figure 2-1 to provide weight-loss professionals and dieters with a quick and simple way to determine healthy weights according to height, for men and women alike.

Find your height in the first column on the left side of the chart, and then move your finger across the graph to a midway point in the healthy weight section to find out approximately how much you should weigh when you're at your healthiest weight.

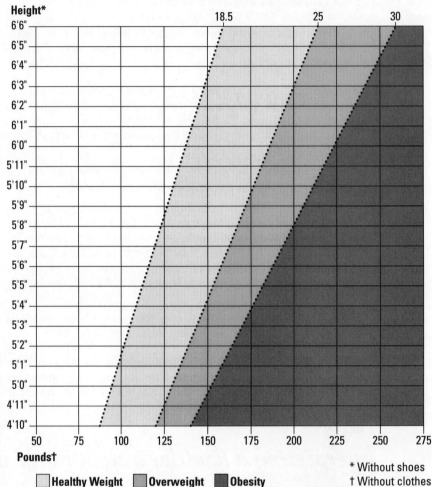

BMI (Body Mass Index)

Figure 2-1:
You can easily determine your best weight with the healthy weight range chart.

* Without shoes
† Without clothes

Source: U.S. Department of Agriculture

Most importantly, this chart shows you a 25-pound weight range for different people who are the same height. Even if you and I are the same height, we may have different amounts of bones and muscles. If you have more muscle and denser bones than me, you may weigh more than I do, but you're not any more overweight than I am. A higher weight within the range probably applies to you, and a lower weight probably applies to me. Men, for instance, often have a higher percentage of muscle tissue and bone mass than women. A younger woman probably has more muscle and bone than an older woman of the same height. Your healthiest and most comfortable weight probably falls somewhere midway in the range for your height.

Just because a healthy weight range chart provides a wide range of healthy weights for your height doesn't necessarily mean gaining weight to the top of your range is healthful. Higher weights are generally considered the norm for men, very athletic women, and anyone else who has a larger frame and more muscle weight.

Computing your BMI

Body Mass Index (BMI) is a slightly more accurate way of measuring yourself than simply looking yourself up on a healthy weight chart. In combination with your waist measurement (which I cover in "Determining your waist-to-hip ratio" later in this chapter), BMI can tell you if your weight is putting you at risk of developing chronic medical conditions.

You can use either the formula or the chart in the following sections to determine your BMI. The formula is just slightly more precise than the chart; I provide the formula for those of you who like doing diet math. The chart is an easy way out for the rest of you!

Using the formula

To compute your BMI mathematically, use the following formula:

(Your weight in pounds) × 704

divided by (your height in inches)

divided again by (your height in inches)

If your weight is within a healthy range, your BMI will be between 19 and 24. A BMI between 25 and 30 is considered overweight, and a BMI greater than 30 means you're obese and may be at risk of developing weight-related health problems. If your excess body weight is from muscle, however, a high BMI may not be indicative of health problems.

For instance, if you weigh 153 pounds and you're 63 inches tall:

153 × 704 = 107,712

107,712 divided by 63 = 1,709.7

1,709.7 divided by 63 = 27.1

In this case, your BMI is 27.1, and you're considered overweight.

Checking out the chart

To use the chart in Figure 2-2, find your height in the first column, and then move your finger along that row until you find your weight. Move your finger straight up that row until you hit your BMI.

	Normal						Overweight					Obese					
BMI	**19**	**20**	**21**	**22**	**23**	**24**	**25**	**26**	**27**	**28**	**29**	**30**	**31**	**32**	**33**	**34**	**35**
Height (inches)	**Body Weight (pounds)**																
58	91	96	100	105	110	115	119	124	129	134	138	143	148	153	158	162	167
59	94	99	104	109	114	119	124	128	133	138	143	148	153	158	163	168	173
60	97	102	107	112	118	123	128	133	138	143	148	153	158	163	168	174	179
61	100	106	111	116	122	127	132	137	143	148	153	158	164	169	174	180	185
62	104	109	115	120	126	131	136	142	147	153	158	164	169	175	180	186	191
63	107	113	118	124	130	135	141	146	152	158	163	169	175	180	186	191	197
64	110	116	122	128	134	140	145	151	157	163	169	174	180	186	192	197	204
65	114	120	126	132	138	144	150	156	162	168	174	180	186	192	198	204	210
66	118	124	130	136	142	148	155	161	167	173	179	186	192	198	204	210	216
67	121	127	134	140	146	153	159	166	172	178	185	191	198	204	211	217	223
68	125	131	138	144	151	158	164	171	177	184	190	197	203	210	216	223	230
69	128	135	142	149	155	162	169	176	182	189	196	203	209	216	223	230	236
70	132	139	146	153	160	167	174	181	188	195	202	209	216	222	229	236	243
71	136	143	150	157	165	172	179	186	193	200	208	215	222	229	236	243	250
72	140	147	154	162	169	177	184	191	199	206	213	221	228	235	242	250	258
73	144	151	159	166	174	182	189	197	204	212	219	227	235	242	250	257	265
74	148	155	163	171	179	186	194	202	210	218	225	233	241	249	256	264	272
75	152	160	168	176	184	192	200	208	216	224	232	240	248	256	264	272	279
76	156	164	172	180	189	197	205	213	221	230	238	246	254	263	271	279	287

Figure 2-2:
The Body Mass Index chart shows you if your weight is normal, overweight, or obese.

Determining your waist-to-hip ratio

If you own a measuring tape, you can measure yourself to determine where you carry most of the excess fat on your body. Calculating your waist-to-hip ratio helps you determine not only where you carry most of your fat, but also how much of a threat your fat actually poses to your health.

Inch by inch

Do you want to figure out where your extra weight is (if you don't already notice it in a mirror?) and if that makes you an apple or a pear? If so, this section can help. Use a tape measure and take the following steps to figure out your waist-to-hip ratio:

1. **Stand in a relaxed position with your feet together and your belly hanging out.**

   (You don't necessarily want to be standing in front of a mirror when you take this measurement.)

2. **Measure your waist at its narrowest point.**

   Write down that number.

3. **Measure your hips at their widest part (midway around your butt).**

   Write down that number, too.

4. **Divide your waist measurement by your hip measurement.**

   The resulting figure is your waist-to-hip ratio.

Your weight is considered healthy if your waist-to-hip ratio is less than 0.8 for women and less than 0.9 for men. If you're a woman and your ratio is between 0.8 and 0.85, or a man with a ratio between 0.9 and 1.0, you may be at moderately high risk of developing health problems associated with being overweight. Higher ratios indicate higher risk.

Nowadays, your waist size gets more attention from health experts than its relationship to your hips. One of the most significant predictors of health problems is a large waist size coupled with a high BMI. If you're a man with a waist size more than 40 inches or a woman with a waist size more than 35 inches, and your BMI is higher than 25, you're at an especially high risk for developing health problems such as high blood pressure, high cholesterol, cardiovascular disease, and diabetes.

Apples and pears

So after you know your waist-to-hip ratio, you can determine what type of fruit shape you are. Apples and pears exemplify two very specific body types.

- An *apple-shaped* person carries his excess weight on the upper half of his body, around the waist. If you're an apple-shaped person, your waist-to-hip ratio is less than 0.8 if you're a woman and less than 0.9 if you're a man. (The formula for figuring out your waist-to-hip ratio is in the previous section.)

- A *pear-shaped* person carries most of her weight below the waist, on the hips and thighs, and in the rear. If you're a pear-shaped person, your waist-to-hip ratio is higher than 0.8 if you're a woman and higher than 0.9 if you're a man.

Apples are at greater risk of developing high blood pressure, heart disease, diabetes, and certain cancers than pears. But if you're an apple, never fear! You can eat less and exercise more to reduce your belly fat and possibly reduce your risk of developing any of these medical problems.

You inherit your basic body shapes, for the most part, and men are more likely to be shaped like apples while women are more likely to be shaped like pears. But no hard-and-fast rule dictates a person's shape because shapes change, and factors like age and alcohol consumption have been known to turn pear-shaped women into apples, with all the associated health risks.

Chapter 3

Working with Guidelines for Healthy Low-Calorie Living

In This Chapter

▶ Doing your diet research

▶ Figuring out your calorie counts

▶ Getting the scoop on low-calorie nutrition

▶ Exploring ways to cut calories

Medical doctors and dietitians have proven again and again that cutting calories and adopting a low-calorie lifestyle, one that includes plenty of physical activity to burn calories, is the only sure way to shed extra pounds and keep them off.

This chapter explains why you need to commit to a low-calorie lifestyle to lose weight, gives you formulas for figuring out your calorie needs, and lays the groundwork for making healthy food choices on a low-calorie diet plan.

Cutting Calories for Weight-Loss Success

Before you start a low-calorie diet, you may want to know why cutting calories is the only surefire way to lose weight and why you need to commit yourself to low-calorie living for long-term success. Understanding the reasons behind what you have to do is a surer road to success than blindly jumping in. In the following sections, I compare past diet trends and explain how you can successfully incorporate a low-calorie diet into your life.

Registered dietitians, licensed nutritionists, doctors with an active practice in weight control, exercise physiologists, and licensed or certified psychotherapists who specialize in compulsive overeating are all in a position to provide sound weight-loss advice or refer you to another expert who can. In addition to having the appropriate educational background and experience with weight loss and weight maintenance, these experts generally stay up-to-date with the latest research and developments. You don't have to get your guidance directly from any of these experts, but you need to be sure that whatever weight-loss advice you follow comes from a reliable source.

Comparing low-calorie diets to other diets

If you've been around for a few years, you've probably seen a ton of popular diets come and go. Even if you're new to the diet scene, you're probably well aware of the many magazine articles, books, infomercials, and Internet pop-ups that bombard you every day with promises of easy new ways to lose weight. If you live long enough, most of these diets and promotions will surface again in some form, making the same old promises to a new audience of overweight people looking for that one magic diet that really works.

Unlike a low-carbohydrate diet, a low-fat diet, or a high-fiber diet, a low-calorie diet focuses strictly on limiting the number of calories you consume. Here's a secret, though: All diets, no matter what nutrients they're high or low in, must restrict calories if they help you lose weight.

Counting calories is the oldest method of intentionally losing weight, going back at least as far as 1918, when Dr. Lulu Hunt Peters defined calories and showed dieters how to count them in her book *Diet and Health with Key to the Calories.* Peters recommended a diet low in fat and high in carbohydrates, and one that averaged 1,200 calories. Calorie counting has gone in and out of fashion since that time, but now, almost 100 years later, it's back. Calorie counting is the only weight-loss method that has stood the test of time.

In the mid-1980s, counting fat grams became the new way to lose weight. The message that dieters heard was that calories don't matter as much as fat. I actually heard people say that you could only get fat from eating fat, or that if you stick to a low-fat diet, you can eat 200 extra calories a day. Of course, these statements may be true if you plan your menus very carefully, but many dieters forgot to factor in calories they were consuming from other sources.

Eventually, dieters tired of counting fat grams, seeking out lowfat foods, and gaining weight as a result of all their efforts. The fat-free fad faded away, and high-protein diets moved in as the new wave in weight control. High-protein diets became very popular when dieters discovered that they could lose weight if they cut back on carbohydrates and ate more high-protein foods at every meal. Increasing the amount of lean protein foods you eat and cutting back on carbs usually does help with initial weight loss. One reason why is: Your body needs extra water to digest and metabolize foods that are high in carbohydrates, especially high-fiber foods. When you start cutting back on these foods, your body no longer holds onto that extra water. So along with any weight you lose by cutting calories the first few weeks of your diet, you lose water weight, which can be motivating when you first start dieting.

However a high-protein diet has some serious downsides. You don't eat much bread on a high-protein diet. No bagels, no muffins, no waffles, certainly no cookies, cakes, or pastries. Some high-protein diets say you can't even have a potato. As a result of these limitations, most people can only stick to a low-carb diet for several months at most.

If you're considering a high-protein, low-carbohydrate diet, you need to know this valuable piece of information. A sugar called *glucose,* which comes from foods high in carbohydrates, is the only fuel your brain can use for energy. Lowering or even eliminating carbs (and not getting enough glucose) affects your body in several ways:

- ✔ Your brain could be in trouble. Your brain can only use glucose for energy, so it can't work without it.

- ✔ In order to protect your brain, your body turns to its muscles, breaking them down to provide your body with substances it can use to make its own glucose.

- ✔ Meanwhile, as your body starts using fat stores for energy (because not enough carbohydrate is available), you develop a condition known as *ketosis.*

    When your body is in a state of ketosis, you're not eating enough food, especially carbohydrates. In response to the ketosis, your metabolism slows down and you stop burning fat. As a result, you only want to view this type of diet as a short-term solution for kick-starting a more balanced diet plan.

Any diet that emphasizes one food group over another or virtually eliminates a whole category of foods is bound to throw your body chemistry out of whack. That's why a nutritionally balanced, reduced-calorie diet that promotes normal, healthy eating habits is the best route to weight control.

For most people, the goals and benefits of following a low-calorie diet are to lose weight, to develop better eating habits, and to maintain weight loss in hopes of reducing the health risks that come with being overweight. Chapter 16 describes these benefits — which include more energy, better sleep, and lower risk for developing medical problems such as high blood pressure and heart disease — in greater detail.

Some experts say that weight cycling — losing weight and gaining weight repeatedly over time — is bad for your health and that it's better to stay at one higher weight than to suffer the ups and downs. The jury is still out though. No one knows for sure if weight cycling is bad for you. (Check out Chapter 2 for more info and how weight cycling affects your overall health.)

Figuring out what a "low-calorie" diet means to you

A low-calorie diet can take different forms for different people, but the one thing common to all successful low-calorie diets is commitment. In the following sections, I explain how you can personalize your low-calorie diet while maintaining a full commitment to your new lifestyle.

Maintaining flexibility

On first glance, a low-calorie diet may seem very rigid, but cutting calories may not be as hard as you think. Sure, you're limited to a rather exact number of calories, which can limit the amount of food you're allowed to eat. But actually, if you choose to eat mostly low-calorie foods, you can eat plenty of them! If you choose to eat higher calorie foods, you have the flexibility of eating whatever type of food you want. You may have to eat smaller portions than you're used to, but no one's going to tell you that you can't have a bagel, a bowl of pasta, or a chocolate cookie.

Most weight-loss experts believe that some rigidity is good when you really want to lose weight because the closer you follow a strict diet, the better chance you have of mastering new eating habits and seeing quicker results. Don't worry; you don't have to eat exactly the same number of calories each day or include any foods in your diet that you don't like, just because you think they're good for you. It simply means that the more committed you are to your low-calorie lifestyle, the better it will work for you.

Even though this book contains one, straightforward, low-calorie diet plan, it's a flexible plan. This plan has plenty of room for personalization because I know that no one-size-fits-all diet plan can work for everyone who wants to lose weight. You have to be happy with your diet or you'll never stick to it.

No matter if you like to cook most of your meals from scratch, if you prefer stopping at a deli or restaurant for take-out on your way home from work each day, or if you keep your cupboard and freezer stocked with convenience foods, you can work any of these eating styles into a low-calorie diet plan that suits your particular lifestyle.

Adopting your new dietary lifestyle

The concept of "going on a diet" fell out of fashion years ago, when both weight-control experts and those who struggle with their weight began to agree that weight-loss diets don't work because they don't keep the weight off in the long run. *Diet* was recognized for what it had become to so many overweight people: a four-letter word.

The reason is simple. If you "go on a diet," the implication is that, at some point, you'll go off the diet. And that's what most people do. As soon as they're off the diet, their excess weight usually returns because they're no longer doing what they did to keep it off.

The new way to diet is to adopt a dietary lifestyle and embrace it as your own. Instead of going on a diet, practice healthier living by eating better, eating less, making sure you get enough physical activity, and reprogramming your thinking so that you can continue these healthier habits for a lifetime.

If ever there was a commitment you need to take seriously, it's the commitment you're making when you follow this low-calorie diet plan. Let it lead you into a healthier lifestyle that can keep you at a healthy weight for the rest of your life. This "diet" is a commitment to never give up on yourself.

Focusing on Formulas for Low-Calorie Living

The first thing any dieter wants to know is "How much food can I eat?," which is the same as asking, "How many calories can I have?" The answer is simple: To lose weight, you have to eat fewer calories than you're eating now. Yes, you can burn some of your extra calories off through physical activity, and in fact you can burn off a lot of extra calories if you're an avid exerciser or plan to become one. But to lose weight, most people also have to cut some, and often, many, calories from their diet.

If you like math, then the formulas you find in this section are for you. Dietitians and other weight experts sometimes use these formulas to help dieters determine a sensible range of calories within which they can safely lose or maintain weight.

You can use these formulas to figure out approximately how many calories you can eat every day to prevent further weight gain or to get to a healthier weight. After you establish your calorie allowance, you can work with the menu plans in Chapter 6, which are also designed to help you work within a range of calories to start losing weight right away. All weight-loss formulas are limited, however, and the results they give are very general guidelines, not absolute numbers to live by every day.

Determining the number of calories you need

Your body needs a minimum number of calories to have enough energy to be healthy, which is called your *resting metabolic rate*. By figuring your resting metabolic rate, you can determine the amount of calories your body needs just to keep your heart pumping, your brain thinking, your kidneys clearing, and all your other body systems operating properly.

1. **Calculate your body's basic calorie needs.**

   To do so, take your healthy weight (if you don't know it, choose a midrange weight from the healthy weight range chart in Chapter 2), or the weight you want to be, and multiply it by 10 if you're a woman or 11 if you're a man. (Men get more calories in their calculations because they tend to be taller and have a higher ratio of muscle to fat than women.)

   (Healthy weight) × (10 or 11) = Your basic calorie needs

   So, for example, if you're a woman who is 5-feet, 5-inches, your weight goal may be 140 pounds. Using the formula, 140 × 10 = 1,400, which amounts to your basic calorie needs for a day.

   Along with your basic calorie needs, the next three steps can help you figure out the maximum number of calories you can eat while you're trying to get to your goal weight.

2. **Figure out how many calories you need for the amount of exercise you get.**

   Read the following descriptions and then multiply your basic calorie needs from the previous section by the percentage that matches your activity level.

   Sedentary (20 percent): You sit, drive, lie down, or stand in one place for most of the day and don't do any type of formal exercise. Multiply by 0.20.

   Light Activity (30 percent): You walk for exercise, up to two hours every day. Multiply by 0.30.

   Moderate Activity (40 percent): You take exercise classes, dance, do a lot of housework, swim, or ride a bicycle most days. You do very little sitting. Multiply by 0.40.

   Heavy Activity (50 percent): You play physical sports, have a labor-intensive job, or engage in heavy workouts at the gym almost every day. Multiply by 0.50.

   (Basic calorie needs) × (Percent activity level) = Activity calorie needs

To continue with the example, take your basic calorie needs (1,400) and multiply that figure by .40. (Just suppose that you take a couple exercise classes a week and go with your kids for a couple of bike rides a week.) Your activity calorie needs are 560.

3. **Figure out how many calories you need for normal digestion and metabolism of food.**

   Yes! It's true! You burn calories digesting and absorbing the food you eat. Add your basic calorie needs from Step 1 and your activity calorie needs from Step 2, and then multiply the total by 10 percent (0.10).

   (Basic calorie needs) + (Basic activity needs) × 0.10 = Calories for digestion

   With the example, your basic calorie needs (1,400) plus your activity needs (560) equals 1,960 calories. Multiply that by 0.10 and you get the calories you burn for digestion: 196.

4. **Add your basic calorie needs, your activity calorie needs, and your calorie needs for digestion.**

   The resulting figure represents your total energy needs in calories.

   (Basic calorie needs) + (Activity calorie needs) + (Digestion calorie needs) = Total calorie needs

   To finish the previous example, your basic calorie needs (1,400) + your activity needs (560) + your calorie needs for digestion (196) = your total calorie needs (2,156).

This number — your total calorie needs — represents the number of calories you can eat every day to maintain a healthy weight at the activity level you've chosen. When you're trying to lose weight to get to a healthy weight, this number is a good guide to the *maximum* number of calories you can eat on any given day while you're dieting. But remember: This number is just a guide. The actual number of calories that works for you depends on how much you exercise as well as other individual factors, such as your age and your individual metabolic rate.

Using another formula for weight loss

If you know exactly how many calories you normally consume each day (and you can figure that out by keeping track of your calories in a food diary, as demonstrated in Chapter 4), use this shortcut to find out how many calories you need to cut from your daily diet. To lose a pound of body weight in a week without doing any additional exercise, you have to cut 3,500 calories from your diet that week, or an average of 500 calories a day. So, if you currently consume about 2,000 calories a day, you have to cut your daily calorie allowance by 500 calories, to 1,500, to start losing a pound a week.

At some point, the number of calories you can eat and still lose weight will get too low and you'll have to stop cutting calories. Your only option at that point is to exercise more. That's why losing weight initially is much easier when you have a lot to lose and much more difficult when you're down to those last 10 pounds and you don't have many calories left to cut.

In the following sections, I give you a couple of strategies, based on the formulas in this chapter, for choosing a calorie range that can help you lose weight or maintain your current weight and prevent more gain.

Finding your weight-loss range

Everyone has a range of calories within which they can lose weight. If, through your calculations, you determine that you can lose a pound or two a week if you stick to a 1,500-calorie diet, you'll find that you can lose that same amount of weight on a 1,400- or 1,600-calorie diet.

Sometimes the best way to find your personal calorie range for losing weight is by trial and error. If you want, you can skip all the formulas and calculations in this chapter, go right to Chapter 6 (featuring a variety of menu plans), and put yourself on a 1,500-calorie-a-day diet plan. That level may or may not help, but it won't hurt you. If you find it impossible to stick with, or if you stick with it and lose more than 2 pounds the first week, you may consider adding 100 or more calories to your days. (A safe limit when you're losing weight is 2 pounds a week. If you lose more than 2 pounds, you're losing too quickly. If you lose too much weight early on, you're more likely to gain back some or all of it.) If you don't lose any weight at all, skip down to a 1,200-calorie plan and see what happens at the end of a week.

After you master the art of eating low-calorie meals and sticking to a prescribed number of calories every day, you may see that you can "cheat" a little on your diet by occasionally indulging in some of your favorite higher calorie foods and still lose or maintain weight. Eventually you can figure out how to balance your calorie intake over the course of several days, or even a week, rather than focusing on one day at a time.

Preventing weight gain

If you've recently been gaining weight, or you're not quite ready to commit to the lifestyle changes required to lose weight, you first want to avoid any further weight gain. Doing so can be a huge accomplishment in and of itself. After you stop gaining and your weight levels off, you can move on to the next stage of your plan, which is to start losing weight.

To stop weight gain in its tracks, use the quickest formula for figuring out how many calories you need to stay at your current weight and possibly start losing weight: Multiply your weight times ten. Stick to within 100 calories of that amount on most days so you can stabilize your weight until you're ready to embark on a sensible, long-term plan.

Understanding the Nutritional Nuts and Bolts of a Low-Calorie Diet

Right now, you're probably thinking more about losing weight than you are about protecting your health while you're following a low-calorie diet. As a dietitian, I have to look at you more holistically. I have to look at the effects of the food choices you make on your current and long-term health. That's why I'm including this primer on all the important nutrients you need in your diet and the foods that provide them. Think of this section as a freshman level course in basic nutrition with an emphasis on calorie control.

Getting the nutrients you need

In the old days, dietitians were trained to say "There are no good foods and no bad foods, just too much of some foods." That's still true to a certain extent, but dietitians know better now. Some foods are much better for you than others and, for many people, some foods seem to have an addictive quality that makes it impossible to resist eating more, after you've had a taste. That quality doesn't make them bad foods, but those foods aren't good for you until you gain better control over the amount you eat.

This section discusses good food sources of all the nutrients that are essential to a healthful low-calorie diet. You also figure out how to make smarter choices with treats and sweets, and how some junk food can still play a role in a healthy low-cal diet.

Carbohydrates

The bulk of your calories — a little more than half, or 55 to 60 percent — should come from foods high in carbohydrates. You may have heard about the two types of carbs — good carbs and bad carbs. The following bulleted list explains each more in-depth and tells you why most of your carbohydrate calories should come from good carbs.

- **Simple carbohydrates:** Foods high in "bad" or simple carbohydrates are candies, cookies, chips, cakes, pies, sodas, and many of your other favorite foods that supply plenty of calories from sugar and refined flours, but not much in the way of good nutrition.

  Simple carbohydrates are just that: simple. They're not as complicated, chemically speaking, as complex carbohydrates. Foods high in simple carbohydrates, for the most part, supply mostly calories and little or none of the good stuff. That's why dietitians refer to these foods as "empty calorie" foods.

- **Complex carbohydrates:** Foods high in "good" complex carbohydrates include whole grains, beans, and vegetables.

Foods high in complex carbohydrates are better for you because they contain vitamins, minerals, fiber, and *phytochemicals* (substances found in plant foods that are neither vitamins nor minerals, but are thought to convey health benefits).

Fruit is the exception to the rule. Fruit contains plenty of simple sugars, but it also contains valuable nutrients, including many of the disease-fighting antioxidant vitamins and phytochemicals. Dietitians and other nutrition experts always put fresh fruit in the "good" carb group.

If you're eating simple carbohydrates such as cookies, pastries, and fried chips in place of healthier foods, or if you're simply eating so many of these foods in addition to healthier foods that you're gaining weight, then junk food is a problem for you. Eating these foods is okay, however, if you only eat them some of the time and in small amounts. In Chapter 15, you can find tips and recipes for fitting simple sugars into a healthful low-calorie diet.

Protein

When discussing protein, you first need to know about *amino acids,* which are the chemical "building blocks" of protein found in food. After you eat the amino acids in say, a hamburger, your body absorbs them via your bloodstream where they spend most of their time connecting and reconnecting with each other to form thousands of different proteins that do thousands of different jobs in your body. Some of the most important roles amino acids and proteins play in your body include

✔ **Antibodies:** These proteins protect you from bacteria, viruses, toxins, and allergens.

✔ **Hormones:** Protein is an essential component of many of your body's most important regulating hormones, including those that regulate food intake and metabolism, such as insulin and leptin.

✔ **Repair:** Protein is essential for mending muscles, bones, and skin, and for pregnancy and growth.

✔ **Replacement:** When you wash your body, comb your hair, or clip your fingernails, you're losing body cells that contain protein that needs to be replaced so that new skin cells, hair, and nails can grow.

Adult women who are at a healthy weight need approximately 45 to 60 grams of protein in their daily diets; most men who are at a healthy weight need at least 60 to 65 grams. Because most foods contain some protein, reaching or exceeding those amounts from day to day is easy. Meat, poultry, fish, egg whites, and reduced-fat dairy products are all especially good sources of high-quality protein in a low-calorie diet, but vegetarians and near-vegetarians have nothing to fear about getting enough protein. Legumes, nuts, breads, pastas, and soy foods are also good sources, and even most fruits and vegetables, which are almost pure carbohydrate, contribute a gram or two.

Check out Table 3-1 for a list of some common foods and their protein scores.

Table 3-1	Protein Counts in Common Foods
Food	*Protein (grams)*
Turkey, light meat (4 ounces)	34
Hamburger, lean (4 ounces)	32
Flounder (4 ounces)	27
Tuna, canned in water (3 ounces)	22
Yogurt (8 ounces)	12
Tofu (½ cup)	10
Milk, skim (8 ounces)	9
Black beans (½ cup)	8
Peanut butter (2 tablespoons)	8
Cheese, reduced fat or part-skim (1 ounce)	8
Cheese, regular (1 ounce)	7
Pasta, cooked (1 cup)	7
Soy milk (8 ounces)	7
Bagel (3½-inch diameter)	7
Oatmeal (1 cup)	6

Fat

There are many different types of dietary fats and some act very differently in your body than others. If all you care about are calories, then the type of fat or oil you use to prepare or flavor food doesn't matter, because they all contain 9 calories per gram or approximately 100 calories per tablespoon. But if you're concerned about your overall health, and I hope you are, then the type of fat you use matters very much.

The most healthful fats are in liquid form. Olive oil, canola oil, corn oil, and other liquid fats are thought to be best because they can help keep your blood cholesterol and blood fats at acceptable levels. The fats to watch out for are the *hydrogenated fats* (oils that have been chemically converted to solid fats), which are listed on the ingredient labels of many processed foods such as crackers and pastries, and the saturated fats found mainly in animal products such as meats, butter, and whole-milk dairy products. In the case of animal foods, you can easily trim away excess fat from meats and choose leaner cuts of meat and reduced-fat dairy foods.

Your body needs some fat (at least 20 grams) to help absorb and transport fat-soluble vitamins, such as vitamins A and E; your skin and hair need fat to look alive; and your brain and nervous system need fat to function effectively. But eating too many foods that are high in any type of fat can, and probably will, cause you to gain weight and affect your health. Medical experts say that no more than 30 percent of your daily calories should come from fat and many recommend even less. On a 1,500-calorie diet, 30 percent is about 50 grams of fat. The smart thing to do, overall, is to eat small amounts of the right types of fat.

Don't be fooled into thinking that all lowfat foods are low in calories. Some are, but many aren't. Check and compare the calorie counts on the labels of similar products to be sure you're getting a lower-calorie food. For instance, many reduced-fat cheeses contain one-third to half the amount of calories of their full-fat cousins. But the same can't be said for some flavored yogurt products and other foods, like peanut butter or cookies, that may have the fat removed but are sweetened with enough sugar to make up the calorie difference.

Vitamins and minerals

Each and every known vitamin is essential to good health and you need them all in your diet, but you only need them in small amounts. That's good news for low-calorie dieters who are only eating small amounts of food!

Vitamins comprise the two following categories:

- **Water-soluble vitamins:** These include vitamin C, all the B vitamins, and beta carotene, which your body converts to the fat-soluble vitamin A. To ensure you get plenty of vitamin C and beta carotene, eat a variety of fruits, veggies, and whole-grains. Meat and dairy products supply the B vitamins.

- **Fat-soluble vitamins:** These include vitamins A, D, E, and K. You get D from egg yolks and dairy foods, E from vegetable oils, nuts, and wheat germ, and K from leafy green vegetables such as spinach and broccoli. You get vitamin A from yellow, orange, and dark green vegetables.

You don't get energy from vitamins; you can only get energy from carbohydrates, fats, and proteins. But your body uses vitamins, specifically the B vitamins, to metabolize carbohydrates, fats, and proteins and produce energy. Like protein, vitamins also play a huge role in the growth, maintenance, and repair of most of your body cells.

Like vitamins, minerals help keep your body healthy by keeping your bones dense, your heart pumping, your immune system strong, and all other body systems functioning properly. Scientists know of 22 minerals that are essential for good health. You can find some minerals, such as iron and zinc, in meat and seafood, others such as calcium and magnesium in dairy products, and still others, such as potassium and selenium, from fruits, vegetables, and grains. Minerals are just another reason to eat a varied diet!

Fiber

Fiber is a carbohydrate found in whole grains, fruits, and vegetables, but it's a unique type of carb that your body can't digest. You eat it and it passes out of your body unchanged. Because of the way fiber works (or doesn't work) in your body, it keeps your digestive system healthy and also helps regulate blood cholesterol and sugar levels. Those contributions are noteworthy for a substance that, technically, isn't even a nutrient.

Fiber also has other benefits. It can help you shed excess pounds. And as soon as you lose weight, fiber can help you maintain the loss. It's sounding better and better all the time, isn't it? High-fiber foods can help you stick to a low-calorie diet and make that diet work for you. Do you want to know how? Read the following list:

✔ High-fiber foods are bulky so you feel satisfied after you eat them.

✔ High-fiber foods take longer to digest than other foods, so they stay in your stomach longer, helping to prevent hunger from striking too soon again.

✔ High-fiber foods are naturally lowfat, and fat contains more calories than carbohydrates and protein.

Nutrition experts recommend that adults get at least 25 grams of fiber each day. In Table 3-2, you see how some foods stack up in terms of their fiber content. In Chapter 7, you can find a full-day's menu that emphasizes fiber at each meal. In Chapter 12, you can find a list of high-fiber foods commonly eaten for breakfast.

Table 3-2	Fiber Amounts in Common Foods
Food (½ cup cooked)	*Fiber (grams)*
Beans (such as kidney, black, pinto)	7 to 10
Barley	5
Bulgur	5
Lentils	5
Pear, medium	4
Broccoli	3
Winter squash	3
Brown rice	2
Strawberries (½ cup raw)	2

If you plan to increase the amount of fiber in your diet, do it slowly! Adding too much, too soon, can wreak havoc on your digestive system in the form of gas, cramping, or diarrhea. Your best bet is to add a gram or two of fiber at a time, every few days over a period of several weeks, and be sure to drink plenty of extra water as you go along. Fiber soaks up liquids like a sponge in your stomach, and if you don't have enough extra water to help move it along, your plumbing will jam up.

Water

Water is calorie-free. No other natural substance can make that claim, so drink up! When you're trying to lose weight or maintain a healthy weight, you certainly don't want to waste precious calories on other drinks.

Of course you also need to drink plenty of water for other reasons. For one thing, you can't live long without it. You need a constant flow of water coming in to replace the water that goes out through breathing, perspiration, and excretion. Water keeps your muscles moving, your blood flowing, and your joints bending. Even your bones need water to stay healthy.

Drinking more water is a matter of developing new habits. The following are just a few ways to bring more water into your life on a regular basis:

- Keep a bottle of water nearby at work.
- Carry a water bottle with you wherever you go.
- Whenever you see a water fountain, take a sip.
- Always ask for water when you sit down at a restaurant. Not only does asking help you fill your water needs, but it also can help fill your tummy and curb your appetite as well.

Most people need to aim for 8 to 10 cups of water a day. If your diet is high in fiber or sodium (salt), you may need more. If your diet is high in watery foods like lettuce, tomatoes, oranges, watermelon, milk, and yogurt, you can probably drink less because the water from these foods counts toward your daily requirement.

Phytochemicals

When phytochemicals first came on the nutrition scene in the early 1990s, many people thought they were miracle substances. They weren't vitamins or minerals. Health experts described *phytochemicals* as non-nutrients found in fresh foods that could help prevent and fight cancer and other life-threatening diseases. Scientists estimate that hundreds, if not thousands, of them exist in foods, most commonly in fruits and vegetables.

Researchers still have a lot to discover about phytochemicals and their specific roles in fighting disease. The jury is also out as to whether or not phytochemicals work when they're isolated from foods and put into a capsule or pill and sold as supplements. What experts do know is that many health-promoting substances are found in foods, some with rather unnatural sounding names like lycopene, flavanoid, indole, genestein, and carotenoid, that may save or extend your life. When you're following a low-calorie diet, eating a wide variety of fruits and vegetables is important to ensure you get as many phytochemicals into your diet as you can.

Keeping your energy high and your diet interesting

What's different about low-calorie nutrition and regular nutrition, you may ask? When you're on a low-calorie diet, you need to make smart food choices because getting all the energy and nutrients you need from food is more difficult than when you're consuming more calories.

Creating balance

A nutritionally balanced meal contains mostly carbohydrates from grains, fruits, and vegetables; some protein from meat, poultry, fish, dairy products, beans, nuts, or eggs; and a small amount of fat. With the exception of most fruits and vegetables, most foods have at least a little bit of fat, so you're automatically getting some fat in a balanced meal. Small amounts of added fat also help balance the meal.

You can easily determine if you're eating a balanced meal. When you look at your plate, more than half needs to be covered with foods that are high in carbohydrates, and less than half with foods high in protein.

Balance is particularly important in a low-calorie meal plan because a balanced diet helps ensure sustained energy as your body absorbs different types of foods and different combinations of foods and converts them to energy at different rates. Foods that are high in simple sugars move more quickly into your system and are metabolized and converted to energy more immediately. Foods that are digested more slowly, such as some complex carbohydrates and fats, provide energy later in the day.

Eating a variety of foods

After you balance the major food groups, choosing a variety of different foods within those groups helps ensure a good balance of vitamins, minerals, and other substances in food that keep you healthy.

One way to know whether or not your diet contains enough variety is to look at the colors on your plate. The more colors you see, the better variety of nutrients you're getting from your meal. Eating a variety of foods also helps keep your low-calorie diet more interesting and more appealing so that you stick with it.

Using Proven Strategies for Cutting Calories

When it comes to healthy weight control, *how* you eat is just as important as *what* you eat. The "what" is all about the actual food that's on your plate and in your mouth. The "how" is all about how much you actually eat, how many calories are in the types foods you choose, and how to make low-calorie choices within different food groups to ensure a nutritionally sound diet.

Controlling portion size

If you can control the portion sizes of the foods you eat, you can eat anything you want. For example, if you can eat one small piece of chocolate or one small scoop of ice cream or one handful of chips, you can eat those foods every day and not worry about gaining weight from them. Right now, you're probably saying, "Yeah, right!" because you can't imagine being able to eat such small amounts of your favorite indulgence foods and feeling satisfied. Don't worry. It's a process you have to discover; it doesn't usually happen overnight.

The menu plans in Chapter 6 call for very specific amounts of foods, or in other words, *portion control.* When you prepare meals using these menus for guidance, you figure out how to eyeball a specific amount of food and know that it's an appropriate amount to eat on a calorie-controlled diet. The portion sizes represent an average number of calories for each food group. In other words, you may see 1 cup of broccoli on one menu and 1 cup of mini carrots on another. You're free to ignore both suggestions and substitute a cup of snow peas or a cup of asparagus. That's because, as a group, a portion of one vegetable contains approximately the same number of calories as the same portion size of another vegetable. For more information on calorie counts by portion size within the different food groups, check out Appendix B.

In addition to helping you lose weight, a good weight-loss plan shows you how to eat in a way that you'll eventually be able to maintain your weight loss without being on such a strict diet. You won't always have to struggle with concepts like portion size, after you figure out what eating a reasonable amount of food means. The plus side to controlling your portion sizes is that by limiting the amount of each individual food you eat, you can eat several different types of foods. Eating different types of foods not only helps ensure you're getting a balance of essential nutrients, but it also helps keep your low-calorie diet from getting boring. (See "Keeping your energy high and your diet interesting," earlier in this chapter, for more about balance and variety in a low-calorie diet.)

However, you can go overboard, even with the good stuff. On a low-cal diet, you can eat too much of the good stuff, such as fruit and vegetables, because all foods supply calories and even the most nutritious foods add excess calories to your diet if you eat too much of them. As a result, you need to know how to control your portions when you're on a mission to lose weight.

When you're home, you can portion out your food with measuring cups and spoons as a way of teaching yourself what a serving size looks like. When you're eating out, the easiest way to figure out portion control is by using visual aids for standard serving sizes. Picture this:

- ✔ A 3-ounce serving of meat or poultry is about the size of a deck of cards or the box that holds a cassette tape.
- ✔ A standard muffin is about the size of a tennis ball (not a softball!).
- ✔ An ounce of cheese is about the size of a pair of dice.

An even easier strategy for measuring just about any type of food is to count on your fingers. You can use your hand to measure your favorite foods at home and to gauge your portion sizes when you're away from your own kitchen. For instance, a standard portion of meat is about the size of the palm of your hand. Make a fist, and you're looking at a cup of vegetables or pasta. From the tip of your thumbnail to its second joint is about the size of an ounce of cheese. The more average-size your hand, the more accurate these measurements are. But if you're a large person, with large hands, you need to eat a little more food anyway, so this strategy still works for you. See Figure 3-1 for an illustration of this hands-on approach.

Eating "free" foods

On a low-calorie diet, you don't always have to eat low-calorie foods. But if you want to eat large quantities of food, then you have to make low-cal choices. That's the premise behind any diet that says you can eat great volumes of food and still lose weight. After all, if I give you permission to eat all the spinach or romaine lettuce you want on this diet, you couldn't possibly eat enough of either of those foods to make a dent in your diet. At the same time, you could fill up on them or other leafy greens to cut your appetite and to make sure there's not enough room left in your stomach to fill up on too much of anything else. That's why eating a big salad (with just a little light dressing) at lunch and dinner works as a weight-loss strategy for so many people.

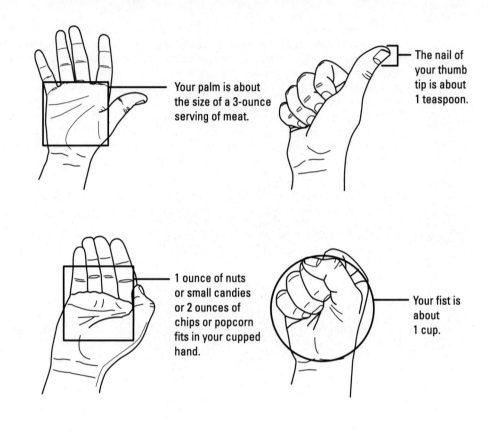

Your palm is about the size of a 3-ounce serving of meat.

The nail of your thumb tip is about 1 teaspoon.

1 ounce of nuts or small candies or 2 ounces of chips or popcorn fits in your cupped hand.

Your fist is about 1 cup.

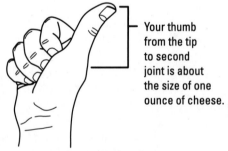

Figure 3-1: You can use your own hand to guesstimate portion sizes of most foods.

Your thumb from the tip to second joint is about the size of one ounce of cheese.

The same basic concept applies when you're choosing foods for meals and snacks and you want to eat larger quantities of food. That's when you have to make low-calorie choices at the level of individual foods. You can choose to use up your 100-calorie snack allotment by eating a small handful of fruit-flavored gum drops or jellybeans, or, for the same number of calories, you could eat half of a pineapple, five plums, or two cups of steamed green beans with a spoonful of light salad dressing for a dip.

Of course, if what you want to eat is a handful of jellybeans, then don't force yourself to eat fruit or vegetables. But these examples serve to show how choosing lower calorie foods on a regular basis can make room for those occasional indulgences.

When you're dieting to lose weight, sitting down to a large quantity of food is certainly more satisfying and less discouraging than sitting down to a plate that contains only small portions. Whenever you need more than your calorie limit allows or you need to "cheat" on your diet for any reason, feel free to choose foods from this list to help fill up your plate:

- ✔ Bouillon or fat-free broth
- ✔ Cabbage
- ✔ Celery
- ✔ Cucumber
- ✔ Green or red onions
- ✔ Greens: escarole, mustard, collard, dandelion
- ✔ Lettuce (any kind)
- ✔ Mushrooms
- ✔ Plain coffee or tea, including herb teas
- ✔ Radishes
- ✔ Seltzer, club soda, sparkling water, or other calorie-free drinks
- ✔ Spinach
- ✔ Unsweetened pickles, such as dill, "new," or half-sour
- ✔ Zucchini or yellow summer squash

To add flavor to "free" foods, use "free" condiments such as mustard, horse-radish, soy sauce, Worcestershire sauce, hot sauce, lemon juice, lime juice, or vinegar, or sprinkle your free foods with fresh or dried herbs and spices. Garlic, onion, and hot peppers go a long way toward seasoning steamed vegetables without adding any notable calories.

Watching calories from carbohydrates, proteins, and fats

After you decide a low-calorie diet is for you, you probably need to cut calories where you most indulge. For example, do you eat a big bowl (or container) of ice cream every night? Are you snacking too often on crackers and chips between meals? Does your sirloin steak take up your entire plate? Your excess calories probably aren't coming from big bowls of salad, unless you're filling your salad bowl with cold cuts and topping it off with gobs of dressing. And you're probably not gaining weight from vegetable side dishes, unless the only vegetables you choose are the starchier, more caloric ones like French fried potatoes and buttered corn.

Look at your diet to examine your food preferences and figure out if you overindulge when it comes to a particular food group. Keeping a food diary (see Chapter 4), and reviewing it with this purpose in mind, may yield some surprises about just how much of a particular type of food you actually eat.

The number of calories a food supplies depends on the amount of carbohydrate, fat, or protein in that food. That amount is shown in grams, which is a measure of weight.

- ✔ A gram of carbohydrate supplies four calories.
- ✔ A gram of protein supplies four calories.
- ✔ A gram of fat supplies nine calories.

Keep in mind that a gram of alcohol supplies seven calories, which makes it closer in calories to fat than to protein or carbohydrates. Cutting back on calories from alcohol can help you lose weight.

When you compare carbohydrates or protein to fat, you can see that, gram for gram, fat supplies more than twice as many calories. That's why cutting back on fat works for some people as a diet tool. But cutting fat is strictly a tool for people who are eating too much fat to begin with; it can't work alone as a strategy for losing weight or maintaining a healthy weight.

The following sections explain how to save calories and where to cut calories from carbohydrates, fats, and protein.

Choosing the best carbs

Contrary to some popular diet myths, cutting carbohydrates from your diet will only help you lose weight in the long run if you're eating too many carbohydrates to begin with! If you know you overdo it when it comes to cakes, cookies, pies, and even breads and pastas, then you probably already know you have to change your diet to trim some of those carbs for a better balance.

Cup for cup, starchier vegetables — potatoes, winter squash, corn, and green peas — are much higher in calories than other vegetables, but that doesn't mean you have to avoid them. You just need to watch your portion sizes when you choose these foods as side dishes.

On a low-calorie diet, the best carbohydrates are fresh or frozen fruits and vegetables, and high-fiber grain foods. For instance, if you like to eat pasta, choose whole-wheat varieties. You can mix whole-wheat pastas with regular pasta if you don't want to go completely whole-grain. You can also mix brown rice with white rice or mix rice with grains such as barley and cracked wheat to boost the fiber.

Increasing protein

If you eat a lot of one type of food on a calorie-controlled diet, you have to eat less of another food to stay within your calorie limit. Because fat is already limited in most sensible diets, the choice becomes whether to increase protein and decrease carbohydrates, or to eat more high-fiber carbs and fewer foods that are high in protein. A balanced diet gets 15 to 20 percent of its calories from protein. On a 1,500-calorie diet, that translates to at least 56 grams.

The best sources of protein on a low-calorie diet are seafood, poultry, lean meats, reduced-fat dairy products, and vegetarian sources such as soy foods and grain products. Chapter 5 contains plenty of information for making healthful protein choices at the supermarket.

If you tweak your low-cal diet to include more protein, know that it's a short-term solution for weight control. Like other trendy diets, a high-protein plan (a diet that gets more than 20 percent of its calories from protein) doesn't help you control your weight in the long run and can have a negative impact on your long-term health (see "Comparing low-calorie diets to other diets," earlier in this chapter, for more info on how it impacts your health).

Trimming fat

Fat supplies more than twice as many calories as either protein or carbohydrates, so if your diet is high in fat, you can start cutting there. You can make the cuts in more than one way. To cut down on the amount of fat in your diet, you can

- **Choose naturally reduced-fat and fat-free foods.** In addition to naturally lowfat foods like fruits, vegetables, and leaner cuts of meat, you can take advantage of lowfat dairy products and other foods that may be lower in calories because they've been modified to reduce the amount of fat they contain. (Just be careful to compare labels to make sure lower-fat foods are also lower in calories.)

- **Eat a wider variety of foods so that fat takes up less space in your diet.** Fill up on naturally lowfat foods, such as salads, broths, fruits, vegetables, legumes, and grains, so that you're not tempted to satisfy your hunger with higher fat foods.

- **Control your portion sizes.** Doing so ensures that you're not getting too much fat from any one food. For instance, eat ¼ of a bag of French fries, not the whole thing!

Part II

Getting Started: The Four-Week Plan and Beyond

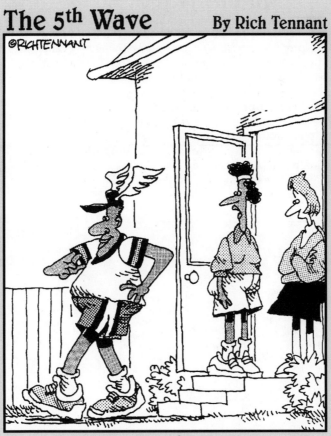

The 5th Wave   By Rich Tennant

"He's lost 12 pounds on his low-calorie diet. Now if I can just get him to lose that hat."

In this part . . .

*T*his part is the heart of the book. It tells you how to prepare yourself for low-calorie living by evaluating your habits, setting up your kitchen, choosing menu plans, keeping your diet life interesting, and figuring out the type of ongoing physical activity that fits into your lifestyle. In this part, you set goals, keep journals, and figure out how to adjust your attitude along with your eating habits. And you can find out how to make it all happen with positive thinking, mindful eating, and self-monitoring along the way. You can see how this part quickly became the biggest part of the book — you have a lot to do here!

Chapter 4

Kick-Starting Your Low-Calorie Plan

In This Chapter

▶ Assessing your habits

▶ Taking active steps to change your ways

▶ Gearing up with a good attitude

▶ Monitoring your progress with handy tracking tools

▶ Being mindful of your new lifestyle

You're probably familiar with the expression, "You can't teach an old dog new tricks." It's a cousin to the saying, "Old habits die hard." No matter how you say it, change doesn't come easy to most people, and yet change is essential to weight-loss success. My attitude is this: I can teach anyone some new diet tricks, but some people take more time than others to get it right. And although breaking old habits isn't always easy, if you work hard enough to replace them with new, healthier habits, doing so is certainly possible.

In this chapter, you assess your eating and exercise habits, establish your short-term and long-term weight goals, check your attitude, set up a monitoring system, and mentally prepare yourself to live a low-calorie lifestyle. This chapter is the essential groundwork you need to map out a plan that can ensure your long-term success because it prepares you for making necessary changes in your eating, exercising, and thinking patterns.

Examining Your Current Diet Habits

You may be very open-minded, and consider yourself to be quite flexible, but still, deep down, you may not be completely comfortable with the idea of changing your diet, which is normal. Change comes hard to most people because it usually means giving up something. In this case, you're giving up precious calories. Some change is necessary and inevitable, though, if you're going to break free once and for all from unhealthy behavior patterns like overeating, underexercising, and thinking self-defeating thoughts.

In the following sections, I show you how to recognize your unhealthy behaviors and typical dieting styles.

Recognizing problem behaviors

Sometimes you may do something for no reason other than you've been doing it that way for so long. You form habits — good and bad —by repetition. You may have acquired your earliest habits first from family members and later from friends, but they became embedded in your lifestyle by years of repetition.

The types of food you eat, your eating patterns, your exercise routine, the way you think about yourself, and the way you view the world around you, are all habits you've developed by eating the same foods, making the same choices, coming up with the same motivations and the same excuses, and thinking the same thoughts, over and over again, throughout your life. These behaviors shape who you are. They also help determine your shape!

Know thyself

Your first step toward developing healthier habits is to look inward and think hard about changing your ways. Thinking about change is an important part of the process of enacting real change, so if all you can do right now is think about it, you're still on the right track. For more about making healthy changes, see "Giving Yourself a Lifestyle Makeover," later in this chapter.

You're probably wondering why you need to do all this soul searching. Why not just skip straight to Chapter 6 and go on a low-calorie diet? You need to search inside because a successful weight-loss plan is about making lifestyle changes, and you can't change what you don't know or understand. The better you know yourself, the better your chances of getting to the root of your weight problem to conquer it once and for all.

Breaking your bad habits

It wasn't a banana that made you overweight. It wasn't your grandmother's lasagna, the slice of chocolate cake at a birthday party, or that double cheeseburger you devoured on your way home from work. No individual food is possibly responsible for your weight gain, but your habit of overeating some of these foods probably did you in.

Which of these behaviors contribute to your bad eating habits? Check the ones that apply to you.

❑ I eat randomly.

❑ I eat too much food at once.

❑ I eat when I'm sad.

❑ I eat out often.

❑ I routinely skip meals.

❑ I eat on the run.

❑ I eat at fast-food restaurants.

❑ I eat when I'm lonely.

❑ I eat too quickly.

❑ I eat when I'm not hungry.

❑ I eat when I'm bored.

❑ I eat late at night or just before I go to bed.

❑ I eat snacks all the time.

❑ I wait more than four or five hours before eating.

❑ I eat a lot of high-fat foods.

❑ I eat a lot of high-calorie foods.

❑ I eat when I'm angry.

The habits you checked are the eating habits you need to focus on when you're thinking about the lifestyle changes you have to make to accommodate your low-calorie lifestyle.

Eating, exercise, and other lifestyle habits don't change overnight. You can't just suddenly cut your calorie intake in half without some mental preparation. You can't just get up one morning and run a marathon if you haven't been training. Changing the thinking patterns that dictate your behavior takes time, patience, and a fair amount of retraining.

Playing diet games

Everyone I've ever counseled about weight control has admitted to some type of self-defeating behavior. One time it was a woman who secretly snacks on the types of foods she knows will kick off a binge. Another time it was a guy slacking off on the exercise routine that was just beginning to show results. If you know your own weakness, you can renew your commitment to change the behavior that's blocking your weight-loss success.

When making a commitment to losing weight, some people play destructive mind games with themselves. Here are some examples:

- ✔ **The "if only" game:** "If only I had a faster metabolism." "If only I had enough money to go to a spa." "If only I were taller and could carry more weight." "If only I had more time, I'd go to the gym more often." These excuses really don't fly, however, because getting fit isn't about daydreaming. It's about being determined, taking action, and staying motivated. No one stays in shape without having to work at it.

- ✔ **The blame game:** This game really is a trap that prevents you from taking responsibility for yourself and your weight. Here's how it goes: "I had a fight with my husband so I ate a large bag of potato chips." "My kids drove me crazy all day so I devoured a pint of ice cream after they went to bed." Sound familiar?

- ✔ **The "pity me" game:** Feeling sorry for yourself helps you avoid committing to a fitness plan because you can just point at everything that's wrong with you and decide you're not worth helping. "It's too late." "It's too hard." "Why bother?" In some ways, you may even enjoy the attention you get for being "poor you" and may be reluctant to give it up.

Your diet personality is probably a lot like your overall personality with respect to how easily you make commitments and motivate yourself to approach difficult tasks. If you answer "yes" to any of the following questions, you may be standing in your own way of getting to a healthier weight:

- ✔ Do you think someone else is responsible for the way you eat?

- ✔ Do you believe other people lose and maintain weight easier than you?

- ✔ Do you look for quick-fix solutions?

- ✔ Do you live a life of deprivation, eating foods you don't like and avoiding those foods you do in an attempt to lose or maintain weight?

- ✔ Does the prospect of following a diet and losing weight overwhelm you?

- ✔ Do you try to lose weight on your own, without ever seeking help?

- ✔ Do you give up easily?

- ✔ Do you feel like a failure when you fall off the food wagon and eat too much?

The best fitness plan is one that you fine-tune to fit your personality and lifestyle. After you answer the preceding questions, ask yourself the following questions so you can tailor the plan in this book to suit your diet personality.

- ✔ Are you a joiner, or do you like to go it alone?

- ✔ Are you a grazer who nibbles all day long, or do you normally sit down to three full meals and a formal snack or two?

✔ Do you want someone to tell you what and when to eat in a prescribed plan, or would you rather have a flexible diet that allows you to make on-the-spot food decisions?

Giving Yourself a Lifestyle Makeover

The more you know about who you are as an individual and the better you identify your habits, the easier making those necessary changes and committing to a lifelong plan of healthier eating and living will be. The following sections help you start a low-calorie lifestyle today.

Making changes one step at a time

When you're clear about which aspects of your life actually need to be changed, you can begin taking real steps to enact those changes.

The best place to start is with a commitment to yourself. Promise yourself that you're never going to give up on yourself. Acknowledge now that cutting back on the amount of food you're used to eating won't be easy. At the same time, keep telling yourself you can do it! Be your own cheerleader. Promise yourself that you won't kick yourself when you fall off the food wagon. Successful dieters don't scold themselves or give up. They give themselves a pep talk and jump right back on.

Make small changes, one at a time, at your own pace, and allow yourself to get used to one change before moving on to the next. For example, your first change may be to switch from regular salad dressings to low-calorie dressings. Or, you may decide to steam vegetables instead of stir-frying them to save calories from added fat. If both of those changes appeal to you, make one change today and the other tomorrow.

When a person takes real-life steps to make permanent lifestyle changes, scientists call it *behavior modification.* The following examples of eating behavior modification techniques can help you start your low-cal lifestyle:

✔ **Eat before you go food shopping.** When you're hungry, you're more likely to make impulse purchases of foods you don't really want to eat.

✔ **Make a shopping list when you go to the grocery store and stick to the list when you get there.** Don't allow yourself to buy "indulgence" foods likes snacks and junk food that aren't on the list. In Chapter 6 you find low-cal menus that you can work from when writing up your list.

✔ **Don't buy "indulgence" foods or any calorie-laden foods.** These foods can contribute to overeating when you're first starting a new diet. (See Chapter 5 for more tips on shopping for a low-calorie diet.)

✔ **Keep healthier foods on hand and ready to eat in your refrigerator and cupboards.** Doing so gives you options other than junk food when you're looking for an easy snack or a quick meal.

✔ **Prepare strict single portions so you aren't tempted to overeat (and consume more calories) if you're cooking for yourself only, and not following a recipe.** When you're cooking for yourself from a recipe that makes more than one serving, wrap up the additional servings and put them in the fridge or freezer as soon as possible so you're not tempted to go back for seconds.

✔ **Use smaller plates.** Low-calorie meals tend to look lost on larger plates and may make you feel deprived.

✔ **Always sit down when you eat, even if you're just having a quick snack, so that you pay attention to how much you eat.** You can easily forget about the calories you consume when you eat on the run.

✔ **Leave the table when you're finished eating what's on your plate.** Doing so reduces the temptation to go back for more food.

✔ **Don't skip meals.** If you do, you may overeat at your next meal or snack too much in between.

In the section "Using Tracking Tools As You Get Started," later in this chapter, you discover how to document and evaluate your eating habits and identify those that need changing. At that point, you can figure out where to make small changes in your diet and begin to shift the eating behavior patterns that are working against you.

Knowing your diet limits

When you go to your favorite south-of-the-border restaurant, do you order the steamed fish and vegetable special? Do you get a baked potato on the side and top it with a lowfat yogurt–sour cream blend? No? I'm not surprised because, frankly, I don't know anyone who does. Everyone I know who enjoys Mexican food goes for the gusto — the cheese nachos, the beef tacos, the chile rellenos, not to mention the margaritas and the lime-infused brew. How do you handle that on 1,000 calories a day? Very carefully, I'd advise, or not at all until you feel confident that your can order sensibly.

Some people can eat just one. No matter what they're offered, whether it's a tortilla chip or a chocolate chip cookie, they take a small sample and never go back for more. However, most people aren't like that. If you're watching your weight, you may need to avoid most convenience food stores, your supermarket's snack section, and all Mexican restaurants.

Adjusting your food plan through the seasons

Just as you need a change of wardrobe when summer gives in to early fall, you may need to change your food plan when one season fades into another. Food availability changes with the seasons and so might your physical needs. You may be more active in spring and summer than in winter, and you may cook more in the winter than in the summer or crave heartier foods. You may routinely take your vacations midsummer and late fall, and these vacations may be opportunities to enjoy new and different foods. These seasonal, and temporary, lifestyle changes can affect the way you eat.

For many people, a change in seasons also means a change in mood. If you suffer from winter blues, your diet may suffer, too. The best way to prepare for any seasonal changes in your lifestyle that affect your diet is to look ahead and have a plan in place.

Remember, too, that some things *don't* change with the seasons. You need to drink as much water in the winter as you do in the summer, and your body needs good nutrition and a good physical workout all year round.

When you know you won't be satisfied with small portions of your favorite foods, stay away from them until you're feeling stronger. Never say "never," but definitely figure out how to say "not right now."

Even if you're an independent operator and you're used to making decisions on your own, don't be afraid to admit if you can't handle this one alone. You can find a diet buddy or an exercise buddy, join a gym, join a weight-loss program, or seek professional counseling. Whatever it takes for you to start and stick to your low-calorie lifestyle, do it. (See Chapter 11 for more information and advice on asking for and getting the right type of help.)

Keeping your diet fresh

Initially, you have to make all sorts of changes in your diet and perhaps other areas of your life. Then what? In time, your new low-cal lifestyle will get old and you'll have to reevaluate your plan to keep it from getting stale.

Boredom is a common trigger for overeating. Sometimes, feelings of boredom are actually a habit of your mind. You're in the habit of telling yourself that you're bored, so you feel bored on a regular basis. If that's the case, you have to make a huge effort to push past those thoughts as soon as they enter your mind and find something interesting to do.

If you spend too many nights sitting around eating and can't think of anything else to do, sign up for an evening cooking class (preferably a healthy cooking or low-cal cooking class). With a class, you can still eat but you'll be spending most of your time learning about food and preparing food in a social setting. You may even discover something new that can help keep your diet interesting. (For more ideas on how to keep your new diet and lifestyle fresh, check out Chapters 7 and 9.)

Checking Your Attitude

When following a low-calorie diet and controlling your weight, attitude is everything. Well, almost everything. To succeed, you definitely need a positive attitude and a good, steady supply of resolve. That means paying as much attention to what's in your head as you do to what's on your plate.

In the following sections, you find tips you can use to help keep your attitude happy, healthy, and in check.

Finding and maintaining your motivation

Different things motivate different people to start a low-calorie diet and stick to it. You have to find your own best personal motivators by figuring out what matters most to you and what makes you feel good about yourself. Do you want to be healthy, look good, live longer, and feel the tremendous sense of accomplishment that comes from breaking bad habits and developing good ones? The motivators you believe in are the ones that will work for you.

For example, if you believe that eating a low-calorie diet is an essential part of a healthy lifestyle, and you want to be healthy, then good health is a motivator that works for you. When you're tempted to eat that second piece of cake, you can remind yourself that eating double helpings of dessert isn't a healthy habit because the fat in that cake may raise your cholesterol levels. Or if you're driven by a desire to look your best, you can remind yourself that double helpings of dessert end up as double helpings of fat on your thighs.

Loosening up

Yes, following a low-calorie diet takes a good deal of determination and self-discipline, especially if you have a great deal of weight to lose and plan to stay on your diet for some time to come. You have to be strict about the amount of food you eat, and willing to follow a new set of lifestyle rules.

But at the same time, changing your thinking, eating, and exercise patterns takes flexibility and open mindedness. Be open to new ideas. After all, whatever you've been doing up until now hasn't been working for you, so clearly you need to try something new.

You can help yourself adjust to the idea of change by challenging yourself in small, nonthreatening ways. For instance, if you normally eat the same breakfast every day, try something new, just for one morning. (You can find plenty of ideas in Chapters 6 and 12.) Think of ways you can be open-minded that have nothing to do with food, too. Buy a shirt in a color you don't normally wear but that you think looks good on you and wear it. One of the things you're teaching yourself with these types of challenges is that you can survive change, and you may even enjoy it. After you open up your mind to these smaller, temporary changes, you may feel more confident approaching the larger lifestyle changes with a low-calorie lifestyle.

Staying positive

With the right attitude, your chances of succeeding, sticking to your plan, and losing weight greatly increase. A negative attitude, on the other hand, only prevents you from pushing on and moving forward in your new lifestyle. If you have trouble replacing negative thoughts with positive thoughts, the section "Thinking mindfully," later in this chapter, can help.

Are you ready? If all or most of the following statements are true for you, then what are you waiting for? Start managing your weight today.

✔ I can make a commitment to myself to follow through on my diet, no matter what else is going on in my life.

✔ I can make the necessary changes in my diet and exercise program.

✔ I can spend time at the beginning of each week planning my meals and exercise routine for that week.

✔ I can continue to find ways to stay motivated until I reach my goal weight.

✔ I can assess my plan from time to time to make sure it's still working for me.

✔ I can figure out how to accept lapses and setbacks as opportunities to come up with new goals and strategies, not to use them as excuses for giving up.

Any "false" answers point out the areas that need special attention. To work on those areas, use the goal-setting tools in the next section.

Using Tracking Tools As You Get Started

One benefit of using a self-help weight-loss method like the plan in this book is that you have plenty of flexibility within the plan, and you don't have to answer to a nutritionist, a group leader, or a weight-loss counselor. But because you're going it alone, you have to do a little more thinking for yourself. You have to set yourself up on a personalized program and to do that, you need to use the same tools any professional would use to set that plan up for you. These tools include goal setting, journaling with a food diary, and keeping track of your weight.

You don't have to use every tool in the book or answer every question in every quiz, but the more you discover about yourself and your eating habits, the better your chances of developing a plan that works for you.

Establishing your weight goals

The amount of weight you want to lose, the lifestyle changes you're willing to make to help you lose it, and all the little steps you'll take along the way make up your long-term, intermediate-term, and short-term goals. (Before you settle on your goals, you can use the formulas in Chapter 2 to figure out how much weight you want to lose.)

- ✔ **Long-term goals:** Your first long-term goal is the total amount of weight you want to lose, or, if you prefer to put it another way, the final weight you want to reach. Your primary long-term goal may also be a normal Body Mass Index (BMI), which is a measure of weight for height that may be a little more accurate than most standard weight charts. (Flip to Chapter 2 for more about BMI.)

- ✔ **Intermediate goals:** These goals are the ones that you establish and change along the way. Right now, one of your intermediate goals may be the weight you hope to be when you're halfway to your long-term goal. For example, if you want to lose 60 pounds by this time next year (a very reasonable long-term goal for someone with 60 pounds to lose at the recommended rate of 1 to 2 pounds a week), then two of your intermediate goals may be to lose 15 pounds in the next three months and 30 pounds six months from now.

Unless your weight seriously compromises your health, for example if your BMI is 30 or higher or if your doctor has told you that you're already at risk for developing obesity-related medical problems, your goal needs to be gradual weight loss, which means losing 1 to 2 pounds a week. If your weight is putting you at immediate risk of health complications, you may want to consider faster weight loss in a medically supervised program. Speak to your doctor about your health risk and to find out what type of weight-loss program is right for you. (See Chapter 11 for more on medically supervised programs.)

✔ **Short-term goals:** These goals are immediate goals you focus on from day to day. For example, you can set a goal to lose 1½ pounds this week.

Establishing mini-short-term goals to help you reach your short-term goal and to satisfy any need you may have to do something about your weight right now is a good idea. For instance, deciding to eat steamed fish for dinner tonight is a mini-short-term goal that can help lead to your 1½ pound weight loss goal for the week. Another mini-short-term goal may be to buy a pocket-size calorie count book today, make copies of the calorie counter pages in Appendix A and Appendix B, or locate calorie-count information on the Internet so you have it available wherever you are.

Setting up your lifestyle goals

In addition to your weight goals (see the previous section), several other types of goals are essential to the long-term success of a low-calorie lifestyle plan. They include your

✔ **Food goals:** These goals are the changes you want to make to your diet, such as how much you eat, the types of food you choose to eat, and the amount of calories you consume.

- Your long-term food goal is to make a low-calorie diet plan part of your permanent lifestyle.

- Your intermediate-term food goal may include preparing and eating more low-cal meals at home.

- In keeping with these far-reaching goals, one of your short-term food goals may be preparing a low-calorie dinner tonight. (See Chapter 14 for several ideas.)

✔ **Behavioral goals:** When your long-term goals include eating better and permanent weight loss, behavior modifications are necessary for those goals to become permanent changes.

- Your long-term behavioral goal may be to eat mindfully, that is, pay more attention to what and how you eat (see "Eating mindfully," later in this chapter for details).

- One intermediate-term goal may be to take your time and eat slowly.

- A short-term behavioral goal toward that end may be to start practicing putting your fork down between bites at your next meal.

See "Giving Yourself a Lifestyle Makeover," earlier in this chapter for more about changing your overall eating habits.

✔ **Psychological goals:** If you're going to change the way you eat forever, you probably have to change your emotional relationship with food.

- Your long-term psychological goal may be to avoid emotional eating and overeating, the type of eating you do when you're sad, angry, or lonely.

- Your intermediate-term goal may be to find something else to do other than eat when you're not happy or to seek professional help to make changes you can't make alone.

- Your short-term goal may be to dig out those knitting needles, paintbrushes, or toolbox, and get to work right away on a new project that can keep your hands busy tonight.

See Chapter 9 for more about adjusting your mindset.

✔ **Exercise goals:** If you're going to supplement your low-calorie diet with increased activity, exercise goals can help you pace yourself.

- Your long-term goal may be to swim 15 laps at least four times a week.

- Your intermediate-term goal may be rearranging your schedule so that you have time to add that much swimming to your exercise routine.

- Your short-term goal may be joining a gym that has a pool or to start using the pool at the gym you already attend.

See Chapter 8 for advice about how to work more physical activity into your daily life.

When setting your goals, keep these two important points in mind:

✔ **Make sure your goals are realistic.** You want to be able to complete your goals within the timeframe you give yourself. For example, if you say you're going to cook a low-cal dinner tonight, be sure you have the ingredients on hand when you get home. If you find that any goal is unrealistic, don't stress out. Redefine the goal.

✔ **Make sure your goals are as specific as possible.** The clearer your goals, the easier it is to measure your progress along the way. For example, you don't just want to be thinner; you want to lose 60 pounds. You don't want to simply cut back on the number of calories you consume; you want to stick to a 1,200-calorie plan.

Putting your goals in writing can help you clarify them. Make a goal organizer, something like the one in Figure 4-1, to jot down your long-term, intermediate-term, and short-term goals in each lifestyle category.

Focus	Goal	Time Frame	Steps to Take	Date Reached
Food	Eat less chocolate	Short	Give away the rest of the truffles	
Food				
Food				
Food				
Behavior	Skip my morning snack	Medium	Stay away from the snack cart at work; start by skipping every other day	
Behavior				
Behavior				
Psych	Positive attitude about self	Medium	Wake up every day and say out loud: "I can do it!"	
Psych				
Psych				
Exercise	Start jogging	Short	Buy new running shoes this week	
Exercise	Start jogging	Short	Get up earlier to jog before work every day	

Figure 4-1:
Writing down your goals can help you keep track of where you stand.

These pointers can help you use your organizer to its fullest potential:

✔ Separate your goals into food, behavioral, psychological, and exercise categories. Write down any steps you can think of, big or little, that you can take to reach that goal.

You can write down as many goals as you want, but remember, you don't have to work on them all right now! Your goals reflect the changes you're going to make over the next few days, weeks, months, and, in some cases, years.

✔ As you reach each goal, write down the date. Doing so helps motivate you when you look back over your goals and see what you've accomplished.

> ✔ Review your goals weekly to remind yourself which areas still need work. As you reach your current goals, you may want to establish new ones and write them down in your goal organizer.

Keeping a food diary

Whenever I counsel new clients, I ask them to keep a *food diary* (a record of all the food they eat) for at least three days before their first appointment. At this point, I'm asking you to do the same. Your food diary doesn't have to include three consecutive days, but it needs to cover three days that honestly represent the way you eat. I usually suggest documenting at least two weekdays (workdays) and one weekend day (one day off).

Most people think they eat less food than they actually do, and if that's the case, the number of calories that shows up when they start keeping track surprises them. They also think they eat less fat, sugar, and salt than they actually do. A food diary is such an important tool because it helps you see all this information. In the following sections, I show you how to keep a food diary and what you can find from the information you gather from having one.

If you start your food diary before you start your diet, you'll use it to assess your current eating habits and figure out where you have room for improvement. At the end of the day, when you look at your diary, you'll have most of the information you need to set behavior goals, reshape your diet, refigure your calorie allowance, and keep track of your progress.

How to keep a food diary

You have several ways to keep a food diary, and how you do it depends on how much you enjoy documenting your own life and how much time you can devote to record keeping. When you're busy, a food diary can be as simple as a scrap of paper on which you write down everything you eat and how much of it you eat. You can carry a piece of paper in your wallet for each day you maintain a record.

A better way, however, is to buy a special pad or notebook and fill it with as much information as you can about what, when, why, and how you eat. The more time you spend documenting and reviewing your diet now, the more you can discover about yourself and your diet and the less necessary it will be to write it all down as time goes on.

Each page in a proper food diary has a minimum of five columns. (See Figure 4-2 for an example.) Write the day and date at the top of the page. Then fill in your diary entries every time you eat, as soon as you eat, whether it's a full, sit-down meal or a snack. (You can fill in the actual calorie counts at the end of the day or whenever you find time.)

Time	Food	Amount	Calories	Reason
6:45 a.m.	Raisin bran with	½ cup		Breakfast
	skim milk	½ cup		
	Coffee with	1 cup		
	skim milk	¼ cup		
	Nectarine	1		
10 a.m.	Plain bagel	½		Snack cart arrived
	Coffee with	1 cup		
	skim milk	¼ cup		
1 p.m.	Roasted peppers	1 cup		Lunch from salad bar
	3-bean salad	½ cup		
	Water	16 oz.		
5 p.m.	Tiny pretzel sticks	10		Hungry
7:30 p.m.	Grilled salmon steak	4 oz.		Dinner at restaurant
	Steamed green beans	1 cup		with Cindy
	New potatoes	3 small		
	Wine	1 glass		
10 p.m.	Chocolate truffle	1		Wanted chocolate

Figure 4-2:
A page in a food diary lists five columns of important information.

If you wait until the end of the day and try to remember what you ate, you may not remember everything from every meal or snack. You may forget about food you ate on the run.

The following list details the five columns in a food diary and explains what you need to record.

- **The first column is for the time.** Here you write down the time you started eating.

- **The second column is for listing the food you eat, as specifically as possible.** Don't forget to include drinks. You can even include water and other noncaloric drinks so you can get a sense of how much fluid you drink each day. Try to separate the components of foods. For example, instead of cheese sandwich, enter whole-wheat bread, cheddar cheese, tomato, and mustard. Doing so makes it easier for you to figure out the calorie counts on some foods.

- **The third column is for guesstimating the amount of food you ate.** Write down the size, quantity, volume, or weight of each food you listed in the previous column. Using your cheese sandwich as an example, you may put 2 slices next to the bread, 2 ounces next to the cheese, 4 thin slices next to the tomato, and 1 tablespoon next to the mustard. You can refer to Chapter 3 for help figuring out the portion sizes of different types of foods.

✔ **The fourth column is for approximating the number of calories provided by those foods.** Obviously, the more you know about weights, measures, and calorie counts, the more accurate you can be with this information. Appendixes A and B are full of calorie count info.

✔ **In the fifth column, write your reason for eating and any other relevant information such as whom you ate with and how you were feeling when you ate.** For example, if you're eating simply because it's lunchtime and you're hungry, then you can just put "hungry" or "lunchtime" in the reason column, or nothing at all. But if you're eating because you don't want to offend your grandmother or because you're angry with your boss, then noting the reason why you ate is important so that you can work on finding other ways to deal with emotional situations. (Chapter 9 covers these types of "trigger" situations and provides suggestions for how to deal with them.)

While you're keeping an initial food diary:

✔ **Eat normally; that is, eat what you ordinarily eat throughout the day.** Don't try to make changes in your diet or eating habits while you're keeping your initial food diary. At this point, you're simply assessing your current eating habits and food preferences, many of which can be incorporated into your new low-calorie plan and can actually help make the new plan work better for you. For example, if you love chocolate, don't avoid it. Write it down, and later on you can figure out how to enjoy chocolate without sabotaging your diet.

✔ **Write down everything you eat.** This point is important both for calculating your total calorie intake and for helping to determine how you can better balance your diet in the future.

✔ **Put as much information in your diary as you can.** The more you discover about your food habits, the better you can help yourself devise a low-cal plan that's sure to work for you.

The beauty of having a formal food diary is that, in addition to the five basic columns, you can use the same book in which you list your foods to also record your goals, your progress, your exercise log (see Chapter 8 for details), tips and advice you collect, and all your thoughts and feelings about everything you're doing to lose weight and get to a healthier state of mind and body. You can divide your book into different sections for each of these areas or let some of them overlap. For instance, you can create a separate section in the back of your book for your thoughts about the weight-loss process, or you can write your thoughts in the margins on the same page where you record your goals or your exercise progress. Get used to writing in your diary every day. Eventually you'll stop writing down every bit of food you eat and every mile you log on the treadmill, but until you meet your weight-loss goals, you're sure to have something to add to your journal. For now and for the future, you have all your personal weight control material in one place.

What your food diary tells you

When you examine your food diary, look for patterns. You'll discover that you have specific food habits, some good, and some not so good. Answering the following questions allows you to see your eating patterns more clearly and helps you focus on those areas that need improvement.

- ✔ Are you actually hungry when you eat?
- ✔ Do you eat too often?
- ✔ Do you eat too much?
- ✔ Do you skip meals?
- ✔ Are you an emotional eater?
- ✔ Do you eat a balanced diet?
- ✔ Do you routinely snack?
- ✔ Do you sit down to regular meals?
- ✔ Do certain situations trigger you to eat when you're not actually hungry?
- ✔ Do you undereat earlier in the day and overeat later on?
- ✔ Do you choose too many high-calorie or high-fat foods?
- ✔ Do you overeat from one particular food group?

Keep a food diary for as long as you find it helpful. Some people keep a food diary for weeks, or even months, using it to monitor themselves every day. Eating less is easier when you're writing down and are aware of every bite. If keeping the food diary becomes problematic, put it down for a while. Don't throw it away; just put it away until you feel like using it again. You may never write in it again, but you may want to look at it from time to time and use it for motivation or as a reminder of how far you've come.

Weighing in on a regular basis

Most people who are concerned about their weight own a bathroom scale. Weighing in is one way of monitoring yourself and assessing your progress. It can also be a good motivating tool, giving you the push you need to work a little harder on your goal, as long as you don't become a slave to your scale.

The following sections tell you when to weigh yourself and how to maintain a weight-change chart.

Knowing when to weigh yourself

A scale is a useful tool for tracking weight changes and documenting progress. Weighing yourself allows you to keep a record of how far you've come and how far you have to go to reach your goals.

When you weigh yourself, remember that your weight can fluctuate up to several pounds for any number of reasons, including hormonal changes, a rise or dip in your level of body fluids, and the type of food and drinks you consumed that day. These weight fluctuations have nothing to do with your true weight. For that reason

✔ Weigh yourself no more than once a week.

The numbers on a scale generally don't lie, but they may not always be an accurate reflection of your true body weight. Don't be alarmed if the numbers move up or down in inexplicable ways. A certain amount of weight fluctuation is normal from week to week or day to day, even from hour to hour, which is why you don't want to weight yourself too frequently.

✔ Always weigh yourself on the same day of the week, at the same time of day. Morning is probably best for motivation, because you haven't eaten yet and weigh less than you will at any other time of day.

✔ Weigh yourself when you're naked and dry. You could add up to several pounds of false weight from clothing or wet hair.

Filling in a weight-change chart

A weight-change chart (see Figure 4-3) graphs your weight loss (or gain) from week to week so you can monitor your diet and exercise changes and be sure they're working for you.

You may also begin to see a pattern of slight weight gain from time to time, and you'll also be able to see that this weight gain levels out again after such periods. When you see the repetitive pattern on paper, you'll be better able to accept these fluctuations as naturally occurring events and trust that they have nothing to do with real weight.

Use the following steps when using your weight-change chart (shown in Figure 4-3):

1. **Begin by filling in your current weight (starting weight), in the space provided, a few lines down from the top of the chart.**

2. **One week from now, weigh yourself.**

   Go to week number 1 at the top of the graph.

3. **If you've lost weight, move down the graph until you reach the row for the number that represents your weight change for this first week.**

   Put an *X* in the appropriate column.

   For example, if you lose 2 pounds, stop at the –2 row and put an *X* in the Week 1 column.

4. **If you gain weight, move *up* the graph until you reach the row for the number that represents the number of pounds you gained.**

Week	1	2	3	4	5	6	7	8	9	10	11	12	13	14	15	16
+5																
+4																
+3																
+2																
+1																
0																
Start Weight ___																
-1																
-2																
-3																
-4																
-5																
-6																
-7																
-8																
-9																
-10																
-15																
-20																
-25																
-30																

Figure 4-3:
A weight-change chart is a handy, easy-to-use tracking tool.

5. **If you gain or lose a half pound, draw a diagonal line through the center of the appropriate box.**

6. **Repeat each week, graphing the total number of pounds you've lost since Week 1 or since the last time you gained weight.**

   If you continue to gain, graph the total number of pounds you've gained since you stopped losing weight. If you don't gain or lose any weight during a given week, check the 0 row for that week.

   For example, if you lost 2 pounds during Week 1 and 2 more pounds during Week 2, mark the –4 row in the Week 2 column. If you gain 1 pound the following week, mark the +1 row in the Week 3 column. If you lose 2 pounds the following week, mark the –2 row again in the Week 4 column. (But if you gain another pound during Week 4, mark the +2 column in Week 4.) Continue this way for several months to see if your weight fluctuations have a pattern. What you may find is that you lose weight steadily for a period of time, only to gain a pound or two whenever your normal schedule is interrupted or when you experience hormonal changes.

   If you're really into graphing, use dots instead of *X*'s, and connect the dots for a more graphic representation of your weight fluctuations. *Note:* This chart doesn't graph your actual weight or your total weight loss, only the number of pounds you lose (or gain) each week and how your weight sometimes fluctuates.

Practicing Mindful Low-Calorie Living

If you're a Buddhist or you're familiar with Buddhist philosophy, then you already have some idea about what it means to live mindfully. If you're not familiar with mindful living, that's okay. You don't have to join a monastery to understand the concept. *Mindful living* simply means paying attention to what's going on in your life right now, in this moment. That's a no-brainer, right? What's difficult for many people, however, is the actual practice of mindfulness. For most people, it's a practice that takes practice.

Mindful living incorporates many useful guidelines for low-calorie living. Some of these guidelines deal directly with eating behavior and provide practical tips for changing that behavior, and others help with the psychological aspects of overeating, such as changing your thinking patterns to help ensure success.

Eating mindfully

Mindful eating is all about being aware of what and how you eat. It means thinking about your food and paying attention to your eating habits. It's the opposite of *mindless* eating, which is actually easier because it requires no thought whatsoever.

Eating mindfully prevents you from eating too much food at one sitting or putting food into your mouth all day long without even realizing that you're eating. Perhaps the best thing about mindful eating is that it has no negative after-effects and no guilt involved. You can't say the same about eating mindlessly!

Here are the basic steps of mindful eating to follow every time you eat:

1. **Pay attention to the way you prepare your food.**

2. **Prepare your food carefully and thoughtfully.**

3. **Prepare your dining table with care and attention.**

4. **Pay attention to the amount of food you put on your plate.**

5. **Relax as you sit down to eat.**

6. **Look at your food, smell it, be aware of it as you eat.**

7. **Eat slowly.**

8. **Avoid interruptions and stressful conversations while you eat.**

9. **Pay attention to your body's hunger level as you eat.**

10. **Eat no more than you need to eat to feel satisfied.**

11. **Spend a quiet minute or two reflecting on your meal when you've finished eating.**

Thinking mindfully

How often have you said to yourself, "I'm too fat" or "I hate my thighs" or even "I'll never be able to stop eating"? Mindful thinking encourages you to pay attention to this type of negative "self-talk" and the effect it has on your self-esteem and motivation.

When you think mindfully, you catch yourself in negative self-talk and allow yourself a moment to change it to something positive. Mindful thinking allows you to listen to your own brain chatter and ultimately replace negative and destructive thoughts with something more affirming.

Self-supporting statements such as "I am loving and capable" are called *affirmations.* They're nothing more than soft and fluffy thoughts that are help- ful for giving yourself a lift and keeping yourself motivated when the dieting gets tough. If you're not in the habit of using affirmations, you may want to come up with a few affirmations that have meaning for you and start using them to replace the harsher thoughts you sometimes have about yourself. For instance, if you're ready to give up before you even begin your diet, you may say to yourself, "There's no point; I'm never going to lose weight." Because that type of thinking doesn't help, having an opposing affirmation handy, per- haps one that says "I'm not giving in to failure," or at least, "I'm going to give this my best shot," can be beneficial.

Some people think affirmations are silly and are completely turned off by them. If you're one of those people, try to suspend your judgment and prac- tice using affirmations in your daily life. See if they help bring you back to a positive frame of mind when you're slipping into negative waters. See if they help you maintain a better outlook throughout the day. You may not always feel on top of your world, but at the very least you may be able to muster up something like, "I've had worse days" when you hit a roadblock and are tempted to give up.

Whether you're looking in the mirror or searching your soul, focus on your best personal traits and on your successes, not on your failures. Use the fol- lowing affirmations to replace negative thoughts in a variety of situations.

Instead of:	*You Can Say:*
I'm going to be fat forever.	It took a while to get here; it'll take a while to get back.
I hate my body.	My body's getting healthier every day.
I'm starving.	I'm looking forward to eating healthier foods.
This diet is too hard.	Just wait. Good things take time.
It's going too slow.	If I'm patient, I'll be successful. I can wait as long as it takes.

Instead of:	You Can Say:
I'm going to buy a candy bar.	I'm strong enough to say "no" this time.
I feel sick all the time.	I'm getting stronger and healthier every day.
I'm so ashamed of the way I look.	I'm so proud of myself for setting weight goals.
I can't do this.	I can't wait to see the new me.
I'm going to fail again.	Every day is a new beginning.

Come up with some affirmations that work for you. Write them down and carry them with you wherever you go until you get in the habit of speaking to yourself in a more positive tone. Affirmations are especially useful in situations that trigger overeating. When you face a trigger situation, you encounter a choice (to eat or not to eat in response to the situation). The decision you make at that moment is crucial to the success of your day. Those deciding moments are also crucial to the success of your diet.

Chapter 5

Cooking in a Low-Calorie Kitchen

- -

In This Chapter

▶ Preparing low-cal foods according to new guidelines

▶ Making the best choices at the supermarket

▶ Equipping your kitchen and considering low-cal cooking techniques

- -

*I*n the practical arena of your kitchen, the foods you buy and the techniques you use to prepare them bring your low-calorie diet to life. You make some of the most important decisions affecting the success of your diet from day to day in your kitchen.

Following a healthful low-calorie diet starts with your food choices, but it doesn't end there. At home, you also have to make choices about how you're going to prepare your food and which utensils and cooking techniques to use. At its best, low-calorie eating means eating simple foods that don't require much fuss and bother.

This chapter helps you buy and prepare the best food for your low-calorie diet. You discover a little bit about stocking your kitchen with low-calorie cooking tools and appliances, many of which you probably already own. Finally, I explain how to utilize the best cooking techniques for your new low-calorie lifestyle.

Gearing Up for Low-Calorie Meals

Combined with the general basics of good nutrition found in Chapter 3, this section can help you decide exactly which foods you want (and don't want) to keep in your low-calorie kitchen. Don't forget that the object of this low-calorie diet is not only to help you lose weight but also to show you how to eat better. I want you to come away from this plan leaner, healthier, and much more knowledgeable about living a lower-calorie lifestyle.

In the following sections, I tell you how to incorporate the latest dietary guidelines into your diet, compare different types of foods you can eat, and explain the importance of making a shopping list so that you can stick to your food selections.

Following dietary guidelines

The U.S. Department of Agriculture (USDA) recently updated its dietary guidelines and released them in early 2005. For the first time ever, the guidelines include the specific recommendation that overweight people gradually reduce their calorie intake and increase their physical activity for slow and steady weight loss.

In addition to eating fewer calories and becoming more active, the new guidelines say that most Americans can benefit from making smarter food choices and balancing their daily diets to include an average of the following:

- 2 cups of fruit
- 2½ cups of vegetables
- 3 or more 1-ounce servings of whole-grain products
- 3 cups a day of fat-free or lowfat milk or the equivalent in dairy products such as cheese and yogurt

  Note: Dairy alternatives such as soy and rice beverages and products made from these beverages can take the place of milk and milk-based foods in a healthy diet if they're enriched with nutrients such as calcium, vitamin D, and B vitamins normally supplied by dairy foods.

The amounts of food in the previous bulleted list are recommended on a standard 2,000-calorie diet, which government nutritionists generally use as a reference point. On a low-calorie diet plan, you may or may not meet these recommendations every day, and aiming for a little less in each category is okay. What's most important is that you recognize that variety and balance are essential to the long-term success of a low-calorie diet and that these foods play essential roles in your long-term health. (See Chapter 3 for details on the importance of balance and variety in a low-calorie diet.)

Other recommendations in the guidelines that are more general but still very important to low-calorie dieters include

- **Vary your protein choices with more fish, beans, peas, nuts, and seeds.** Meat isn't your only choice for good sources of protein. Replacing some of the meat in your diet with seafood and non-meat sources of protein reduces fat and adds fiber and other nutrients not found in meat.

✔ **When selecting meat, poultry, dry beans, and milk or milk products, make choices that are lean, lowfat, or fat-free.** Most meat and dairy products that are lower in fat are also lower in calories than their higher-fat counterparts.

✔ **Choose fiber-rich fruits, vegetables, and whole grains as often as possible.** When you buy rice, pasta, breads, and cereals, check and compare the fiber content listed under "Total Carbohydrate" on the Nutrition Facts labels. (You can find more information about fiber and how much you need in Chapter 3 and more on the Nutrition Facts label in the "Reading the labels" section, later in this chapter.)

✔ **Get the most nutrition out of the calories you consume.** If you use your calories on a few high-calorie foods instead of dividing your calories among a variety of lower-calorie foods, you probably won't be getting many of the nutrients your body needs to stay healthy.

You can read more about the USDA's dietary guidelines and pyramid eating plan on its interactive Web site at `www.mypyramid.gov`. This site shows you how to personalize the general recommendations for eating well and balancing your diet. The site also gives suggestions for incorporating more exercise into your daily routine as a way of cutting calories.

Because the dietary guidelines now recommend that overweight people lose weight, they also say if you have a chronic medical condition or if you regularly take medication, you need to consult your physician before embarking on any weight-loss program.

Deciding which foods to eat

When you change your way of eating, especially when you're cutting calories to lose weight, you have many food choices to make. Do you prefer to cut calories by eating low-calorie and calorie-free food products? Do you want to continue eating the same way you've been eating, knowing that you have to limit the amount of some of your favorite foods? Maybe you can reach a compromise and decide to do a little of both. For instance, you may decide that you don't want to eat the calorie-controlled entrees available in your supermarket's freezer section in favor of "real foods," but you do want to save calories by using artificial sweetener in your coffee.

In the following sections, I explain the use of calorie-modified and full-calorie foods in a low-calorie diet, and the advantages and disadvantages of using each kind.

Faking it with commercial diet products

Many weight-loss programs and food companies sell packaged, calorie-controlled and nutritionally enhanced food products such as shake mixes, frozen and shelf-stable entrees, light salad dressings, and calorie-free sweeteners (see the nearby "Substituting artificial sweeteners to reduce calories" sidebar) to help dieters stick to a low-calorie plan by providing both convenience and structure. Many of the modified foods and meal replacement beverages available in supermarkets and health food stores come with a calorie-controlled diet plan of their own.

Often, you have few decisions to make when you use these products because they have been packaged to fit into a prescribed plan similar to the menu plans in Chapter 6. Having fewer decisions certainly simplifies everything because if you decide to use these products, you can interchange them with the menu plans in this book.

Even if you decide to use modified foods in your diet plan, make sure one of your long-term goals is to return to real food. Most meal-replacement products sold in supermarkets and drugstores and through commercial diet programs are fine for the short term if they help you stick to a calorie-controlled plan. On their own, however, they're generally not considered long-term solutions for weight control because they're not natural foods and they don't contain all the nutritional substances found in natural foods. Keep in mind that your body is naturally designed to digest and absorb whole foods, not pills and potions (unless you're sick). Just as multivitamin pills and other nutritional supplements can help fill nutritional gaps in your diet, meal replacements and other specialized food products can do the same and also help provide structure and convenience. And yes, you can get away with taking some supplements and using some modified food products in your diet for an unlimited period of time. But most health experts agree neither should be considered a complete or permanent replacement for real food (see the next section).

Keeping it real with natural foods

If you're a purist with your food, you're probably not interested in diet foods, such as the calorie-controlled frozen entrees, meal-replacement shakes, artificial sweeteners, and other nutritionally modified food products that many people use to control calories.

If you choose to go the "real foods" route, and eat more natural foods, you'll find plenty of options for creating simple meals in the menu plans in Chapter 6 and the recipes in Chapters 12 through 15. Inevitably, it takes more time to prepare your own meals than it does to simply pop open a can or stick a frozen entree in the microwave oven. But when your low-calorie diet consists of mostly natural foods, you've got a head start on the road back to normal eating.

Keeping a good supply of basic, healthful convenience foods in your pantry can help ensure that you have the makings of a quick, low-calorie meal on hand at all times and perhaps prevent you from eating or overeating less nutritious or more fattening foods. In "Browsing the grocery shelves," later in this chapter, you can find a list of suggested packaged foods to have for preparing "real" and simple everyday meals, along with any specialized low-calorie meals you may keep in your freezer for everyday use or "emergencies."

Substituting artificial sweeteners to reduce calories

If you have an uncontrollable sweet tooth, another way to keep the calories down in your diet is to use sugar substitutes. Artificial, or non-nutritive, sweeteners that have been approved by the Food and Drug Administration (FDA) for sale in the United States include (in order of sweetness):

✔ **Saccharin** (sold as Sweet'N Low, Sweet Twin, Sweet'N Low Brown, Necta Sweet) is 200 to 700 times sweeter than white table sugar and doesn't lose its sweetening power when heated.

✔ **Sucralose** (sold as Splenda) is 600 times sweeter than white table sugar. It can be used in cooking and baking because heating doesn't reduce its sweetening power.

✔ **Aspartame** (sold as NutraSweet, Equal, Sugar Twin) is considered 160 to 220 times as sweet as white table sugar. Aspartame can't be used in cooking and baking because it loses its sweetening power when heated.

✔ **Acesulfame-K** (sold as Sunett, Sweet & Safe, Sweet One) is considered 200 times sweeter than white table sugar, and it can be used in cooking because it doesn't lose its sweetening power when heated.

Other FDA-approved, non-nutritive sweeteners that aren't commonly available for everyday use by consumers but that may be used by food manufacturers to sweeten soft drinks and other beverages, dairy products, frozen desserts, baked goods, candies, chewing gum, and other food products include sorbitol, xylitol, maltitol, mannitol, lactitol, isomalt, and neotame. You may see some of these products listed on the labels of any low-sugar, no-sugar-added, and artificially sweetened products you buy in the supermarket. For more about artificial sweeteners, see Chapter 2.

Making a list and sticking to it

This section is especially important for those of you who can't eat just one of anything. You need to stick very closely to the food shopping list that you create from the menu plans you're using on your diet so that you don't have any extra or "forbidden" food in the house that may tempt you to overeat (see Chapter 6 for more on menu planning). In addition to your weekly list of menus, maintain a written running list as you start to run low on any staples you normally keep in your cupboard and fridge, such as flour and other baking goods, canned soups and sauces, milk, and eggs.

Try to keep your supermarket shopping trips down to once or perhaps twice a week. The less you shop for food, the less opportunity you have to buy impulse and indulgence items, such as snack and dessert foods or anything extra you may be tempted to buy simply because it's on sale. Keep a list on your refrigerator door or anywhere in the kitchen that's handy so you can jot down items you need whenever you think of them.

Earning your favorite treats the low-calorie way

Can't imagine life without ice cream? If not, go ahead and have some, but make sure you earn it. For example, rather than putting ice cream (or another favorite indulgence food) on your shopping list (or sneaking it into your supermarket cart even though it's not on your list), make yourself leave home for it every time you want it. And no, that doesn't mean hopping in the car and driving to the local dairy bar. Walk or ride a bicycle to your ice cream source, and then walk or ride home. This method has two benefits:

✔ First, you're getting some exercise that will help burn off your indulgence calories.

✔ Secondly, you may be less inclined to eat ice cream every night if you have to leave the comfort of your home to get it.

If you must drive for the sake of safety or because the store is just too far away, having to travel for your treats is still better than keeping indulgence foods around the house. You can still make up for high-calorie treats by doing extra exercises another time. Just be sure to impose an "exercise for treats" rule on yourself and follow it!

To get in and out of the supermarket as quickly as possible, organize your shopping list according to your supermarket's aisles and overall layout. Start with the aisle closest to the entrance and end with the last aisle you walk down before heading for the checkout.

Shopping for Low-Calorie Foods

When you think about it, your diet really starts in the supermarket, where you make your final decisions about which foods to buy and bring home. Sure, you plan your menus and make up your shopping list at home, but in the supermarket is where you decide whether or not to stick to your list, choose substitutes, or maybe throw a few "extras" into your shopping cart that aren't even on your list. In the long run, these decisions can make or break your diet.

Amidst the temptations that call out to you at every turn, your supermarket's aisles are actually stocked with more products and tools that can help you stick to your diet than with those that help sabotage it. Use just a few of these helpful tips on your next supermarket trip:

✔ **Focus on the produce section:** The produce section of some of the larger supermarkets chains often takes up a large chunk of floor space devoted to healthful food. You can't go wrong in those aisles!

✔ **Look for the label:** Nutrition labels on every packaged food in the store help you make smart decisions when you're comparing similar foods.

✔ **Search for helpful information:** Very often, supermarkets display free brochures and recipe cards loaded with helpful tips for buying and preparing healthful foods.

In the following sections, I help you shop smart by reading labels and selecting great foods from every part of the supermarket.

Reading the labels

Food labels are a great source of helpful information to low-calorie dieters. Labels tell you the amount of food you're buying, how many servings are in the package, how many calories are in a single serving, where the food comes from, and which ingredients were used to prepare the food. The Nutrition Facts box on the label provides a nutritional analysis of the food, and many labels also clearly display a nutrition description, such as low-sugar, fat-free, or high-fiber, to help you ferret out products that may be helpful on a low-calorie diet.

Deciphering descriptive lingo

The FDA standardized all the nutrition language on food labels, so you can pick up a package of food and feel confident that what you see is what you get. Table 5-1 defines some terms used on food labels:

Table 5-1	Claims on Food Labels
Label Lingo	*Meaning*
Calorie-free	Less than 5 calories per serving.
Reduced-calorie	At least 25 percent fewer calories per serving than a similar food.
Reduced-fat	At least 25 percent less fat per serving than a similar food.
Low-calorie	40 calories or less per serving.
Fat-free or 100 percent fat free	Less than 0.5 gram fat per serving.
Sugar-free	Less than 0.5 gram sugar per serving.
Reduced-sugar	At least 25 percent less sugar per serving than a similar food.
No added sugars	No sugar or ingredient that contains added sugar was used in the preparation or processing of the product.

The words "fat-free," "reduced-fat," and "reduced-sugar" don't necessarily mean that a food product is low in calories. Many products that are modified to reduce fat or sugar do indeed contain fewer calories than similar products that haven't been modified, but you have to check and compare the product labels to be sure. Likewise, "no added sugar" doesn't mean that a product contains no sugar. Many foods contain natural sugars that will be accounted for on the nutrition label (covered later in this chapter in the "Checking nutrition facts" section). Look for these terms when you're shopping for low-calorie foods, but be sure to compare the actual nutrition information on similar products so that you know you're really getting what you want.

Scoping out the ingredients

All packaged foods that contain more than one ingredient have their ingredients listed on the label in descending order by weight. If the first or second ingredient is sugar, sucrose, fructose, corn syrup, or high-fructose corn syrup, then that food is high in sugar. If you try to avoid any type of food, for any reason, the ingredient list is the first place you need to look when buying convenience foods and other prepared products.

Checking nutrition facts

Just about every packaged food product in the supermarket displays a Nutrition Facts label that you can use to check the number of calories and amount of other nutrients found in a single serving. Some produce and other fresh foods also carry Nutrition Facts labels, either on their skins, their packaging, or on a nearby poster or flyer.

The Nutrition Facts label illustrated in Figure 5-1 is typical of what you'll see on most cans and packages of food in the supermarket and health food store.

Figure 5-1:
Calories per serving are listed on the Nutrition Facts label on most food products.

Nutrition Facts

Serving Size 1/2 cup (113g)
Servings Per Container 4

Amount Per Serving

Calories 120   Calories from Fat 15

	% Daily Value
Total Fat 1.5g	3%
Saturated Fat 1.0g	5%
Cholesterol 10mg	3%
Sodium 290mg	12%
Total Carbohydrate 15g	5%
Dietary Fiber 0g	
Sugars 14g	
Protein 10g	10%

The categories on the label are

- ✔ **Serving size:** All the nutrition information contained on the label applies to this amount of the food.

- ✔ **Servings per container:** If, for instance, the package or can contains 2 servings and you eat the entire contents, you must double the number of calories and other nutrients listed.

- ✔ **Calories:** This number is the amount of calories in a single serving of the food.

- ✔ **Calories from fat:** This amount tells you the number of calories in one serving of this food that come from all fats. The closer this number is to the total number of calories in a serving, the higher the food is in fat.

- ✔ **Total fat:** The total amount of all fats, in grams (g), in one serving of the food is listed (along with saturated fat, cholesterol, and sodium) because many people need to limit these nutrients.

- ✔ **Saturated fat:** This is the amount of saturated fat, in grams, in one serving. The recommended daily limit for most healthy people is 20 grams.

- ✔ **Cholesterol:** This is the amount of cholesterol, in milligrams (mg), in one serving. The recommended daily limit for healthy people is 300 mg or less.

- ✔ **Sodium:** This is the amount of sodium (salt), in milligrams, in one serving. The recommended daily limit for healthy people is 3,000 mg or less.

- ✔ **Total carbohydrate:** This is the total amount of all carbohydrates, including sugar and starches, in grams, in one serving.

- ✔ **Dietary fiber:** The total amount of all fibers is listed, in grams, because this nutrient is lacking in many people's diets. Use this information to compare similar products and choose those that are higher in fiber.

- ✔ **Sugars:** The total amount of all sugars, both added and natural, in grams, is listed because many people consume too much sugar. Use this information to compare similar products and choose those that are lower in sugar.

- ✔ **Protein:** This is the amount of total protein, in grams, in one serving of the food.

The **% Daily Value** listed with some of the nutrients on the Nutrition Facts label tells you how one serving of the food contributes to the average daily requirement for that nutrient. The higher the percentage, the more that food contributes to your daily requirement for that particular nutrient. Daily Values are calculated on the basis of a 2,000-calorie diet for general use, but no matter how many calories you consume, you can use them to get an idea of whether a particular food is high or low in a specific nutrient.

Check and compare the calorie contents of prepared foods. When a single serving of any one food contains more than 400 calories, it's a high-calorie food.

When you check the Nutrition Facts label, you can find out what you're getting in the way of nutrients for the number of calories you're consuming. For the best comparison, make sure you're evaluating equal amounts of similar foods. For instance, choose several different types of reduced-calorie or "light" bread with similar calorie counts per slice and compare them to see which loaf has the most fiber per slice. If you need more fiber in your diet, and all other factors, such as calories, are essentially equal, the bread with the most fiber is your best choice.

Going aisle by aisle

Even though you can find the freshest foods in the supermarket around the store's perimeter, on the produce shelves, and in the meat and dairy cases, you can also find healthful, diet-friendly foods in every aisle. You just have to know what to look for and where to find them.

Picking fresh fruits and vegetables

When shopping for fresh produce, buy fruits and vegetables when they're in season. Not only are seasonal fruits and vegetables less expensive, but they also taste better. And if they taste good, you'll be more inclined to eat more of these highly nutritious and comparatively low-calorie foods, right?

Lucky for you, low-cal salad basics, such as lettuce, cucumber, radishes, sweet peppers, mushrooms, and cherry tomatoes, are tasty and available all year around, as are broccoli, cauliflower, carrots, onions, and celery. You can usually always find a pineapple or some variety of citrus fruit. The following short list is a sampling of other fruits and vegetables arranged by peak season:

- **Autumn/Winter:** Apples, pears, tangerines, kumquats, beets, turnips, cabbage, Brussels sprouts, spinach, fennel, winter squashes
- **Spring:** Asparagus, artichokes, peas, green beans, rhubarb
- **Summer:** Corn, tomatoes, okra, peaches, plums, nectarines, grapes, melons, berries

Choosing lean meats and poultry

Leaner cuts of meat and poultry contain fewer calories than fattier cuts. When shopping for meat and poultry, buy these following examples of lean cuts:

- **Beef:** Eye of round, top loin, sirloin, top round, tenderloin, chuck steak or roast, any cut graded select.
- **Chicken and turkey:** Lighter meat from the breast area contains less fat and fewer calories than darker meat from the thighs and legs.
- **Lamb:** Leg, loin, shoulder chop, foreshank.
- **Pork:** Tenderloin, top loin roast, center loin, loin rib chops, lean ham.

Selecting seafood

When purchasing seafood, buy seafood that is absolutely fresh. Check out the conditions in your supermarket's fish department or at your local fishmonger. All seafood needs to be displayed on ice in very clean refrigerated cases.

Fattier fish, such as bluefish, salmon, catfish, fresh tuna, swordfish, and fresh water bass, are higher in calories than leaner fish, such as cod, flounder, pollock, and orange roughy. Most shellfish are low in calories. In Table 5-2, you can see how some common fresh fish and shellfish compare.

Table 5-2	Calories in Different Types of Seafood
Type of Seafood	*Calories (in 3 ounces cooked)*
Scallops	75
Crab	82
Lobster	84
Shrimp	84
Surimi (imitation shellfish)	84
Cod	89
Flounder	99
Oysters	116
Clams	126
Swordfish	132
Salmon	150 to 175
Tuna	156
Mackerel	171

For more on the calorie counts of seafood and other foods, check Appendix A and Appendix B at the back of this book.

Recognizing the right dairy products

For the most part, lowfat means lower calories in the dairy department. Check out Table 5-3 to see how many calories you can save by choosing reduced-fat, lowfat, and fat-free milk products.

Table 5-3	How Calories Add Up in Milk
Type of Milk	*Calories (in 1 cup)*
Whole	150
2 percent fat	121
1 percent fat	100
Skim	90

When choosing dairy products, remember that reduced-fat cheeses and yogurts also contain fewer calories than similar products made from whole milk. Remember to check the labels, however, because some reduced-fat dairy products are sweetened and flavored with added ingredients and the calories from added sugar may well make up for the calories that were lost with the fat.

Surveying freshly prepared foods

Thanks to the wide variety of ready-to-cook and ready-to-serve foods available in the supermarket today, sticking to a low-cal diet in the most healthful way possible has never been easier. You can buy peeled and cut-up vegetables from the produce department to use in your own recipes or pack for lunch and snacks, or buy premixed salads and complete entrees that require nothing more than a reheating in the microwave oven when you get home.

When choosing prepared meals other than plain vegetable salads, select packages that provide a nutritional breakdown per serving. Otherwise you don't know how many calories you're getting or how much of that particular food meets your low-calorie criteria for a single serving.

Opting for frozen foods

Buying and eating frozen foods has its pros and cons, but for the most part, freezing is preferred over canned for nutritional value because the freezing process destroys fewer nutrients. Frozen foods are often your best bet for buying fruits and vegetables out of season.

Another reason to opt for frozen is convenience. Many calorie-controlled foods are available in the freezer case that require nothing more than a whirl in the microwave oven before eating. If that type of fast food helps keep you away from the high-calorie variety, go for it!

When buying frozen foods, check and compare the labels on fish, poultry, fruits, and vegetables before you buy, and, for the most part, stick to plain foods to avoid added calories. Stay away from foods that are sauced, breaded, or fried before freezing. You may find some exceptions in foods formulated to be part of a healthy, lowfat, or reduced calorie diet plan, but again, check the labels to ensure these foods fit your criteria for a low-calorie diet.

Browsing the grocery shelves

Convenience foods — bottled, canned, and boxed food products — make up the bulk of what you'll find in most people's shopping carts, and low-cal dieters are no different. Just be sure you're getting good nutrition along with the convenience by being picky. Many convenience foods, such as canned fruits and vegetables, lose some or all their nutritional value during processing. They also tend to be high in sodium. Check the Nutrition Facts labels and compare similar products to see what you're actually getting in that can, box, or bottle before you buy.

The following list contains some of the convenience foods I recommend most often to anyone who is stocking a pantry for a low-calorie kitchen. Many of these aren't low-calorie foods, but if you're familiar with appropriate portion sizes, or if you use the menu plans in Chapter 6 as a guide to portioning out your meals, these foods provide the makings for a quick, easy, low-calorie meal.

- An assortment of dried herbs, spices, and seasoning blends
- Canned fish such as tuna, crab, sardines, and salmon packed in water
- Canned legumes (beans, lentils, and split peas)
- Canned soups
- Dry pasta and pasta mixes
- Fat-free beef broth
- Fat-free chicken broth
- Flavored vinegars
- Nonstick vegetable cooking spray
- Olive oil (plain and seasoned)
- Plain crackers such as saltines
- Rice and rice mixes
- Rice cakes
- Salsas, chutneys, and other lowfat condiments
- Small bread sticks
- Tomatoes, tomato sauces, tomato paste
- Unsweetened or lightly sweetened breakfast cereals
- Vegetable broth

Low-calorie foods tend to be plain and simple, so to keep them interesting, use seasonings to spice them up. Table 5-4 shows you which fresh or dried herbs and spices are best for brightening up the flavor of plainly cooked poultry, seafood, meats, beans, and vegetable side dishes. Remember: Garlic and onions go a long way toward flavoring most foods without adding a significant number of calories, so don't skimp!

Table 5-4	Seasoning Guidelines
Season	**With**
Chicken or turkey	Basil, dill, oregano, parsley, rosemary, sage, tarragon, thyme, cumin, chili powder, curry
Beef	Basil, oregano, parsley, rosemary, thyme
Pork	Dill, oregano, parsley, sage, thyme
Ham	Rosemary, tarragon, allspice, ginger
Lamb	Dill, oregano, parsley, rosemary, sage, thyme, coriander, cumin
Fish	Dill, parsley, rosemary, sage, tarragon
Shellfish	Oregano, parsley, tarragon, thyme
Beans, lentils, split peas	Dill, oregano, parsley, rosemary, sage, thyme, chili powder, cumin, curry powder
Carrots	Dill, parsley, thyme
Cucumber	Dill, parsley
Potatoes	Basil, dill, parsley
Summer squash	Basil, rosemary
Tomatoes	Basil, oregano, rosemary

Setting Up a Low-Calorie Kitchen

If one mantra applies to all aspects of low-calorie dieting, it's "keep it simple." That statement certainly applies to the food you choose to eat and the tools and techniques you use to prepare your food. The following sections focus on the basic equipment you need in your kitchen and easy low-calorie cooking methods.

Using the tools of the trade

While on a low-calorie diet, you don't need any extra or unnecessary cooking equipment or kitchen gadgets. The following sections narrow everything down to the relatively few "special" utensils and appliances that are actually helpful to anyone who is on a low-calorie diet and wants to cook at home.

Selecting skillets, saucepans, and woks

The type and number of pots and pans you buy depends on your own personal cooking style. If you enjoy cooking and plan to prepare many of your low-calorie meals at home, you may want to have a variety of skillets and saucepans at your disposal.

The best pots and pans for a low-calorie kitchen are coated with a nonstick finish that allows you to cook with little or no added fat. Beyond that, the quality of skillets and saucepans you buy is your choice. Heavy-duty cookware tends to be more expensive than lighter-weight pots and pans, but it cooks food more evenly and lasts longer.

If you cook for a family of three or more, I suggest larger skillets that are 10, 12, or even 14 inches in diameter. You may also want to have at least one smaller skillet (6 to 8 inches) on hand for making individual dishes such as omelets and for general use when cooking smaller amounts of food.

Like skillets, saucepans come in many sizes, and if you cook, you need at least one small (1-quart) and one large (3- to 4-quart) pan. In addition, a very large (a least 5- to 8-quart) saucepot, or Dutch oven, is essential for cooking pasta and large quantities of soups, stews, or vegetables.

In addition to your regular pots and pans, consider buying a wok. No single piece of kitchenware is more versatile than a wok, especially if you cook in a small kitchen where you can only benefit from having one good-size pot that does several different jobs. A wok is used first and foremost for stir-frying (see "Stir-frying" later in this chapter), and thanks to its size and shape, can take the place of almost any size skillet in many different types of recipes. A wok can also double as a steamer and, in fact, a complete wok set includes a steaming rack. You can also braise or simmer foods in a wok, which means you can also use it to make soups, stews, and saucy dishes.

Woks come in different sizes. The size you choose depends on the amount of food you normally cook at one time. Woks are made of different materials. The woks that work best are made from 14-gauge spun steel, anodized aluminum, or cast iron. Avoid stainless steel (unless it's clad with aluminum) because stainless steel poorly conducts heat, and stir-fried food sticks to the bottom and sides of a stainless steel wok. Because woks cook food with a minimal amount of fat, you don't need a wok finished with nonstick coatings. Actually the slippery surface prevents stir-fried foods from cooking properly.

Most wok sets come with a cover, a cooking ring to hold round-bottom woks, and appropriate utensils such as a wire strainer, a ladle, and a wide spatula that can pick up and move larger amounts of food around the wok at one time better than a regular spatula or spoon. Expect to pay as much for a good wok as you would for a good saucepot.

Finding one good knife

A knife is probably more important than any other piece of kitchen equipment because you use it to slice, dice, and otherwise prepare food. A good knife simplifies the work of preparing fresh food from scratch, which in turn can help motivate you to make home-cooked, low-calorie meals on a regular basis.

If you can only afford one good knife, choose an 8- to 10-inch chef's knife. With knives, as with most everything else in life, you get what you pay for, so be prepared to spend as much as $75 or more for a high-quality chef's knife. If you can afford two good knives, choose the chef's knife and a small paring knife.

The best quality knives sold in department stores and culinary supply stores are usually made from high-carbon, nonstaining steel. The blade needs to extend into the full-length of the handle (known as a *full-tang blade*). Ask to hold the knife before you buy it, to make sure it feels comfortable in your hand.

After you own a good knife, it'll last your lifetime if you take care of it properly. Wash your knife by hand and dry it immediately. Store it in its own sheath, in a knife block, or on a mounted magnetic knife strip where it won't get banged around. Use a sharpening stone or electric sharpening machine to keep a fine edge on your blades.

Gathering assorted utensils and bakeware

If you're trying to figure out which basic utensils and bakeware you need in your low-cal kitchen, start with this checklist:

❑ Casserole-type baking dishes — round, square, and rectangular

❑ Cutting boards

❑ Dry measuring cups

❑ Large colander

❑ Liquid measuring cups

❑ Measuring spoons

❑ Mixing bowls — small, medium, and large

❑ Nonstick bakeware — baking (cookie) sheets, 12-cup muffin pan, 9-inch pie plate, 9-inch round cake pans, 8- or 9-inch square cake pan

❑ Nonstick spatulas — flat and spoon-shaped

❑ Nonstick or wooden whisks — small and large

❑ Wooden spoons — various lengths

❑ Wire mesh sieves (strainers) — small and large

If you never bake and never plan to, you don't need much, if any, nonstick bakeware, but certain standard baking items, such as cookie sheets, cake pans, and pie plates, can come in handy for other types of cooking. For instance, if you like to make pita pizzas or cheese nachos, you need a flat cookie sheet. Likewise, you can use a cake pan or pie plate for roasting a small amount of food, such as a single chicken breast on the bone or a pair of baked potatoes.

You can accessorize your kitchen with all types of extra gadgets, but only buy what you'll use on a regular basis. Otherwise, you'll just end up with a cluttered kitchen and an empty pocketbook. Use this checklist as a guide to "extras" often found in a well-stocked low-cal kitchen:

✔ Cheese grater

✔ Citrus reamer

✔ Garlic press

✔ Large kitchen shears for cutting through poultry bones and other heavy-duty clipping chores

✔ Pepper grinder

✔ Pizza wheel

✔ Salad spinner

✔ Small kitchen scissors for snipping herbs and a variety of other tasks

Choosing small appliances

If you watch any of the television home shopping shows, or peruse your local department store's ads, you can see how easy it could be to clutter up your kitchen counters with all kinds of cooking gizmos and gadgets that are supposed to save time and somehow make your life easier. The truth is, you don't need much when it comes to setting up a low-cal kitchen and you probably already own most of the small appliances that are most helpful.

Some helpful small appliances you may already have and may want to continue using in your low-calorie kitchen include

✔ **Blender:** If you're a fan of smoothies and shakes, keep your blender out on the counter, rather than stored away in a cupboard.

If you're not familiar with hand-held immersion blenders, check them out next time you're in a kitchenware department. You can use an immersion blender to mix a smoothie right in the serving glass or to puree a soup or sauce while it's still in the saucepan. (You can find more information about using immersion blenders in Chapter 12.)

✔ **Food processor:** A food processor is a must-have appliance for anyone who likes to make homemade soups and sauces. If you cook in large quantities, invest in a large processor. Small food processors are available if you cook your food in individual servings.

✔ **Rice cooker:** Perfectly cooked rice is always possible when you prepare it in an electric rice cooker. If you eat rice often, this appliance is a worthwhile investment.

Electric rice cookers and pasta pots or lobster pots with perforated draining baskets can often double as steamers. If you own this type of cookware, you probably don't need a separate steamer. You can also improvise your own steamer with kitchen items that you probably already own. (See the next section for more on using a steamer.)

✔ **Toaster oven:** These tiny ovens can do anything a regular oven can do, but only for small amounts of food. They're perfect for cooking or heating up individual portions of food.

A toaster oven does more than toast; it bakes and broils small quantities of food, which makes it a perfect appliance for any low-cal dieter who is cooking for one (or two) and doesn't want to heat up the regular oven. Toaster ovens come in various sizes, and some feature two levels for cooking larger quantities or more than one type of food at a time.

Two additional appliances that are extra handy in a low-calorie kitchen are a steamer and a microwave oven. I give you the full scoop on both items in the following sections.

Getting all steamed up

Because steaming is at the top of the list of good low-calorie cooking techniques (see the "Steaming" section later in this chapter), you may want to get serious about steaming equipment. Collapsible metal steamers that fit inside most saucepans are inexpensive and easy to find. They're best for foods that can easily be removed from the pan with tongs or a fork.

If you're going to get serious about steaming, your best bet is a Chinese-style, stackable bamboo steamer. These multilayered steamers are very efficient because they can cook more than one layer of food at a time so you can steam your entire meal, entree, and side dishes, all at the same time, in the same container.

Making the most of a microwave oven

Everyone knows that microwave ovens were born for reheating leftover food, thawing and cooking frozen entrees, and warming up coffee that's gone cold. What you may not know is that a microwave oven is also a good weight-loss tool because you can use it to cook fresh food with little or no added fat. Microwave ovens are especially good at cooking vegetables. (You can find cooking times for specific vegetables in "Cooking in a microwave oven," later in this chapter.) In fact, any food that can successfully be cooked in a steamer, including fish and poultry, also does well in a microwave oven.

Use these guidelines and tips if you're considering the purchase of a new microwave oven:

- ✔ Most microwave recipes and cooking times in this book and elsewhere are based on 600- or 700-watt full-size ovens set at 100 percent power. Lower wattage ovens cook foods more slowly, and higher wattage ovens cook foods more quickly.

- ✔ Some microwave ovens come with variable power levels. Most foods are cooked at 100 percent power, but you may find that you use half (50 percent) power or less for slower cooking, reheating, melting, and thawing.

- ✔ Microwave ovens often come with optional features such as turntables that automatically rotate food for even cooking, moisture sensors for detecting how much longer a food needs to cook, and one-button controls for thawing, reheating beverages, and popping popcorn. When you're trying to choose between different oven styles, think about which features you're most likely to use.

Brushing up on low-calorie cooking techniques

Some cooking methods fit more easily into a low-calorie lifestyle than others, and you probably know that deep-fat frying isn't one of them! In general, any method that doesn't require adding fat to the pan, such as steaming, microwaving, or poaching, is your best bet. Any method that requires only a small amount of fat, such as sautéing or stir-frying food in a skillet or wok with just a spoonful of oil is your second best bet. Roasting and broiling can both be low-calorie techniques for cooking meat and vegetables, as long as you don't add much fat. I cover these techniques in the following sections.

Steaming

Steaming is the ideal cooking method for low-calorie cooks who are in a hurry because it's a relatively quick and easy way of preparing food that adds no calories and requires very little clean-up.

If you're steaming food, place it on a rack or in a steamer basket. You then put the rack or steamer basket over boiling liquid in a tightly covered container. Don't immerse the food in the boiling liquid; the steam created from that liquid trapped in the covered pot cooks the food.

The method may vary slightly, depending on the type of steamer you use (see "Getting all steamed up," earlier in this chapter), but the following basics apply whenever food is steamed over boiling liquid:

✔ Never overcrowd your steamer pot with food. Work in batches, if necessary, to avoid uneven cooking.

✔ When using a steamer basket inside a pot, bring the liquid to a boil first, and then lower the filled steamer basket into the pot. Doing so helps assure even cooking. You may need to use a kitchen glove or potholder so you don't burn your hands.

✔ To successfully steam a dish, be sure the food sits over, not in, the boiling water or other liquid used to create steam, and that the steamer has enough room for the steam to circulate freely.

✔ Always uncover your steamer with the lid opening away from you. Otherwise, you could get a steam burn on your hands or face.

✔ If you're new to steaming, keep a pot of water simmering, in case you need to replenish the liquid in the bottom of the steamer. If the liquid evaporates in your steamer before you replace it, the cooking process will be interrupted and you may damage your steamer.

To improvise a steamer, fit a metal cooling rack, wire mesh strainer, or metal colander inside a large deep saucepan. Another way to steam food is to invert a small heatproof bowl or custard cup in the bottom of a deep skillet or saucepot large enough to hold a heatproof plate with at least ½-inch open space around the perimeter to allow steam to circulate. Fill the pot with an inch of boiling water or enough to come halfway up the side of the bowl. Place the food to be steamed on a heatproof plate and lower the plate into the pot to sit on the inverted bowl. (See Figure 5-2.)

However you improvise a steamer, be sure you can tightly cover the pot, and be sure to protect your hands, arms, and face from hot water and steam whenever the pot is uncovered. As with all stovetop-cooking methods, keep young children away from the stove while you're steaming.

Cooking in a microwave oven

The most popular uses for a microwave oven may be reheating leftovers and heating up precooked convenience foods, but for low-cal cooks and other healthy eaters, microwave ovens are also excellent for cooking certain foods from scratch, especially fresh vegetables. As with steaming, the vegetables preserve more of their flavor and nutrients when cooked quickly in the very small amount of water required in a microwave oven, and no calories are added.

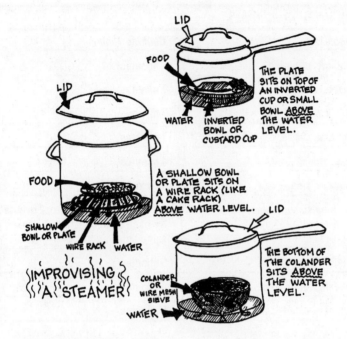

LID

FOOD

THE PLATE
SITS ON TOP OF
AN INVERTED
CUP OR SMALL
BOWL *ABOVE*
THE WATER
LEVEL.

WATER   INVERTED
         BOWL OR
         CUSTARD CUP

LID

FOOD

A SHALLOW BOWL
OR PLATE SITS ON
A WIRE RACK (LIKE
A CAKE RACK)
ABOVE WATER LEVEL.

LID

SHALLOW
BOWL OR PLATE

WIRE RACK   WATER

IMPROVISING
A STEAMER

COLANDER
OR
WIRE MESH
SIEVE

WATER

THE BOTTOM OF
THE COLANDER
SITS *ABOVE*
THE WATER
LEVEL.

Figure 5-2:
A home-
crafted
steamer can
work as
well as one
that's store-
bought.

Use Table 5-5 as a general guide to cooking fresh vegetables in a full power (700 watt) microwave oven. Cooking times vary, depending on the size of the vegetables and the oven. These cooking times are for 1 pound of vegetables cooked in a covered container with 2 tablespoons of water for most vegetables and 3 tablespoons of water for starchier vegetables such as peas and potatoes. Be sure that vegetables are trimmed or cut into equal-size pieces for even cooking. When cooking vegetables or other food in a microwave oven, check halfway through the cooking time and stir or rearrange the pieces for even cooking, if necessary. Most vegetables require a standing time after cooking of 1 to 5 minutes to finish cooking.

Table 5-5	Microwave Cooking Times for Vegetables
Vegetable	*Cooking Time*
Asparagus spears	5 minutes
Beans, green	6 minutes
Broccoli spears	7 minutes
Brussels sprouts	9 minutes

(continued)

Table 5-5 *(continued)*

Vegetable	Cooking Time
Cabbage, chopped	7 minutes
Carrots, sliced	7 minutes
Cauliflower florets	7 minutes
Eggplant, cubed	7 minutes
Peas, green	4 minutes
Potatoes, small	10 minutes
Potatoes, baked	6 minutes for one potato, 2 minutes longer for each additional potato cooked at the same time
Spinach leaves	5 minutes
Squash, winter	8 minutes
Zucchini, sliced	5 minutes

The following tips can help you when cooking foods and making the most of your microwave oven:

✔ If time allows, defrost frozen foods first in the refrigerator before reheating them in the microwave oven. Defrosting food in the microwave can cause *hot spots,* areas where some of the food is actually cooking while other areas are still thawing and/or reheating.

✔ Use only food-safe, microwaveable containers to cook or reheat food in a microwave oven. Any container not designed for use in a microwave oven may melt, explode, catch fire, or impart toxic substances to your food.

✔ Reheat bread and other baked goods at half (50 percent) power to avoid drying out and hardening.

✔ Cook individual boneless, skinless chicken breast halves (cutlets) in a small covered dish with ¼ cup chicken broth or other liquid for about 8 minutes or until the flesh in the center of the breast is opaque. Allow the chicken to cool slightly before cutting.

✔ Cook 1 pound fresh fish in a covered container (no added liquid is necessary) for 5 to 6 minutes or until the fish flakes easily and the flesh in the center of the fish is opaque.

✔ Pregrilling is another good use for the microwave oven because it speeds up the time food spends on the grill. Cook meat or poultry at half (50 percent) power until half-cooked, and then immediately transfer to the grill to finish cooking.

✔ Use only popcorn that is packaged for popping in a microwave oven.

Poaching

Poaching simply means simmering plain food in enough liquid to cover it in a pot or deep skillet. It's a technique that is well suited to low-calorie dieting because it adds no calories to the food being poached.

Poaching is used mainly for cooking whole or filleted fish, shellfish, and boneless, skinless chicken or turkey breasts. Generally, when cooking seafood, use fish stock, and when cooking poultry, use chicken broth. For your cooking liquid, use well-seasoned salt, whole peppercorns, and herbs, and enhance it with seasoning vegetables such as onions, carrots, and celery that cook alongside the seafood or poultry. The food that is poached picks up some of the broth's flavor and, in turn, the broth's flavor is enriched by the food that cooks in it. You can serve the leftover poaching liquid with the food or use it to make a sauce or soup. You can buy special poaching pans, but any pan that's large enough to hold both the food and the liquid will do.

Follow these easy steps when poaching poultry and seafood:

1. **Add the fish or chicken to cold poaching liquid.**

2. **Slowly bring the liquid to a boil over medium heat.**

3. **Reduce the heat to low.**

    Use the following times when poaching certain meats. Remember that poaching time begins when the water just starts to bubble.

    Fish steaks or filets until opaque in center, 6 to 10 minutes depending on the type and thickness of the fish

    Chicken breasts until opaque in center, about 6 to 8 minutes

    Lobster, crab, or shrimp (in their shells) for about 20 minutes per pound

    Increase the poaching time for larger turkey breasts and whole fish accordingly.

Stir-frying

Like steaming, stir-frying is a moist-heat method of cooking that's quick, easy, and, if done properly, light on calories. When you stir-fry in a wok or deep skillet, you stir the food constantly to keep it moving so that the heat of the pan cooks your food without burning it. Using the pan's heat to cook the food allows you to use less added fat than with other forms of frying.

Stir-frying is also similar to sautéing, which is the method most people use to cook food in a skillet with just a teaspoonful or, at most, a tablespoonful of fat, and stirring often to prevent the food from sticking and burning. With stir-frying, you spend most of your time preparing the food by cutting meats and vegetables into bite-size, similar-size pieces for even cooking.

Use these helpful tips for successful stir-frying:

- ✔ Cut and slice all foods and measure and mix all seasonings and sauces in advance of cooking. You usually don't have enough time to cut up food between adding in the next ingredient when stir-frying.
- ✔ Arrange your ingredients in the order in which they'll go into the wok or skillet.
- ✔ Heat your wok or skillet first, and then add the cooking oil. Doing so helps prevent food from sticking.

Roasting, broiling, and grilling

Roasting and broiling are known as dry-heat methods of cooking that are done in a regular oven, a convection oven, or even a toaster oven. When food is broiled, excess fat falls through the broiler rack and into the broiler pan, eliminating many calories. To get the same benefit from roasting, raise your food by placing it on a rack that fits inside the roasting pan.

Baking and roasting are one and the same — no matter what you call it, food that is baked or roasted is cooked by hot, dry air circulating in a tightly closed oven. Traditionally, the word *roasting* was used to describe a method for cooking large cuts of meat, while the word *baking* was used to describe cooking almost everything else in an oven. These days, however, roasting vegetables, garlic, fish, and poultry is more fashionable than it is to bake them, so the term "roasted" is used more often now to describe food cooked in a regular oven.

Making a marvelous marinade

Look for marinade recipes that contain little or no fat. The following teriyaki marinade contains no fat, is relatively low in calories, and tastes absolutely yummy on meat, chicken, or fish:

Stir together ½ cup soy sauce, 3 tablespoons light brown sugar, 2 tablespoons dry sherry or white wine, 2 teaspoons minced garlic, ½ teaspoon ground ginger or ¼ teaspoon Chinese five-spice powder in a small bowl. Yield: about ¾ cup marinade.

Lean meats, poultry, and fish — mainstays in many low-calorie diets — can easily dry out when they're roasted in an oven or cooked under a broiler. To prevent lean meats from drying out and getting tough, marinate the meat (for at least 30 minutes at room temperature or 1 hour in the refrigerator) before cooking and baste it with the marinade or its own pan juices several times while cooking.

Another way to keep lean meats from drying out in the oven is to cover the roasting pan for the second half of the cooking time so that steam is formed, helping the meat to stay moist.

Broiling is usually quicker than roasting and can be likened to grilling because, when done correctly, it quickly browns and crisps the outside of your food while cooking the inside just to the doneness you desire. Be careful if you aren't an experienced cook. You don't want to burn the outside of your food before the inside is done.

To avoid burning your food when broiling, place your meats, poultry, fish, or vegetables 4 to 6 inches from the heating element, as long as you check the food from time to time while it's cooking.

Chapter 6

Planning Low-Calorie Menus: The First Four Weeks

. . . .

In This Chapter

▶ Understanding how this diet works

▶ Planning your meals for four weeks

. . . .

*O*ne problem with many weight-loss plans is that they're too rigid. That rigidity — the strict rules and regulations about what to eat and what not to eat — often causes well-intentioned dieters to lose sight of their goals and give up.

This plan is different because you have more than one way to approach the diet. You can follow it to a "T," or you can make your own rules (within reason, of course). Most importantly, you limit your calories and stay aware of the amount of food you're eating, regardless of which approach you take.

These first four weeks are crucial to the long-term success of your diet because during this time you're getting used to eating fewer calories each day and establishing the habits that can help you eat better throughout your lifetime. This chapter gives you the basics on the number of calories you'll consume and guidelines for sticking to the plan. I also provide you with four weeks of simple, delicious menus, complete with helpful tips and shortcuts.

Preparing Yourself for the First Four Weeks

Before you dive into this chapter, you need to know the basics of starting a low-calorie diet plan: the number of calories you're going to consume, the importance of maintaining the plan, and fun ways to keep the plan interesting.

Going by the numbers

This plan is designed so you can ease into your diet by simply sticking to 1,500 calories for the first few days. To allow you to move gradually into a more restricted plan, the daily menus in this chapter begin at 1,500 calories and taper down to 1,000. If 1,500 calories is too high a limit for you, start off with 1,400 or 1,300 or whatever calorie level feels right.

You can always go back to 1,500 if you feel too restricted. If you're looking to lose only 10 or 15 pounds and want to dive right in and start your diet at 1,000 calories a day, that's okay, too. Just skip the first two weeks of meal plans and start with Day 14. (For more information on determining how many calories you need each day, see Chapter 3.)

If you want to cut back further on calories on any given day or within any of your meals, reduce your portion sizes, rather than eliminate foods. That way, your diet stays as nutritionally balanced as possible.

You can always eat less, if you don't feel hungry on a particular day, but if you eat too few calories one day, you'll likely find yourself ravished and overeating the next day. In general, 1,000 calories is as low as you should go. Remember: No less for long-term success!

Following the rules as closely as possible

If you want structure and don't want to have to think much for yourself, follow each day's menus closely. (I've done all the planning for you!) Pay attention to the serving sizes and variety of foods offered at each meal. Doing so can help you master portion control and nutritional balance. (See Chapter 3 for more about portion sizes.)

Planning is everything when you're living a low-calorie lifestyle. Take the time to plan a week's worth of menus in advance. How do you do that?

- Choose your menus for the week from the selection you find later in this chapter, or use the menus in this chapter as guides to create your own.
- Use the menus to make up shopping lists.
- Shop only for those items you need to prepare your planned meals and snacks throughout the week.
- Stick to your shopping list. Chapter 5 contains plenty of good advice for navigating the aisles of your supermarket.
- Try to get all your shopping done in one weekly trip to avoid having to go back to the supermarket and be faced with the temptation of buying foods that aren't on your original list for the week.

Stick to your calorie limit each day. But remember that your limit is an approximate number and you're working within a range of calories. For instance, if you find you're simply starving at the end of the day, eating an apple or a ½ ounce of cheese that adds 50 or 75 calories won't break your calorie budget for the day. Eating a few extra calories is much better for the overall success of your diet than feeling so hungry and deprived you end up bingeing in the middle of the night.

While you're following this plan, don't worry about the calorie content of individual foods. I've already done the math for you. All you have to do is follow the menu plans and rest assured. The calorie counts for each day are included with the menu plans, so you'll know how many calories you've consumed.

At some point, however, you'll find yourself in situations where you have to deviate from your plan or you'll have questions about how to make substitutions without adding additional calories. When this happens, refer to Appendixes A and B for calorie counts of both individual foods and food groups.

Coffee, tea, water, seltzer, and diet beverages are all "free foods" that aren't tallied against your daily calorie count. (You can find more "free foods" in Chapter 3.) If you use milk in your coffee or tea, take it from the measured amounts of milk or other dairy products allocated at meals. If you add sugar to your drinks, you must take those calories from someplace else. For instance, if you choose to put sugar in your coffee at breakfast, compensate for the calories by eliminating or reducing the amount of pancake syrup, jelly, or other condiment you use throughout the day.

If you choose not to use lean, lowfat, or reduced-fat versions of products, such as milk, yogurt, mayonnaise, and lunch foods, and you choose the higher-fat version instead, cut the amount called for in half to avoid extra calories. And when you're confronted with a choice between small, medium, and large sizes of foods such as whole fruits or breads and other baked goods, opt for small to medium to be on the safe side.

Doing your own thing to keep the plan fresh

Most people who need to lose weight benefit from a disciplined eating plan, one that has you eating three square meals a day and maybe a snack or two, regardless of your personal or work schedule. This type of discipline helps prevent you from losing control over what and how much you eat.

That said, no law says that you can't have spaghetti for breakfast or raisin bran for dinner, just as no law dictates that you must eat your snack at 2 p.m. You can certainly look at your day's menu plans and decide to eat your lunch in the morning, use your dinner menu as a guideline for ordering lunch, and eat your breakfast foods at 8 p.m.

If you get bored with following the menu plans so precisely, or if that simply doesn't appeal to you from the start, you can personalize the menus and rearrange them somewhat to suit your taste. You can do this by:

- **Substituting equal amounts of similar foods.** For instance, you can substitute a pear for a small banana or half an English muffin for a slice of toast.

- **Exchanging menus from day to day.** For instance, you can eat Wednesday's breakfast on Monday, or next Thursday's lunch today. Just be sure you're substituting meals that contribute approximately the same number of calories.

- **Incorporating this book's recipes.** You can add the breakfast, lunch, and dinner recipes and the ideas for snacks and desserts from Part IV into your low-calorie menu plans. Just make sure that the recipe you select fits in with your calorie intake for the day.

Taking the Plunge: Week 1

When you make any significant diet change, you first have to get used to a new way of eating. In this case, even if a 1,500-calorie plan doesn't kick off any weight, it's still a good place to start because you're getting used to the idea of eating a specific amount of food at each meal and a specific number of calories in a day. You're breaking the habit of eating whatever you want, whenever you want, and instead, getting used to structured meals.

Day 1: 1,500 calories

On a 1,500-calorie day, each of the meals — breakfast, lunch, and dinner — provide up to 400 calories, which is 100 calories more per meal than you'll eat on your 1,000-calorie days. You also get two snacks that contribute about 150 calories each or one snack or dessert that provides up to 300 calories, twice what you'll be getting from snacks on your 1,000-calorie days.

Breakfast

½ grapefruit

½ medium bagel

2 tablespoons light cream cheese

2 tablespoons fruit spread

1 cup skim milk

Lunch

1 cup black bean soup

1 cup baked tortilla chips

¼ avocado with lettuce, tomato, and 1 tablespoon light salad dressing

1 medium orange

Dinner

3 ounces skinless roast chicken

½ cup cooked rice

2 cups steamed broccoli

½ cup baby carrots

Snacks

1 cup fresh fruit salad

½ cup regular ice cream or frozen yogurt

Day 2: 1,500 calories

Day 2's menu plan is structured just like yesterday's menu, but with different foods. If you prefer, you can substitute any meal or snack from yesterday's menu for a meal or snack in today's plan.

Breakfast

1 blueberry muffin

½ cup applesauce

1 cup skim milk

Lunch

1 ounce lean deli ham

1 ounce reduced-fat Swiss cheese

2 teaspoons mustard

2 slices light bread

1 cup mini carrots

¼ cup coleslaw

Dinner

Cucumber and radish salad made with ½ cup sliced cucumbers and ¼ cup sliced radishes, sprinkled with 1 or 2 teaspoons white wine vinegar

2 cups tofu and vegetable stir-fry

½ cup cooked rice

Snacks

1 apple

10 thin pretzel twists

Day 3: 1,500 calories

You can eat your snacks any time of the day. If you're not a snacker, you can use your snack calories to add more food at each meal.

Breakfast

¼ cantaloupe

1 cup blueberries

1 cup raisin bran cereal

1 cup skim milk

Lunch

1 fast-food small hamburger, small taco, or regular slice plain cheese pizza

½ small order French fries

Side salad with ½ package light dressing

Dinner

1 cup tomato soup (made with skim milk)

5 large steamed shrimp

½ cup cooked barley or orzo pasta

1 cup steamed green beans

1 tablespoon light salad dressing

Snacks

1 small banana

1 cup lowfat frozen yogurt

1 tablespoon light chocolate syrup

Day 4: 1,400 calories

One good thing about convenience foods, such as frozen waffles and bottled juices, is that they often contain added vitamins and minerals. Eating and drinking these fortified foods is helpful on a low-cal plan because the more you cut back on calories, the more difficult getting all the nutrients you need is. (See Chapter 4 for more about shopping for convenience foods.) On a 1,400-calorie plan, each meal contributes 350 to 400 calories and your snacks contribute 200 to 250 calories.

Breakfast

1 (4-inch) frozen waffle

2 tablespoons light syrup

1 cup cut-up fruit or berries

1 cup skim milk or 6 ounces flavored lowfat yogurt

Lunch

2 slices light bread

2 ounces reduced-fat cheddar cheese

2 teaspoons mustard

1 sliced tomato

1 tablespoon light salad dressing

1 cup watermelon chunks

Dinner

1 cup canned vegetarian bean chili topped with 1½ ounces shredded, reduced-fat cheddar cheese

1 small (2-inch) square cornbread

Snacks

½ banana spread with 1 tablespoon peanut butter

½ cup vanilla pudding with ½ cup sliced strawberries

Day 5: 1,400 calories

Today, your snack calories are being used up by two glasses of wine with dinner. You can substitute a mixed drink or a couple of light beers for the wine, if you prefer, or use those 250 calories elsewhere.

Breakfast

1 bran muffin

2 tablespoons fruit spread

1 cup skim milk

1 orange

Lunch

2 cups tossed salad with 2 tablespoons light dressing

1 ounce soft cheese, such as Brie or Camembert

6 saltine crackers

1 medium apple

Dinner

1 cup pasta with ¼ cup tomato-based meat or seafood sauce

1 cup steamed spinach, arugula, or broccoli rabe

1 small roll or slice garlic bread

Snack

2 (6-ounce) glasses red or white wine

Day 6: 1,300 calories

On a 1,300-calorie day, your meals contribute 350 to 375 calories and your snacks contribute between 150 and 200 calories.

Choose juices that contain no added sugar or corn syrup. Some juices that would normally be too tart, such as cranberry juice, must be sweetened. Choose brands that are sweetened with other types of juices.

Breakfast

½ cup unsweetened pineapple juice

½ cup lowfat yogurt

½ cup fresh blueberries sprinkled with ¼ cup lowfat granola

Lunch

3 ounces tuna packed in water, drained

2 tablespoons lowfat mayonnaise

1 small (6-inch) pita bread

1 kiwi fruit

Dinner

2 cups tossed green salad with 1 tablespoon light dressing

1 cup cooked pasta tossed with 1 teaspoon olive oil, 1 cup cut-up steamed asparagus, 1 ounce shredded provolone cheese, and 1 ounce chopped lean ham

Snacks

1 ounce reduced-fat Swiss cheese

½ cup apple slices

Day 7: 1,300 calories

To jazz up the flavor of plain rice without adding significant calories, add bouillon cubes or seasoning powder to the rice cooking water.

Breakfast

2 small (4-inch) frozen pancakes

½ cup sliced strawberries

1 cup skim milk

Lunch

1 cup minestrone soup

1 ounce deli-sliced chicken

1 tablespoon reduced-fat mayonnaise

2 slices light bread

1 pear

Dinner

5 ounces swordfish, broiled with lemon

1 cup cooked rice

½ cup stewed tomatoes

1 cup steamed sugar snap peas

Snack

6 ounces lowfat flavored yogurt

Whittling Down Your Calorie Intake: Week 2

You're tapered down to 1,300 calories a day, and by the end of this week, you'll be down to 1,000 calories.

Day 8: 1,300 calories

You'll probably never know exactly how many calories are in the prepared foods you pick up from a salad bar. Thus, you need to know how to eyeball cup measurements and concentrate more on portion control. (See Chapter 3 for more details on portions.)

Breakfast

1 cup lowfat yogurt fruit smoothie

1 mini corn muffin

1 tablespoon fruit spread

Lunch

1 cup chicken noodle soup

1 small bread stick

½ cup salad bar rice salad with vegetables

Dinner

1 medium baked potato topped with ½ cup vegetarian (bean) chili, 1 ounce shredded reduced fat cheddar cheese, and ½ cup plain lowfat yogurt

Snacks

1 flavored rice cake

1 orange

Day 9: 1,200 calories

On a 1,200-calorie day, your meals contribute about 350 calories and your snacks contribute no more than 150 calories.

Anytime you see "fruit spread" on the menu, you can substitute a low-sugar or sugar-free jelly, jam, or marmalade.

Breakfast

    1 scrambled egg

    2 reduced-fat breakfast sausage links

    2 slices light bread with 2 tablespoons fruit spread

Lunch

    1 cup split-pea soup with ham

    4 saltine crackers

    ½ slice watermelon (1-inch thick)

Dinner

    2 cups fresh spinach leaves with 1 tablespoon light dressing

    1 small bean burrito (as found in your supermarket's frozen-food section)

    2 thin slices avocado

    ½ cup fat-free salsa

Snack

    ½ cup lowfat rice pudding

Day 10: 1,200 calories

These menus are designed for a general population of calorie counters with varied tastes, so, for instance, butter is allowed on today's breakfast toast but if you're happy with fruit spread or low-sugar jam, which has fewer calories and no fat, go right ahead and substitute an equal amount.

Breakfast

    2 slices light bread

    2 teaspoons butter or margarine

    ½ cup pineapple cubes (fresh or packed in juice)

    1 cup skim milk

Lunch

1½ cups salad bar pasta salad with vegetables and cheese

Dinner

6 ounces steamed or broiled salmon

1 cup steamed green beans

½ cup mashed potatoes with 1 teaspoon butter or 2 tablespoons gravy (See "Day 26: 1,000 calories" for tips on eating mashed potatoes.)

Snacks

½ cup chocolate sorbet

½ cup sliced strawberries

Day 11: 1,200 calories

Instead of commercial fat-free dressing on salads, try a sprinkling of freshly squeezed lemon juice or balsamic vinegar. These options are also good for flavoring plain steamed vegetable side dishes without adding calories.

Breakfast

1 small carrot or raisin bran muffin

6 ounces lowfat yogurt

½ cup orange juice

Lunch

2 cups tossed salad with 1 tablespoon light dressing

Egg salad sandwich: 2 slices light bread, 2 hard-cooked eggs, and 2 tablespoons reduced-fat mayonnaise

Dinner

2 cups green salad with 1 tablespoon light dressing

1 cup cooked ziti or other stubby pasta shape with 1 cup mixed cut-up vegetables sautéed in 1 teaspoon olive oil and topped with 2 tablespoons grated Parmesan cheese

Snacks

1 cup strawberries

½ cup creamy cottage cheese

Day 12: 1,200 calories

When you see cheese on a menu, feel free to substitute the same amount of any type you like. If you substitute a full-fat cheese for reduced-fat, cut the amount in half to stay within your calorie allowance.

Breakfast

> ½ cup pineapple juice
>
> 1 (4-inch) potato pancake
>
> ½ cup unsweetened applesauce

Lunch

> 1 cup lentil soup
>
> 2 slices light bread
>
> 2 ounces lean deli ham
>
> 1 tablespoon mustard
>
> ½ cup sliced cucumber
>
> ½ cup mixed fruit salad

Dinner

> ¾ cup cooked cheese or meat tortellini
>
> ¼ cup marinara sauce
>
> 1 cup steamed broccoli tossed with ¼ cup halved cherry tomatoes

Snacks

> 1 ounce reduced-fat Swiss cheese
>
> 1 small apple

Day 13: 1,200 calories

When sugar is included on a menu in this chapter, the calories have already been factored in. But that doesn't mean you have to use it!

Breakfast

> ½ grapefruit sprinkled with 1 tablespoon brown sugar
>
> ½ cup lowfat yogurt
>
> ¼ cup granola

Lunch

½ cup three-bean salad

1 small (6 inch) pita pocket

2 ounces sliced turkey

1 tablespoon reduced-fat mayonnaise

2 slices tomato

lettuce leaves

Dinner

1 cup Manhattan clam chowder

4 ounces broiled flounder or lemon sole

1 steamed artichoke with lemon juice

½ cup corn kernels

Snacks

½ cup part-skim ricotta cheese sweetened with 1 teaspoon sugar

½ cup sliced strawberries

Day 14: 1,000 calories

On a 1,000-calorie day, your meals contribute about 300 calories each and your snacks contribute no more than 100 calories.

When you're not sure about how much you can eat of a particular food, think small, especially when it comes to snack foods. For instance, if your plan says you can eat 30 pretzel sticks, that doesn't mean 30 thick, braided pretzel rods. It means 30 skinny, little sticks!

Breakfast

1½ cups corn flake cereal

½ cup skim milk

½ cup peach slices

Lunch

½ bagel or small roll, toasted and topped with ⅓ cup tuna salad

2 cups tossed green salad with 1 tablespoon light dressing

Dinner

   3 ounces lean pork loin roast

   ⅓ cup cooked rice

   1 cup snow peas

Snacks

   1 cup tomato or vegetable juice

   30 small, thin pretzel sticks (about ½ ounce)

Making Adjustments: Week 3

Congratulations! You're halfway through your first month of low-calorie living. By now you've adjusted to eating less food, and from now on you'll be following a 1,000 calorie-a-day plan until you reach your goal weight.

Day 15: 1,000 calories

TIP

The light breads called for on these menu plans are based on 40-calorie slices. If your bread has more calories, "borrow" those calories from another food.

Breakfast

   1 kiwi fruit

   ½ toasted English muffin

   1 teaspoon butter

   1 slice tomato

   1 scrambled egg

   ½ cup skim milk

Lunch

   2 cups spinach and mushroom salad with 1 tablespoon light dressing

   Sandwich with 2 slices light bread, 2 ounces lean deli roast beef, 2 tablespoons reduced-fat mayonnaise, 2 slices tomato, and lettuce leaves

Dinner

   3 ounces broiled lean ham steak

   ½ cup mashed winter squash

   ½ cup creamed corn

   ½ cup steamed greens such as kale, collards, or spinach

Snack

1 cup grapes

Day 16: 1,000 calories

The calorie counts of soups, stews, and chilis can vary greatly, depending on where you buy them and how they're prepared. Just stick to the recommended portion size, and you won't go too far off course.

Breakfast

½ cup orange juice

½ medium bagel, toasted and topped with ¼ cup light cream cheese and 1 tablespoon fruit spread

Lunch

2 cups spinach and orange salad with 1 tablespoon light dressing

½ cup chili

1 small (2-inch) square corn bread or ½ corn muffin

Dinner

1 (3-ounce) lean turkey, beef, or veggie burger, 1 hamburger bun with 2 tablespoons ketchup, 2 thin tomato slices, and lettuce leaves

1 cup mini carrots

Snack

1 rice cake topped with 2 tablespoons apple butter

Day 17: 1,000 calories

If you get tired of tossed green salads, go ahead and substitute 1 cup of any raw or steamed vegetable. You can still use the dressing for flavor.

Breakfast

1 cup bran flakes

1 cup blueberries

1 cup skim milk

Lunch

1½ cups Chef's salad (made with lettuce, raw vegetables, and an ounce or two of cold cuts such as ham, roast beef, and turkey)

1 tablespoon light dressing

Dinner

2 cups tossed salad with 1 tablespoon light dressing

½ cup cooked rice

½ cup pinto beans

2 tablespoons shredded reduced-fat cheddar cheese

Snack

6 ounces skim milk with 1 tablespoon chocolate syrup

Day 18: 1,000 calories

Dinner on today's menu is from a Chinese restaurant. Feel free to substitute equal amounts of a light soup, stir-fried meat and vegetables, and rice that you cook at home.

Familiarize yourself with the size of a ⅓-cup serving of food. It's a very handy cup size for low-cal dieters because, very often, ½ cup of a food contains too many calories and ¼ cup isn't enough food.

Breakfast

1 blueberry muffin

½ cup unsweetened applesauce

1 cup skim milk

Lunch

2 slices light bread

⅓ cup chicken salad

1 cup sweet red pepper strips

Dinner

1 cup egg drop soup

2 cups vegetable stir-fry with meat or tofu

⅓ cup cooked rice

Snack

1 cup mixed fresh fruit salad

Day 19: 1,000 calories

One way to stick to your menu plan but cut back a little on calories is to substitute fat-free products for reduced-fat. Just be sure to compare product labels so you know you're really saving calories.

Breakfast

2 (4-inch) whole grain waffles

½ cup mixed chopped fruit

½ cup skim milk

Lunch

2 slices light bread

2 ounces lean turkey pastrami

1 tablespoon mustard

⅓ cup coleslaw

Dinner

Open-face roast beef sandwich: 1 slice light bread, 1½ ounces lean deli roast beef, heated, ¼ cup gravy

1 cup steamed zucchini

¼ cup cranberry sauce

Snacks

½ cup lowfat vanilla pudding

¼ cup blueberries

Day 20: 1,000 calories

On a 1,000-calorie day, you can always use your snack calories for any treat you want, as long as it's approximately 100 calories or less.

Breakfast

1 slice frozen French toast

1 tablespoon light pancake syrup

½ cup sliced strawberries

Lunch

Pasta salad: 1 cup small pasta shapes, ¼ cup roasted peppers, ½ ounce light mozzarella cheese, and 1 tablespoon light salad dressing

Dinner

2 cups mixed baby greens with 1 tablespoon light dressing

2 ounces broiled flank steak

1 small baked potato topped with ¼ cup plain lowfat yogurt

1 cup steamed broccoli

Snack

½ cup fat-free frozen yogurt

Day 21: 1,000 calories

Lentils, beans, and split peas are pretty much interchangeable, so when you see, for instance, a lentil salad on the menu, don't think twice about substituting a salad made with any of these other legumes.

Breakfast

2 (4-inch) pancakes

2 tablespoons reduced-calorie pancake syrup

1 cup raspberries

Lunch

1 cup vegetable soup

½ cup lentil salad (from salad bar)

¼ cup olives

1 small breadstick

Dinner

4 ounces scallops, steamed or broiled with lemon juice

½ cup cooked rice

1 cup zucchini with stewed tomatoes

Snacks

1 ounce Swiss cheese

1 plum

Watching Your Weight Drop: Week 4

By now you're used to following a 1,000-calorie diet plan, and if you've followed this diet plan for three weeks, you've probably experienced an initial weight loss of about 4 to 6 pounds. This progress can help motivate you to continue on your 1,000-calorie diet plan if that's the calorie level you feel works best for you.

Anytime you feel that you can't stick to a 1,000-calorie day, follow a menu plan that allows 1,200 or 1,300 calories. If you stop losing before you've reached your goal weight, you can try cutting back to 1,000 calories a day.

Day 22: 1,000 calories

To maintain your calorie limit when making pasta substitutions, choose shapes and sizes similar to what's on the menu plan. If the menu calls for a short, stubby pasta, such as shells, stick with other short stubby shapes, such as elbows, radiatorre, wheels, and so on, when making substitutions. If you want a substitute for spaghetti, think about linguine, fettuccine, and other long thin pasta shapes.

Breakfast

1 cup cut-up cantaloupe and raspberries

1 cup oatmeal with 2 teaspoons sugar

½ cup skim milk

Lunch

2 ounces lean sliced ham

½ cup potato salad

1 small orange

Dinner

1 cup pasta shells with ¼ cup clam sauce

1 cup steamed broccoli

Snack

½ cup lowfat yogurt

Day 23: 1,000 calories

Light (low-calorie and reduced-fat) salad dressings can help make your diet life a little more exciting by acting as dips and sauces for vegetables.

Breakfast

½ cup lowfat yogurt

½ cup mango chunks

¼ cup fat-free granola

Lunch

Turkey wrap: 1 (6-inch) fat-free tortilla, 1 tablespoon reduced-fat mayonnaise, 2 ounces thin sliced turkey, 2 thin slices tomato, and soft lettuce leaves

8 baby carrots with 2 tablespoons light ranch dressing

Dinner

2 cups spinach salad with 1 tablespoon light dressing

5 ounces salmon, steamed or broiled

½ cup cooked couscous mixed with 1 diced tomato

Snack

2 cups light popcorn

Day 24: 1,000 calories

When you don't know the calorie counts of the prepared foods you buy from delis and salad bars, and you have a choice, go for the lower-fat version. You're more likely to be saving calories than if you choose the classic dish.

Breakfast

½ cup orange juice

1 scrambled egg

1 slice light bread, toasted

2 teaspoons butter

½ cup skim milk

Lunch

1 cup mozzarella and tomato salad (from salad bar)

6 baby carrots

Dinner

4 ounces skinless roasted or broiled chicken breast

½ cup corn kernels

½ cup roasted pepper strips

1 cup steamed zucchini

Snack

1 cup melon cubes drizzled with ¼ cup lowfat yogurt

Day 25: 1,000 calories

Check the labels on frozen desserts such as sorbets and ice creams to be sure they come in under 100 calories for a ½ cup serving.

Breakfast

1 slice cinnamon raisin toast with 2 tablespoons peanut butter

½ cup skim milk

Lunch

1 cup black bean soup topped with 1 ounce shredded reduced-fat cheddar cheese

6 baked tortilla chips

½ cup sliced cucumber with 2 tablespoons plain lowfat yogurt

Dinner

1 cup cooked pasta with 1 tablespoon pesto sauce

6 large steamed shrimp

1 tomato, sliced, with 1 tablespoon light dressing

Snack

½ cup raspberry sorbet with ¼ cup fresh raspberries

Day 26: 1,000 calories

On this menu you find mashed potatoes, one of those foods that can be pre-pared a hundred different ways and come out with a hundred different calorie counts. No worries. Add-ins like milk and butter have been factored in, so just stick strictly to the ½ cup portion size and you won't stray far from your calo-rie allowance, regardless of how your potatoes are prepared. The same is true for the meatloaf on this dinner menu. No matter how you make it (or buy it), any type of meatloaf is okay.

Breakfast

½ English muffin with 2 tablespoons apple butter

½ cup lowfat yogurt

1 tablespoon granola

Lunch

2 cups tossed salad with 1 tablespoon light dressing

1 cup mushroom barley soup

4 saltine crackers

Dinner

½-inch slice meatloaf

¼ cup gravy

½ cup mashed potatoes

½ cup steamed green beans

Snack

½ cup lowfat rice pudding

Day 27: 1,000 calories

When the menu on a low-calorie diet plan says "muffin," you can be sure it doesn't mean Texas-size muffin. It means a normal-size muffin, like the type of muffin you make at home in a standard muffin pan. Sorry about that!

Breakfast

1 small corn muffin

1 tablespoon strawberry fruit spread

½ cup skim milk

1 small orange

Lunch

2 ounces lean ham

½ cup macaroni salad

1 sliced tomato

Dinner

1 cup cooked pasta wheels with 1 lean Italian-style turkey sausage link

¼ cup tomato sauce

Snack

½ cup lowfat chocolate pudding

Day 28: 1,000 calories

A small banana means a 4-inch baby banana. If you can't find one, split a regular banana in half and save the other half for a smoothie on another day. (I provide delicious smoothie recipes in Chapter 12.)

Breakfast

1 cup shredded wheat cereal

1 cup skim milk

1 cup mixed fruit

Lunch

1 cocoa rice cake

2 tablespoons peanut butter

1 small banana

Dinner

3 ounce lean turkey or beef burger with 1 slice American cheese, 1 slice tomato, lettuce leaves, and 1 hamburger bun

1 piece (6 inches) corn on the cob

Snack

⅓ cup salsa

12 baked tortilla chips

Chapter 7

Pulling through Your Plan's First Few Months

. . . .

In This Chapter
▶ Updating your goals and planning your next steps
▶ Staying motivated
▶ Trying new menus

. . . .

*I*f you've been following the low-calorie menu plans and diet advice included in this book, then pat yourself on the back. You've not only lost some weight or, at the very least, managed to stop gaining weight, but you've also figured out that living a low-calorie lifestyle means more than eating less food. That lesson is the most important one a dieter can discover! (If you haven't been following the low-calorie menu plans, don't worry. Just go to Chapter 6 to get started.)

Read this chapter after you've been on a low-calorie diet plan for at least a month and you're ready for your next steps. After a month or so, you can pause and assess your plan to see if you're satisfied with the results.

If the plan is working for you, if you have no complaints, and you're happily losing weight, you may not need this chapter yet. Stick with what you're doing and just remember that this chapter is always here when you need it. Come back to it when you start to get restless, bored, frustrated, or concerned that your diet just isn't doing it for you. You can find solutions here.

If you're starting to fall off track, this chapter provides plenty of new ways to approach your diet day to day. You also find ideas for rewarding yourself for a job well done and for distracting and entertaining yourself when you're tempted to overeat. These pointers can help you to avoid falling back into your old routine of overeating and underexercising.

Reassessing Your Low-Calorie Plan

You've prepared yourself in every possible way to live a low-calorie lifestyle now and forever, and to lose weight by following the food plan in Chapter 6. Are you happy with your plan? Is it working out for you? You've stayed on the plan for at least one month, and now is a good time for a self-check! If you can answer, "yes" to all or most of the following questions, then you're definitely on the road to weight control.

✔ **Have you been meeting your short-term goals?** Keep in mind that a short-term goal can be as simple as getting into the habit of carrying a water bottle or working out for 5 extra minutes. Be realistic and keep your goals doable. Check out Chapter 4 for details on setting goals.

✔ **Are you sticking to your menu plans?** If you need more interesting or more focused menu plans, you can find them in the "Getting into Fun Menu Plans" section, later in this chapter.

✔ **Are you eating nutritionally balanced meals?** Why live a low-calorie lifestyle if it isn't healthy? You'd just end up skinny and sick! If you want to review what eating a balanced low-calorie diet means, flip to Chapter 3.

✔ **Have you replaced unhealthy eating habits with healthier new ones?** For long-term weight loss, you need to understand that consuming fewer calories isn't enough. You must change your eating habits, which includes everything from eating more regular meals, to eating more slowly, to making sure you sit down every time you eat. You can find more information on paying more attention to how you eat, otherwise known as mindful eating, in Chapter 4.

✔ **Have you been exercising as much as you promised yourself?** Your exercise goals need to be as realistic as your other goals, or they'll never come to fruition. Chapter 8 is full of exercise info.

✔ **Have you found nonfood ways to deal with stressful emotions such as anger, anxiety, and disappointment?** Many overeaters eat in response to their emotions. If you're an emotional overeater, you can find help in Chapter 9.

✔ **Are you maintaining a positive attitude toward your low-cal lifestyle?** If you're having attitude problems, check out Chapter 4 for more on positive, or mindful, thinking.

✔ **Have you developed a reliable support network?** Asking for help is part of taking care of yourself. If you need more help than you're getting, turn to Chapter 11 for advice on reaching out.

✔ **Do you still feel resolved to follow a low-cal diet plan and lose weight?** If you need a motivational lift, you may find it by reading the section "Motivating Yourself, Bit by Bit" later in this chapter. If you need more help, review Chapter 4.

Review your plan at least once a month during the first six months of following a low-cal diet to be sure that your eating, exercise, and behavioral patterns are in line with your original goals. Revisit your goals (as described in the next section) and, if necessary, update some of your goals to reflect any adjustments you need to make to your plan.

The following sections contain tips and advice on adjusting your original goals, evaluating your diet's makeup, and making any changes necessary to ensure that your low-calorie plan is compatible with your lifestyle.

Revisiting your goals

Many health experts believe that your best weight is whatever weight you can maintain by eating approximately 2,000 calories a day — a little less for most women and a little more for most men — and exercising often. That weight may be something other than what you have in mind for a long-term goal. Just for now, think about a time when you were at a comfortable weight and make that weight your goal. Even if that weight is at the top of your healthy weight range or outside your healthy weight change, it's still a good goal for now. (To find your healthy weight range, check out Chapter 2.) When you reach that goal weight and you're able to maintain that weight for several months, then consider setting new goals for losing a little more.

Chapter 4 shows you how to set weight goals, food goals, fitness goals, behavior goals, and psychological goals. You may choose to focus on one goal at a time or you may decide to dive in and reset any number of goals. Either way, you'll be updating your goals from time to time because they'll change for all kinds of reasons. You'll reach your short-term and intermediate goals and have to set new ones. You may be too ambitious when you establish your goals and find that they're impossible to meet within the timeframe you've given yourself. If your goals turn out to be unrealistic, change them.

While you're revisiting your initial goals, now may be a good time to think about what's realistic for you. Are you trying to get to a weight you were at 20 years ago? Are you trying to get to a weight you can't remember staying at for more than a couple of days? You may not realistically be able to get to the weight you were in your teens, twenties, or even your thirties. Sticking to the very low calorie level required to get to that weight may be impossible. Even if you do reach your desired weight, staying there may be next to impossible. You may even be jeopardizing your health by trying.

What about other goals? Have you been too hard or too easy on yourself when it comes to exercise? Have you been paying as much attention to your eating habits as you have been to the food you eat? If you've already established goals in those areas, update your goals. If you've been taking it slow and focusing only on your diet, now may be a good time to switch gears and set some exercise goals. (You can get some help in Chapter 8.) If you're having trouble setting or reaching behavioral goals or psychological goals, flip to Chapter 9 for some help. And if you feel you simply can't lose weight alone, Chapter 11 can guide you toward the right kind of help.

Taking stock of your diet

This section focuses strictly on your low-calorie diet. Taking stock of your diet means pausing to look at your diet, questioning what you're doing and how you're eating, and determining whether or not you need to carry on the same way or if you still need to take steps to improve your diet plan.

The following questions can help you reevaluate your diet so that you can be sure it leads to long-term weight loss success.

- ✔ **Are you watching your serving sizes?** Portion control is key to a successful low-calorie diet. In Chapter 3, you can find tips for measuring and eyeballing standard serving sizes of different types of food.

- ✔ **Do you feel you're eating enough food?** If not, perhaps you need to plan your diet to include more low-calorie vegetables and other foods that you can eat in larger quantities on a low-calorie diet.

- ✔ **Are you eating often enough?** Eating every three to five hours is important to keep your energy levels up and to prevent hunger and overeating at your next meal. If you find yourself getting hungry in between meals, try breaking your menu plans down into mini-meals you can eat more frequently throughout the day. (You can use the "Grazing day" menu plan later in this chapter as a guide.)

- ✔ **Are you enjoying the food you're eating?** If not, you may need to add more variety to your diet by experimenting with new foods and new recipes. Perhaps you need to find a way to include more of your favorite foods in your low-calorie diet. Check out the alternative menu plans in the "Getting into Fun Menu Plans," later in this chapter for some variety. Chapter 3 also has info on the importance of keeping your diet balanced and varied.

- ✔ **Are you losing 1 to 2 pounds a week?** If you're losing more, your calorie allowance is too low for the amount of exercise you do every day. Although you may find it motivating to lose more than a pound or two a week, the faster you lose weight, the less likely you are to keep it off. If you're not losing at least a pound a week most weeks, cut back on the amount of calories you consume. (You can also consider increasing your physical activity; see Chapter 8 for exercise info.)

Making changes to fit your lifestyle

The closer your diet plan fits to your lifestyle, the better the chance you'll stick to it, so when your lifestyle changes, your diet and exercise plan may have to change, too. For instance, if you get promoted, you may not have time to work out on your lunch hour anymore. If you move or get a new job, you may be shopping in different supermarket chains, frequenting new delicatessens and convenience food stores, and eating in different restaurants. If you get married, you may be spending more time eating with your in-laws or more time eating "real" meals at home. The food routines you've established so far on your low-calorie plan may have to change.

If what you're doing is working for you, keep doing it. If the overall plan you've set up for yourself feels good and shows promise, don't change anything. And if you've stopped doing something that was successful in the past, start doing it again. For instance, if you were watching your diet, and at the same time you were walking for half an hour every day on your lunch hour, and you lost or maintained weight, then that combination worked for you. If you've stopped walking or you're still walking but not watching your diet as carefully, get back with that same program! You may want to add more exercise to your day to lose more weight, but don't stop doing what you were already doing to keep your weight under control.

On the flip side, if you've started doing something that doesn't help you lose weight, stop doing it! If you joined a weight-loss program and you're not following the program, quit. Now is probably not the right time for you to take that approach, so why waste time and money? If you're down to 1,000 calories and you're so hungry that you're driven to distraction, come up with a new plan. Add a couple of hundred calories to your menu plan and try to do ten more minutes of exercise every day.

Motivating Yourself, Bit by Bit

If, in the first six months of your plan, you've lost some of the initial motivation you felt when you started thinking about losing weight, or you can feel that motivation starting to slip away, first remind yourself why you wanted to lose weight in the first place. Then figure out why your motivation is slipping. Are you hungry all the time? Are you bored? Are you tired of going at it alone? Get to the root of the problem and tackle it right away.

In the following sections, I show you how to reward yourself, create diversions to avoid overeating, and get help from family, friends, and diet buddies. Chapter 9 has additional info to help you battle long-term challenges and everyday frustrations.

Reaping rewards for sticking with your plan

The biggest and best rewards for losing weight and getting fit are your own good health and the sense of accomplishment when you lose weight. Ideally, those rewards would be enough to keep you motivated to continue until you reach your long-term goals. But, hey, you're only human. Everyone needs tangible rewards once in a while to keep going. You can try giving yourself a hug, but if you're anything like me, that won't cut it.

Reward yourself for changes in your behavior, attitude, and weight. For instance, if you exercise ten minutes longer, or you start substituting positive thoughts about yourself and your diet for any negative, self-destructive thoughts that have been blocking your success, then celebrate!

Many dieters reward themselves with fabulous new clothes to fit their fabulous new bodies after they've lost a substantial amount of weight. But you certainly don't have to wait until the end is in sight before you start giving yourself motivational rewards. Think about other nonfood rewards, big and small, that you can look forward to and bestow upon yourself along the way. Give yourself a reward every day, if it helps you stay motivated.

Refer to the following list whenever you feel you need some added incentive or when you reach a milestone (otherwise known as a goal) and feel like celebrating. You can also add your own ideas to this list. (Just scribble your thoughts in the margins; you can write in this book!)

- Pick up a bouquet of flowers or a flowering houseplant.
- Get a manicure and a pedicure.
- Get a massage.
- Have a facial.
- Pick out a new piece of jewelry.
- Buy a fashion accessory, like a trendy scarf or belt.
- Splurge on beauty products.
- Find an attractive blank book for keeping your journal.
- Look for an interesting cookbook that features foods that are naturally low in calories.
- Buy a newly released, bestselling book.
- Hire a cleaning service.
- Buy yourself a new wallet.
- Buy a fun magazine.

Match the size of your reward to the specific accomplishment, so you don't run out of ways to reward yourself. If you think small at first, you can reward yourself for achieving the many short-term goals you set early on. A small reward may be as simple as a long bath or a day without housework, or it can be a little bit bigger such as a piece of costume jewelry. As the months go by, and you start to reach your intermediate and long-term goals, you can start thinking about that new dishwasher or car, that gold bracelet, or that African safari you've always wanted to take.

Most likely, you'll also want to come up with a few rewards that don't challenge your budget, such as taking a mental health day or attending a free concert. Another free reward is to let yourself spend some time planning bigger rewards you can redeem when you reach some of your longer-term goals.

Carry a wish list in your wallet or someplace where you can always find it, to remind yourself of the rewards that lie ahead and to keep yourself motivated. A list is handy for those in-the-moment decisions you often have to make about whether or not to eat a particular food, or to spend an extra ten minutes at the gym, or even to eat or exercise at all. If you have your list on hand, you can choose a reward that provides the most motivation, in that moment, to help you make the best diet and exercise choices.

Even though rewarding yourself for a job well done is great, the opposite doesn't hold true. Don't punish yourself for sneaking a snack or even going on an all-out eating binge. Forget about your backslide! Guilt is a very common form of self-punishment employed by dieters. If you want to make amends with yourself, eat a little lighter the next day or bike an extra mile. What makes the most sense is just starting again wherever you left off, getting back on track, and moving forward. Anything else just gets in the way of your long-term success.

Finding diversions to avoid overeating

After a while, you'll probably find that you don't need as many rewards to stay motivated as you did. Instead, you may need distractions to help prevent you from eating when you're not really hungry. Instead of buying yourself something, you may want to try new activities and hobbies that provide the diversions you need.

The following list may not provide any revolutionary new ideas. However, I include it to remind you of the many things you can do with your time instead of eating, thinking about eating, or handcuffing yourself to the bathroom door so you don't eat. I include this list because sometimes, when your mind is so narrowly focused on food, you can't think of a single thing to do except eat. You probably know you could go for a walk instead of eating, pop in an exercise video, or go out and discover how to play a new sport, but you can't spend every spare minute exercising. Some of the rewards listed in the previous section can double as diversions. In addition, the activities in the upcoming list can distract you from overeating. When you get other ideas, add them to this list.

- Plan a weekend getaway.
- Get away for a weekend.
- Set up a fish tank.
- Clean your fish tank.
- Plant a garden.
- Weed your garden.
- Legally download some new music.
- Go for a drive and listen to some new music in your car.
- Read up on how to take better photographs.
- Take pictures of your kids.
- Take pictures of your pets.
- Write in your journal.
- Start a scrapbook.
- Visit a museum.
- Take a guided tour at a museum.
- Browse in a bookstore.
- Browse in a library.
- Buy or borrow a good classic book that takes awhile to read.
- Take a painting class.
- Paint a self-portrait.
- Paint a portrait of your mate.
- Sneak out to the movies by yourself (avoiding the food concession).
- Buy a new address book and fill it in.
- Give your dog a bath.
- Wash your car.
- Call a friend.
- Take up knitting, crocheting, or another form of needlework.
- Brush and floss your teeth.
- Chew gum or suck on a mint-flavored hard candy.

You need diversions to get you through moments of temptation so that you don't make choices you'll regret. If the temporary distractions you're using aren't enough, take time to master some relaxation techniques to help control your moods and impulses. Turn to Chapter 9 for information on mind-body exercises, such as yoga, t'ai chi, and pilates, that can help you relax and ultimately cope with the emotional issues that often underlie overeating.

Using the buddy system

The motivation you need to stick to a low-calorie diet and build a lifestyle around it ultimately has to come from within you. You're the only one who can really drive yourself to do whatever it takes to reach and maybe even exceed your weight-loss goals. But you can still reach for outside help to maintain your motivation along the way. Family and friends who are familiar with and support your weight-loss efforts can help you stay motivated by giving you positive feedback and new ideas to help you reach your goals. Ask them for help when you need it.

One of the reasons a buddy system works so well for dieters is that you may be more motivated to stick to your diet or get out and exercise if someone else is counting on you to keep them on track. If you don't already have a diet buddy, think of the people you know in your neighborhood or at your job and ask someone if he or she is interested in a team approach. When you have an official "buddy," you have someone to share diet and exercise tips with, help you get through your low points, and celebrate your successes.

You can find out more about finding a buddy in Chapter 11. And in Chapter 17, you find a great example of how the buddy system worked for two teachers who dieted together and helped each other stick to a low-calorie plan.

Getting into Fun Menu Plans

Fad diets — especially the ones that encourage you to eat a lot of one type of food or avoid another —usually aren't nutritionally balanced, and they don't teach you anything about normal eating. You won't stay healthy if you stay on this type of fad diet for a long time, and if you can't stick to a diet for the long term, it won't work.

Another reason fad diets don't work, even some of the healthier ones, is because you can only eat so much of any one type of food without getting bored and restless. How long has anyone ever stayed on a cabbage soup diet? Not long, I assure you. How many days can you eat lean meat and salad without having a piece of bread or a potato on the side? Some very determined dieters may go for several months or even years, but most people, including myself, wouldn't make it through one day.

If you take the following "fad" diets for what they are — one-day diets — then they aren't that bad. Just stay on them for a day at a time, just for the fun of it. For instance, you may hear that dairy products can help you lose weight. No single type of food can help you lose weight, but you may be interested in following a dairy diet anyway, because you love dairy foods and because, for most people, there's no reason not to include reduced-fat dairy foods in a low-calorie diet.

All of the following menu plans provide 1,000 to 1,200 calories a day, and, for the most part, they're as nutritionally sound as possible for that calorie level. These menus can help you take a "one day at a time" approach toward your diet and provide ever-changing themes. (And you don't have to wait until you've followed every menu plan in Chapter 6 before you try some of these menus!) They let you try out different types of fad diets without committing to any of them, and they may inspire you to come up with theme menus of your own, just for the fun of it. Diet plans that focus on specific themes also give you an opportunity to discover how to include just about anything you like to eat or drink on a low-calorie diet, as long as you stay within your calorie limits. With that kind of flexibility, how can you go wrong?

Whenever you're on a low-calorie diet plan, however, especially a plan that eliminates any food groups or focuses on one food group in particular, consider taking a multivitamin and mineral supplement that supplies up to 100 percent of the daily requirement for most nutrients.

High-protein day

This day mimics the many high-protein diets that promise fast weight loss. In this case, even though every meal has high-protein foods, these menus are still balanced with a variety of low-calorie carbohydrates.

Breakfast

    2 scrambled eggs

    ½ cup skim milk

    ½ cup blueberries

Lunch

    2 slices light bread

    2 ounces lean ham

    2 ounces reduced-fat cheese

    1 roasted red pepper

Dinner

 3 ounces smoked turkey

 1 cup steamed spinach with garlic and lemon

 1 cup tomato salad with 1 tablespoon light dressing

 1 mini breadstick

Snack

 ¾ ounce (2 generous tablespoons) dry roasted peanuts

High-fiber day

Chapter 3 gives you plenty of reasons to fill up on fiber from whole grains, fruits, vegetables, and legumes. This menu plan provides more than 30 grams of fiber, which is a bit more than the minimum amount that nutrition experts recommend for healthy people to consume each day.

At each meal, you can easily add extra fiber to your diet by sprinkling foods you normally eat with wheat bran or oat bran, adding more fresh fruits and vegetables to your diet, and combining high-fiber, whole-grain foods with lower-fiber, processed grain foods.

Breakfast

 1 cup oatmeal sprinkled with 2 tablespoons wheat bran

 1 sliced pear

 ½ cup skim milk

Lunch

 1 cup mixed fruit salad over 2 cups salad greens

 1 tablespoon light poppy seed dressing

Dinner

 1 cup cooked whole-wheat spaghetti mixed with regular spaghetti (½ cup whole wheat and ½ cup regular)

 ¼ cup marinara sauce

 1 cup steamed broccoli

 ½ cup orange sections

Snack

⅓ cup bean dip

¼ cup salsa

8 baked tortilla chips

Dairy day

Dairy substitutes, such as soy milk, soy cheeses, soy yogurts, and rice and almond beverages that have been fortified with calcium, vitamin D, and other nutrients normally supplied by dairy products, can easily fit into the plan for this day. This day supplies more than 1,600 mg of calcium, which is more than the daily requirement for many people.

In these menus, you can find plenty of good examples of how to boost the amount of calcium you get at every meal. These menus include not only dairy products but also other good sources of calcium, such as canned fish that has been processed with its bones intact and certain leafy green vegetables.

Breakfast

1 cup honeydew melon cubes

1 cup lowfat coffee-flavored yogurt sprinkled with ¼ cup high-fiber cereal

Lunch

2 slices light bread toast

2 ounces reduced-fat cheddar cheese or 3 ounces sardines canned in water, broth, or tomato sauce

1 cup broccoli florets

Dinner

1 cup cooked pasta tossed with 1 teaspoon olive oil and topped with 1 ounce grated Romano cheese

2 cups steamed kale with lemon

Snack

½ cup chocolate pudding or chocolate-flavored yogurt

Fruit fast day

This day isn't exactly a day of fasting, but just a fruit-filled day that shows you a variety of ways fresh fruit and fruit products can add flavor to other foods and be served at every meal.

Breakfast

¼ cantaloupe

1 slice light whole-grain toast with 2 tablespoons apple butter

½ cup fruit-flavored lowfat yogurt

Lunch

½ cup fruit salad

½ cup pineapple cottage cheese

6 wheat crackers

Dinner

2 cups spinach leaves topped with ½ cup grapefruit sections

3 ounces pork loin chop or chicken breast simmered in ¼ cup orange juice

½ cup unsweetened applesauce

1 cup steamed broccoli

Snack

1 cup sliced banana and blueberries

Grazing day

Today you break your calorie allowance up into 6 mini-meals, eating the same amount of food you normally eat, but eating more often than usual. Doing so is a good solution if you find yourself getting hungry and tempted to overeat in between meals.

Breakfast

1 cup raisin bran

½ cup skim milk

Snack

2 mini blueberry muffins

½ cup skim milk

Lunch

2 ounces reduced-fat cheese

½ apple, sliced

4 wheat crackers

Snack

1 cup snow peas or green beans

1 tablespoon light ranch dressing (for dip)

Dinner

1 cup beef vegetable soup

1 thin slice Italian bread

2 cups green salad with 1 tablespoon light dressing

Snack

3 cups light popcorn

½ cup cranberry juice diluted with 1 cup seltzer or club soda

Snack day

Unlike the grazing day in the previous section, where you plan to eat six mini-meals instead of three regular meals, this day consists of normal sized meals designed to include chips, dips, crackers, and other favorite snack foods. This day shows how you can fit a few potato chips and a frozen fruit pop into a low-calorie diet plan.

Be careful with this day! It only works when you have enough willpower to eat small amounts of snack foods. Even if you're feeling strong enough to meet the challenge, don't tempt yourself by buying big bags of junk food and leaving them around the house. When you shop for this day, buy only individual-size bags of snack foods, or portion out what you need and give the rest away — immediately!

When you choose the more sensible snack foods that are available — potato chips that are baked instead of fried, chips and puffs that are made with healthier fats (such as canola oil or olive oil), air-popped popcorn instead of oil-popped, canned fruits packed in juice or light syrup rather than in heavy syrup, frozen fruit bars instead of fruit-flavored ice pops — you can easily justify including them in a low-calorie diet. Just remember that these munchies are still snack foods and they generally don't contribute any important nutrients to your diet. That's why nutrition experts recommend that you eat them in small amounts.

The key to including snack foods in your diet is to have enough other, healthier foods available and ready to eat so you're not as tempted to eat more than a small serving of less nutritious foods. Make sure you have a glass of water with your meal because it helps fill you up as well. The less room you have in your stomach by the time you get to the chips, the less tempted you'll be to overindulge.

Breakfast

> 1 cup dry cereal
>
> ½ cup skim milk
>
> ½ cup canned mandarin oranges

Lunch

> 2 ounces sliced honey-baked ham
>
> ⅓ cup coleslaw
>
> 12 baked potato chips

Dinner

> 1 cup tomato soup topped with ½ cup air-popped or light popcorn
>
> 3 ounces lean beef
>
> 1 cup steamed zucchini

Snack

> 1 frozen fruit pop

Shake it up day

If a liquid diet appeals to you, today is your day! You can enjoy delicious shakes and smoothies from morning to night. The recipes yield a single serving, but you can make double, triple, or quadruple batches if you're sharing with family or friends, or you want to keep a second serving on hand for the next day. (See Chapter 12 for additional smoothie recipes.)

Breakfast

Orange Creme Eye Opener: In a large glass, stir together ½ cup orange juice and ½ cup lowfat vanilla yogurt until blended. Add ice, if you prefer.

1 small corn muffin

Lunch

Berry Good Shake: In a very large glass, stir together 1 cup cranberry-raspberry juice, ½ cup apple cider, and ⅓ cup lowfat plain yogurt.

3 wheat crackers

Dinner

Tangy Tomato Smoothie: In a blender, combine ¼ cup lowfat plain yogurt and 1 cup stewed tomatoes or seasoned, diced tomatoes in juice. Whirl until smooth. Serve over cracked ice.

3 ounces skinless roast chicken breast

½ cup cooked rice

1 cup steamed asparagus with sweet red peppers

Snack

Mocha Freeze: In a blender, combine ½ cup cold coffee, 1 tablespoon "light" chocolate syrup, ½ cup skim milk, and a couple of crushed ice cubes. Whirl until smooth.

The New York dieter's special

If you happen to have grown up in or around New York City, you know what a chocolate egg cream is, and it may even be on your list of all-time favorite soda-fountain foods. To the uninitiated, however, an egg cream can be off-putting, tasting like nothing more than watered down, carbonated chocolate milk. I've heard that opinion, and respect it, but as a New Yorker who grew up drinking chocolate egg creams, I'm thrilled to have discovered this 100-calorie version. Try it and see what you think.

In an 8-ounce glass, stir together ¼ cup skim milk and 2 tablespoons "light" chocolate syrup until well mixed. Slowly, fill the glass with seltzer or club soda. There you have it!

For anyone who drinks diet sodas, you can make an egg creamlike drink that many chocolate-loving dieters seem to favor. Pour 1 cup of skim milk into a very tall glass. Fill the glass with diet chocolate soda. Enjoy!

Salad day

At each meal you have a salad, but this day isn't an all-green day! Breakfast is a mix of fresh fruit, and lunch is Greek salad, which is usually sprinkled with feta cheese and sometimes served with olives and stuffed grape leaves. For dinner, the usual fare is tossed together to make a salad of warm sliced meat served over cool crisp greens with tomatoes and onions. You don't even need salad dressing. Try the same thing another night with roast pork, shrimp, or poultry.

Breakfast

1 cup mixed fruit salad

1 small pumpkin raisin muffin

Lunch

1½ cups Greek salad

1 mini breadstick

Dinner

3 ounces grilled steak over 1 cup shredded romaine lettuce greens with ½ cup finely chopped tomato and ⅓ cup sliced red onion

1 thin slice Italian bread

Snack

¾ cup cucumber-yogurt salad

International food day

You can handle this day in several different ways. You can eat out or eat in. You can stick to one cuisine all day or mix it up, as in the following menu. The idea is to have fun with it. This menu includes a Mexican breakfast, Middle Eastern lunch, Asian snack, and an Italian dinner. These are some of America's favorite ethnic foods.

Breakfast

1 serving Huevos Rancheros (see Chapter 12 for the recipe)

½ cup sliced mango

Lunch

1 cup lentil soup

⅓ cup hummus

1 toasted mini (4 inch) pita

Dinner

1 cup minestrone soup

1 cup linguine with clam sauce

Snack

2 small almond cookies

1 cup jasmine tea

Dessert day

Years ago, I saw a chocolate lover's cookbook written by a physician who had what I considered a brilliant strategy for chocoholics trying to lose weight. According to his plan, you could eat something chocolate and low-cal about half an hour before each meal. The doctor's rationale was that you never deprive yourself, you get your chocolate fix three times a day, and eating the chocolate half an hour before a meal allows enough time for your stomach to send a signal to your brain that you've been fed, so you're not ravishingly hungry when it comes time to eat your meal and you're more satisfied with the amount of food you're limited to on a low-calorie diet.

Following the good doctor's lead, this menu plan puts something sweet into every meal. You can decide whether it makes more sense for you to have it before or after your meal.

Breakfast

6 ounces hot chocolate

1 small (4-inch) pancake

1 tablespoon light syrup

½ cup sliced strawberries

Lunch

2 chocolate drop candies

1 large vegetable salad with 2 tablespoons light salad dressing

Sandwich with 2 ounces sliced turkey, 2 slices light bread, and 1 tablespoon reduced-calorie mayonnaise

½ cup baby carrot sticks

Dinner

1 thin (2-inch) slice angel food cake

½ cup raspberries

1 cup cooked pasta with 2 teaspoons pesto sauce

1 cup tomato salad with 1 tablespoon light salad dressing

Snack

1 small oatmeal-raisin cookie

½ cup skim milk

Wine with dinner day

By using your snack calories and borrowing a few calories here and there from each meal, you can fit an alcoholic drink or two into a low-calorie diet plan from time to time.

Breakfast

1 small toasted bran muffin

2 teaspoons fruit spread

½ cup skim milk

Lunch

2 cups mixed green salad with 1 tablespoon light dressing

2 ounces reduced-fat cheddar cheese

2 saltine crackers

½ cup orange sections

Dinner

1 (5-ounce) glass red or white wine

4 ounces broiled salmon

1 cup steamed broccoli tossed with ½ cup chopped tomato

1 mini breadstick

Most health experts believe that drinking alcoholic beverages in moderation — defined as one drink a day for women and two for men — probably won't harm your health and may even help. If you enjoy a glass of wine with dinner, a beer when you're eating outdoors, or a cordial at the end of a long day, your low-calorie diet doesn't have to get in the way. You can use your snack calories. In Table 7-1, you find out what counts as one drink, and how many calories that drink accounts for.

Table 7-1	Calories in Common Alcoholic Drinks
Alcoholic Beverage (standard serving)	*Number of Calories*
Beer, 12 ounces	150
Beer, light, 12 ounces	100
Wine, red, 5 ounces	100
Wine, white, 5 ounces	100
Champagne, 5 ounces	110
Vodka, gin, rum, whiskey	100 to 125
Martini (2½ ounces)	155
Screwdriver (7 ounces)	175
Daiquiri (4½ ounces)	250
Pina colada (4½ ounces)	260

You probably don't need me or anyone else to tell you what's wrong with drinking too much alcohol, but just remember that too much alcohol can increase your risk of developing liver disease, high blood pressure, heart disease, certain types of cancer, and brain damage. You're also at higher risk of having an accident, getting arrested, and dying from any number of causes. You also increase your chances of gaining weight from alcohol and some of the mixers used to flavor it. If you substitute alcohol calories for food calories, you may not gain weight, but you'll miss out on some very important nutrients and you're likely to become ill.

Fast-food day

This menu plan is based on the types of food found in most fast-food restaurant chains so that you can go into any chain in your area and choose food that fits into your diet. This menu shows you how any meal at a fast-food restaurant can fit into your low-calorie diet plan if you limit the amount of food you eat.

Choose water or another calorie-free beverage to have with your meal. (If you add milk to your coffee or tea, keep it to a splash!) If you think you'll give in to the temptation to eat more, pick up your food to go.

The best tip I can give you overall for making smart choices in fast-food restaurants is this: "Think small!" Many fast-food main dish salads, such as chicken caesar, chef, or BLT salads, contain between 600 and 800 calories per serving and sometimes more. One way to enjoy this type of salad, or other higher-calorie fare like fried fish and chips, a large hero sandwich, a deluxe double burger with the works, or any larger entree that comes in one-size only, is to split a single serving with someone else and have a side salad with light or fat-free dressing on the side.

Breakfast

1 egg on a muffin, biscuit, roll, or half bagel

Coffee or tea with just a splash of milk

If you want egg and cheese, discard half the bread, whether it's a biscuit, roll, muffin, or toast and eat your breakfast sandwich open-face.

Lunch

1 slice pizza or 1 taco or 1 soft taco or 1 small grilled chicken sandwich or 1 small hamburger

Keeping score at fast-food restaurants

The only people who go to fast-food restaurant chains to eat veggie burgers and tossed salads are people who wouldn't be there to begin with if they weren't accompanying small children or hungry friends and relatives who aren't watching their weight. If you're headed for one of the chain restaurants by your own choice, you're either going to cheat on your diet or you've been starving yourself and banking calories all day to earn that superburger you're about to devour. (Unless, of course, you're strictly following the fast-food menu plan in this chapter.)

Most fast-food chains provide nutrition information in their stores and on their Web sites, so if you really want to know the specific calorie count of the double deluxe cheeseburger you're craving, check the nutritional listing. Ask for the information and look at it before you order. It may make you think twice. (For calorie counts on select fast-food fare, flip to Appendix A.)

Unless you're sharing, watch out for any burger, sandwich, or other entree with the words Market Fresh, Ultimate, Deluxe, Whopper-size, Thick, Triple, Supreme, or Meat Lover's in its title, or any food that's served in a basket. The same goes for anything that resembles a shake, malt, doughnut, biscuit, or curly fry. When it comes to condiments, ask for reduced-calorie sauces, mayonnaise, and salad dressings.

If you want to eat a cheeseburger, discard half the bun and eat the burger like an open-face sandwich.

Dinner

> 1 small (3-inch) piece batter-dipped fish or chicken breast
>
> 3-inch corn on the cob
>
> 1 side salad with light or fat-free dressing

If you're in a fast-food restaurant that only serves fish sandwiches, discard the bread or choose grilled fish over batter-dipped.

Snack

> ½ cup soft serve ice cream

Convenience food day

Unlike a fast-food day, where you go out to fast-food restaurants to get your meals, a convenience food day is a day when you're cooking your meals at home, but you don't really feel like cooking. On this day you can take advantage of canned, bottled, frozen, packaged, and fresh-prepared foods found in any supermarket. Check out the listings in Chapter 5 for other convenience foods that fit into a low-calorie diet plan.

Breakfast

> 1 cup skim milk mixed with 1 package breakfast powder mix
>
> 1 cup cut-up watermelon

Lunch

> 1 cup cheese tortellini
>
> 2 tablespoons marinara sauce
>
> 2 mini breadsticks

Dinner

> 2 ounces rotisserie chicken
>
> ½ cup spinach soufflé, from frozen
>
> ½ cup baby carrots

Snack

> ¾ cup pears in light syrup

Chapter 8

Working Out and Working the Weight Off

"Do I *have* to?" are words I hear more often than not when I recommend more exercise to someone who wants to lose weight. Some people even make faces at me and beg for menu plans low enough in calories that they can deal with their weight strictly by dieting. Sorry for the bad news, but diet and exercise go hand in hand. Unfortunately, you can't have one without the other.

Many people certainly try to lose weight with only diet or exercise, but you probably won't have any long-term success with weight control unless you pay attention to both the number of calories you consume and what you do to burn off those calories. That's why you need to incorporate both diet and exercise into your new low-calorie lifestyle.

You can live a low-cal lifestyle to maintain a healthier weight throughout your life, but unless you're an especially tiny person, you can't stay on a strict low-calorie diet (of less than 1,200 to 1,500 calories) forever. And you shouldn't. The point of your new lifestyle isn't to eat less and less food or spend the rest of your life worrying about how many calories are in one food or another. Nor is the point to exercise yourself into a state of exhaustion to try to make up for an eating binge. Doing so is almost impossible anyway, because it can take hours of exercise to work off the calories from that pint of ice cream or triple deluxe cheeseburger that took only minutes to eat! And who has the time anyway? Your higher goal is to discover how to enjoy eating by finding a comfortable balance between the amount of food you eat, or the calories you consume, and the activity you do on a regular basis to burn those calories.

If you haven't already developed an exercise plan, or if you need to improve on your usual routine, this chapter can help you form better physical habits. Just remember that this chapter is a fitness overview. It doesn't include everything you need to know about working out and staying fit. However, you can find solid, basic information and the encouragement to kick-start an exercise routine. For more complete information on exercise and its role in weight control, pick up a copy of *Fitness For Dummies* by Suzanne Schlosberg and Liz Neporent (Wiley). If ever there was a good "companion" book to this one, that's it.

If you're older than 40, if you have any type of health problem, or if you plan to intensify your current program, check with your doctor. Even if you haven't been diagnosed with a medical condition, you need to alert your doctor of any chest pains, back or leg pains, dizziness, or wheezing or breathlessness you experience during or after any mild exertion.

Recognizing the Advantages of Different Kinds of Exercise

Exercise boosts your *metabolic rate,* or the rate at which you burn calories. Burning calories is especially important when you're on a low-calorie diet because, when you start to eat a lot less food than you normally eat, your body goes into a state known as *starvation mode.* Your metabolic rate slows down because your body doesn't know you're on a low-calorie diet. For all your body knows, you could be about to starve. In fact, your body is trying to conserve energy in case it doesn't get enough fuel, and thus it's not able to burn calories as efficiently. Exercise helps counter this effect.

Physical activity helps keep you fit, and when you're fit, you look and feel your best. The more fit you are, the better you're able to work, play, think, and even relax. When you're healthy and in good physical and mental shape, you often feel as though you have energy to spare and you're better able to focus on everything you do and enjoy every aspect of your life.

In the following sections, I explain the two basic types of exercise and tell you about the physical and psychological benefits of each one.

Distinguishing between aerobic and anaerobic exercise

Exercise helps you lose weight and maintain weight loss because it uses up excess calories that would otherwise be stored in your body as fat. Obviously, the amount of exercise you need to control your weight depends on the amount of food you eat as well as the amount and type of exercise. To lose weight, and then to maintain your weight loss, you have to find your own balance between the amounts of food you eat and your amount of exercise. The more rigorous the activity, the more calories you'll burn. However, don't think you have to knock yourself out with intense exercise every day just to stay in shape. Intense workouts help burn fat while you're exercising, but in the long run, steady, moderate exercise is more effective at burning calories than super-intense workouts because moderate activity burns a higher percentage of calories overall.

There are two types of exercise: aerobic and anaerobic.

- ✔ **Aerobic** means "with oxygen." Aerobic exercise, such as running, biking, stepping, spinning, and fast dancing, helps get necessary oxygen into your body cells. While you're doing aerobic exercises, you're burning excess calories.

- ✔ **Anaerobic,** or nonaerobic, means "without oxygen." Anaerobic exercises, such as slow walking, bowling, or strength training with weights, are important to your overall fitness level, but they generally don't help your body burn excess calories while you're performing the exercise.

Different types of exercise affect different parts of your body and have different effects on your health. That's why *cross training,* or incorporating a variety of exercises into your workout routine, is so important. In that way, exercising is similar to eating: You want as much balance and variety in your daily life as possible. Different types of exercise affect different body parts, and each plays a role in losing weight and maintaining a healthy weight. (See "Putting Together a Safe and Effective Exercise Plan," later in this chapter for more details.)

Exploring the physical benefits of exercise

Exercise does a ton more for you than just burn excess calories to help you lose weight. Aerobic exercises have terrific cardiovascular benefits, while anaerobic exercises benefit your muscle groups, bones, and joints. Some of the benefits also cross over. For instance, both aerobic and anaerobic exercises help you sleep better and reduce your blood pressure. Both play huge roles in weight control.

Following are many of the potential physical benefits of aerobic and anaerobic exercise.

Aerobic exercises improve your health by

- Boosting your energy level by building cardio-respiratory endurance
- Conditioning your heart
- Controlling your appetite
- Reducing your risk of developing certain types of cancer and other chronic diseases
- Regulating your hormones
- Lengthening your life

Anaerobic exercises improve your health by

- Bolstering your posture, joint health, and flexibility
- Building up muscle strength and endurance
- Helping you sleep better
- Reducing your blood pressure
- Strengthening your bones

Examining the psychological benefits of exercise

Over time, regular aerobic and anaerobic exercise can have as many positive effects on your mental health as it does on your physical health. The following are some of the benefits:

- Building confidence
- Diffusing anger
- Encouraging other positive lifestyle changes
- Enhancing your ability to deal with stress
- Improving your overall sense of well-being
- Increasing your self-esteem
- Lessening anxiety
- Lifting depression
- Reducing the effects of stress
- Stabilizing your moods

Fitting Exercise into Your Life

The No. 1 excuse people give for not exercising is lack of time. They say they don't have time in their hectic schedules to go to a gym on a regular basis, and they don't have time to work out at home. However, don't you find it funny that although many people can't find enough time to work out, they always find time to eat?

 What you really have to find is the motivation to make a commitment to some type of regular exercise. When you're motivated, you find the time. To get yourself on a path to fitness, use the same motivators you use to stay on a diet (see Chapter 4 for more about finding motivation). To start with, focus on the many ways exercise can improve your health and make it easier to stick to a low-cal lifestyle. Include the way it will make you look and feel about yourself.

 Before you actually start an exercise program, remember this: Everyone's appropriate level of fitness is different, depending on age, gender, heredity, health condition, and individual eating and exercising habits. To improve your fitness level, you have to focus on the factors that you can control, such as your eating and exercise habits and your attitude toward food and physical activity. That's where you have the power to make significant changes. People who don't have weight problems and people who are successful at losing weight and maintaining that weight loss are usually people who not only watch what they eat, but also get some type of exercise on a regular basis.

 In order to get yourself on track and stay there, you need to analyze your life and how exercise can fit into it. The following tips can help.

- ✔ If you join a gym, be sure it's convenient to your home or workplace.

- ✔ If you need other people to help you stay motivated, find a gym buddy or a running partner or join a group exercise activity.

- ✔ When you can't do any type of formal exercise, try to walk more, use the stairs more, and generally move about more throughout your day. Vary your exercise routine and challenge yourself from time to time to keep it interesting.

- ✔ Use the reward system. (Flip to Chapter 7 for ideas on how to reward yourself for a workout well done!)

- ✔ Hire a certified personal trainer through a local gym or a personal referral. Until you become more accountable to yourself, you may need to report to someone else. A professional trainer knows just how far to push you and can help you push yourself. A trainer can also instruct you how to be most efficient with your workout time.

In the following sections, I give you tips on setting up a regular workout schedule, increasing your amount of exercise, and adding some activity to your daily routine.

Easing into an exercise routine

Just as you manage your low-calorie diet by setting goals for changing your eating habits and losing a certain number of pounds in a certain period of time, you need to manage your fitness program by setting exercise goals. (You can read more about goal setting in Chapter 4.) Your first short-term goal may just be to sit down and start setting goals. After that, your goal may be to join a gym this week or to take your first brisk walk tonight after dinner. After you establish the type of exercises you're going to do and when, your next set of goals needs to focus on how much time you want to spend on each exercise, how many repetitions you want to do, how fast you want to go, and so forth.

To help turn sporadic attempts at exercise into a real fitness routine, start by picking a time of day that's best for you to exercise. For most people, that time means early in the morning, during a lunch hour, or right after work. You can start off exercising just two or three days a week, if that's all you can manage.

If you're new to formal exercise, start slow and work in a few more minutes of activity every day until you build up to a full routine. Start with a 10-minute walk, a 10-minute swim, or 10 minutes on the stair climber. If it's 10 minutes more than you were doing before, then you're making a great start! Later that same day, see if you can fit in another 10 minutes of similar activity.

A good long-term exercise goal is to get 30 minutes or more of steady, moderate exercise at least 5 days a week. At times, however, you may have to break those 30 minutes up and get your exercise in 5- or 10-minute spurts throughout the day. That's better than no exercise at all, and in fact, some researchers now think that shorter bouts of activity repeated throughout the day can have at least an equal effect on metabolism as one continuous exercise session, especially in people who don't exercise on a regular basis.

Too much exercise too soon can be more harmful than helpful, so if you haven't been exercising recently, start slow. Normally sedentary people who suddenly get up and exert themselves are among those at high risk of dying from a heart attack. Gradually build up your fitness level. Walk before you run, and bike slowly before you race. Do 10 minutes of exercise a day the first week, build up to 20 minutes the second week, and so on.

Organizing your workout schedule

After you have established some sort of exercise routine, and you feel comfortable adding to it, you can start setting your sights a little higher. A good workout schedule includes

✔ Ten minutes of warm-up exercises at the beginning of every workout

✔ Thirty minutes or more of ongoing aerobic exercise at least three times a week

✔ Twenty minutes of weight lifting at least twice a week

✔ Thirty minutes of calisthenics, sit-ups, push-ups, pull-ups, and weight-bearing exercises at least three times a week to build up muscular endurance

✔ Ten minutes of cooling-down exercises at the end of every workout

✔ Ten minutes of gentle stretching, which can follow your warm-up exercises or be incorporated into your cooling-down exercises

For more about these workout elements, see "Putting Together a Safe and Effective Exercise Plan" and "Exercising Additional Workout Options," later in this chapter.

Interval training, which means alternating between high intensity and low intensity activity, is a great exercise technique when you can't fully commit to an aerobic exercise. You burn extra calories because you boost your metabolic rate during short bursts of intense exercise without having to commit to a full hour of high sweat. For example, say you're walking or riding a bike for your daily exercise. First you warm up at a slow pace for about 10 minutes. Then you move into a brisk walk or speed up your cycling for a minute or two, and then slow down to a more moderate pace until you fully catch your breath. Repeat this cycle at regular intervals, taking as much time to catch your breath before you go back to full speed. Remember to cool down when you're done. Besides helping you burn more calories, interval training helps you work up to more intense activity and it can alleviate boredom, which can help keep you exercising longer.

Although some people have a problem with overexercising (and you can read more about exercising too much in "Knowing How Much Exercise Is Too Much," later in this chapter), many more have a problem with not exercising enough. Studies have shown that people who say they have a hard time losing weight tend to overestimate their amount of exercise by as much as 50 percent (and at the same time, underestimate the amount of food they eat by almost as much). That's why consistent record keeping is an important weight-loss tool.

To keep consistent records, you can use an exercise log like the one in Figure 8-1 in two different ways:

✔ You can create an advance workout plan for the week and write down your exercise goals (see Chapter 4 for more about setting these goals).

✔ You can simply keep a record of how much exercise you do each day and track your progress.

Day/Date		Exercise	Type of Exercise	Reps/Time Spent
Monday	1/23	In-line skating	Aerobic	1 hour
Tuesday	1/24	Push-ups	Strength/tone	24
		Sit-ups	Strength/tone	12/2x
		Treadmill	Aerobic	20 minutes
Wednesday	1/25	Yoga	Strength/flex/tone	1½ hours
Thursday	1/26	Sit-ups	Strength/tone	12/2x
		Push-ups	Strength/tone	24
Friday	1/27	In-line skating	Aerobic	1 hour
Saturday	1/28	Treadmill	Aerobic	35 minutes
Sunday	1/29	Treadmill	Aerobic	30 minutes

Figure 8-1:
A daily exercise log helps you keep track of your physical activity.

Figure 8-1 gives you an idea of what a basic exercise log looks like. The following easy steps can help you fill out your own daily exercise log.

1. **In the first column, write down the date.**

2. **In the next column, write down the actual exercise you did or plan to do.**

3. **Next, write down the category that particular exercise falls into.**

   Knowing this information helps you make sure your exercise plan has enough variety to cover different muscle groups and different body parts throughout the week.

4. **In the last column, write down how long you exercised, how far you went, how fast you went, or how many sets or repetitions you completed.**

You can add additional columns, such as a column for calories burned with each aerobic exercise if you have that information, steps walked if you use a pedometer, or even a column for jotting down any motivational tips or workout advise you come across.

Increasing activity in your everyday routine

Are you a little intimidated by all the muscleheads and sweaty 20-somethings in your local gym? Don't worry. You don't have to set foot inside a gym to incorporate more exercise into your lifestyle. The following are just four examples:

✔ **Turn your commuting time into exercise time.** If you normally drive or take public transportation to work or school, consider walking, cycling, scooting, or skating.

- **Get a dog.** Dogs need to be walked several times a day, and if you get the right kind of dog, he'll need to run as well. Take him to the park and run with him.

- **Do it yourself.** The price you pay for hired help may be higher than you think. Housework, gardening, lawn maintenance, and home repairs are all calorie-burning, strength-building, and flexibility-increasing activities. The more physical work you do around the house, the more calories you burn and the more fit you'll be.

- **Take fitness vacations.** Next time you plan a trip, consider a fitness option. You can choose from any number of spa vacations, hiking trips, mountain climbing trips, yoga retreats, and cross-country skiing vacations, to name just a few fitness-oriented escapes.

Putting Together a Safe and Effective Exercise Plan

When you exercise to lose weight, you're trying to hold on to calorie-burning muscle while you lose unwanted fat. In order to accomplish this, you need to exercise all your body parts and not just the ones that you don't like! The more muscle mass you have, the higher your metabolic rate, the stronger you are, and the easier it is to stay active and become even more active.

Sticking to an exercise plan is much easier if you choose activities you enjoy. If you like group activities, you can choose numerous activities including taking classes at a gym, joining a bowling league, playing other team sports, finding a tennis partner, or joining a bike club or hiking group. If exercise time is time you'd rather spend alone, then walking, jogging, swimming, and bike riding may be more your style. The best exercise for you is the one that you'll actually do!

In the following sections, I explain the importance of warming up before you exercise and cooling down afterwards, give you more details about aerobics, and provide a few ideas on strength-building activities to try.

Warming up, cooling down, and other workout essentials

The point of exercise is to get and stay healthy, not to hurt yourself! Warm-up exercises such as walking, slow jogging, slow biking, and arm and leg rotations reduce your risk of injury by sending blood to your muscles and connective tissue to literally warm up these areas before you go into full-blown activity. The additional blood flow increases the temperature in these areas and provides additional oxygen needed for exercise. Warm up for at least 10 minutes with body motions similar to those used in the type of exercise you choose, so that you're warming up the same muscles. For instance, swim a couple of slow laps before swimming at full speed or work up to a fast walk or slow jog before running.

A cooling-down period is just as essential to a good workout as a warm-up. Cooling down, or gradually reducing the intensity of your workout, allows your heartbeat to drop slowly back to a normal rate. Instead of stopping suddenly, you simply continue with your same workout at a slower rate. That means bringing your run down to a slow jog, lowering the speed on your treadmill, or slowing down your rowing action for at least 5 or 10 minutes before you call it quits.

When you're exercising, don't forget to breathe regularly because holding your breath can adversely affect your blood pressure. If you have a tendency to hold your breath while exercising, get into the habit of frequently reminding yourself to exhale. Most people get a little winded from working out, but you don't ever want to find yourself gasping for breath.

One of the most essential pieces of workout equipment you can own, regardless of what type of exercise you're doing, is a water bottle. Carry one with you at all times and drink from it often during your workout. Drinking water throughout your workout not only prevents you from becoming dehydrated, but it also fills you up on a calorie-free fluid.

Burning more calories with aerobics

In Chapter 3, I discuss the magic number for losing a pound a week, which is 3,500 calories. That is, you have to consume 3,500 fewer calories, or burn 3,500 more calories than you normally do in a week to lose one pound that week. In numbers that are easier to swallow, you have to cut 500 calories a day from your diet or burn 500 more calories a day through some sort of physical activity.

But actually it doesn't have to be an "either/or" situation. You can compromise. For example, you can cut 250 calories from your daily diet and add enough exercise to burn the other 250. Or you can cut 100 and burn 400. Or come up with any other combination that suits your needs for the day. That's the beauty of dieting and exercising at the same time. If losing weight by cutting calories means you have to be on a 1,000-calorie plan but you'd be happier with 1,200 or 1,300 calories, no problem! Just add 300 calories worth of exercise to your day.

Aerobic exercise is a surefire way to burn plenty of calories. The following sections tell you how to aim for the correct heart-rate range as you work out, show you different aerobic exercises that you can try, and give you the scoop on just how many calories you can burn with different exercises.

Targeting the right heart rate range

More important than anything else, calorie counts included, is the safety and effectiveness of your workout. The way to measure it is simple. It's in the palm of your hands. Well, not quite in the palm, but up a little farther, in your wrist. It's called your pulse. Your pulse measures your heart rate, or your heartbeats per minute (bpm). Your normal, resting heart rate, which is your bpm in the morning when you first get up and before you begin your day's activities, needs to be between 60 and 90 bpm, give or take a few beats. Your *target heart rate,* or training heart rate, may be twice that, or more. You need to figure out this number so that when you do aerobic exercises, or any exercise that gets your heart beating faster, you can determine if your workout is safely and effectively helping you burn calories to lose weight.

Everyone has a safe and effective *heart rate range* (which is the number of beats per minute your heart should be beating during intense exercise) within which to work out. This range is 50 to 85 percent of your maximum heart rate, or the fastest your heart can beat. To estimate your maximal heart rate, you simply subtract your age from the number 226 if you're female or 220 if you're male. So, for example, if you're a 37-year-old woman, your estimated maximal heart rate is 189. Your target heart rate range, then, is between 95 (50 percent) and 161 (85 percent). That information is useful but you now have to figure out if you're working out at a rate that puts your heartbeat in that range.

The most accurate and convenient way to determine if you're within your target range is with a heart monitor. (See the sidebar "Using exercise gadgets and gizmos," later in this chapter, for more information on this exercise tool.) If you don't have a heart monitor, you can count your own heartbeat. To do so, stop exercising and immediately take your pulse at your wrist or your neck, counting the beats for 15 seconds. Multiply that number by 4 to find your beats per minute. If your heart is beating faster than the high end of your target heart rate range, slow down. If it's beating slower than the low end of your range, you can work yourself a little harder.

For example, if you're the same 37-year-old woman in the previous example, and your target heart rate is between 95 and 161, then your beats per minute must be less than 161.

When you first start a new exercise program, and especially if you're out of shape, you may not even be in your target heart range. At that point, your goal is to get your heart rate up to the low end of your range (50 percent). Your next goal is to work to the top of the range as you get fit.

Surveying aerobic activities

Any activity that brings your pulse up into your target heart rate range and keeps it there for at least 20 minutes is an aerobic exercise. If you stop and start again, as you do when you play basketball, you're not getting a true aerobic workout because your heartbeat doesn't stay in your target range long enough.

The following list includes activities such as running and bicycling that are considered aerobic exercises under the right circumstances, as well as activities such as tennis and boxing, which aren't actually aerobic, but can provide a rigorous workout that promotes weight loss.

- Bike racing
- Boxing
- Cardio-stepping
- Climbing the stair climber/ step platform
- Cross-country skiing
- Cycling
- Fast dancing
- Fast walking
- Jogging
- Jumping rope
- Playing the following:
  - Handball
  - Racquetball
  - Squash
  - Tennis
- Riding a stationary bike/ recumbent bike
- Rowing
- Running
- Skating
- Spinning
- Swimming
- Using elliptical trainers
- Walking on a treadmill

Any aerobic exercise that involves running, jumping, or heavy stepping is considered a high-impact activity that can eventually take its toll on your knees and other joints. Exercises like swimming, cycling, rowing, and skating, on the other hand, are low-impact aerobic workouts that provide great cardiovascular benefits and burn a significant amount of calories without putting stress on your bones and joints.

Calculating the number of calories you're burning

Aerobic activities burn anywhere from 5 to 15 calories per minute, depending on how much you weigh and the exercise's intensity. The more you weigh, the harder it is to perform aerobic activities, so if you weigh more, you'll burn more calories working out for the same amount of time than a person who weighs less.

Table 8-1 shows the approximate number of calories burned per hour for various activities performed by someone who weighs approximately 155 pounds. If you weigh less, you'll burn somewhat fewer calories performing the same activity for the same period of time; if you weigh more, you'll burn a few more.

Table 8-1	Calories Burned with Aerobic Activities
Activity	*Calories Burned (per hour)*
Stretching exercises	180
Weight lifting (light)	220
Walking (3.5 mph)	280
Bicycling (<10 mph)	290
Light gardening/yard work	330
Golf (walking/carrying your own clubs)	330
Dancing	330
Hiking	370
Weight lifting (vigorous)	440
Heavy yard work (chopping wood)	440
Playing basketball	440
Walking (4.5 mph)	460
Aerobic exercise	480
Swimming (slow freestyle laps)	510
Running/jogging (5 mph)	590
Bicycling (>10 mph)	590

Building your strength

Aerobic exercises increase your metabolic rate while you do them, and therefore increase your capacity to burn calories while you're working out, but they don't necessarily build up your muscles. The more lean, healthy muscle tissue you have in your shoulders, arms, legs, back, chest, midsection (abdominals), legs, and butt, the more effective your body will be at burning calories all the time. The way to build bigger and better muscles is with strength training. Any type of exercise that involves weight resistance, either from lifting free weights, working out on weight machines, or using your own body as a weight, will result in better muscle health, which in turn results in a higher metabolic rate and more efficient calorie burning.

A strength-training routine becomes more important as you get older and your metabolism naturally begins to slow down. If you don't build up your lean muscle tissue, it starts to wither away and becomes less metabolically active in the process. When that process happens, you start gaining weight even if you're not eating any more than you ever did. Your body can no longer burn calories at the rate it did when you were younger so if you don't work out, you have to eat less food to prevent weight gain.

Different types of strengthening exercises work out different muscle groups. Squats and lunges work your legs and butt, while abdominal crunches strengthen your midsection and back. A good goal is to exercise each muscle group at least twice a week. Because your muscles need to recuperate after weight training, skip a day between sessions.

The following are all considered strength-training/muscle-building exercises:

- Abs, butt, thighs classes
- Body ball exercises
- Body sculpting/strength-building sessions
- Elastic band or tube exercises
- Free weights
- Sit ups, pull ups, push ups
- Weight machines
- Yoga, pilates, t'ai chi

Fighting cellulite

Most women older than 35 are on intimate terms with cellulite. But you may be surprised to discover that the lumpy, bumpy, jiggly stuff on your thighs and butt isn't really much different from any other fat in your body. It just looks worse. Cellulite is much more common in women than men because body fat is distributed differently in women. Nature took care of that, in an effort to make fat more readily available for quick energy if needed during pregnancy and breastfeeding. With aging and lack of exercise, skin also loses much of the elasticity and firmness it once had to hold that layer of fat smoothly in its place.

The only way you can fight cellulite is by maintaining a normal weight and exercising; no cream or scrub will do it. I'm sorry, but you can't deal with cellulite in any special way, and no special therapy is available to make it disappear. You can't get rid of your cellulite without removing fat from your body, but you may be able to diminish its pitted appearance by dieting to lose some of your body fat, doing aerobic exercise on a regular basis to burn stored fat, and building up your muscles with weight training to help hold your skin more taut.

Whether you work out at home or at a gym, always enlist the aid of a trainer for at least several sessions when you first start weight training, to guide you in proper form, check your breathing, verify that you're using the appropriate amount of weight, provide safety precautions, and make sure you get the best benefit from your workout. Ultimately, you'll be able to gauge for yourself whether you're lifting the right amount of weight by evaluating the effort it takes to lift a certain weight at least eight times. Generally, if you have to give up before you get to eight, you're lifting too much. If you get to 12 repetitions and feel you could easily continue, you probably need to add more weight. Somewhere in between lies the appropriate amount of weight. To help prevent injury and make your workout easier, always remember to warm up and cool down before and after strength training, just as you do for aerobic exercise. See "Warming up, cooling down, and other workout essentials," earlier in this chapter for more details.

Exercising Additional Workout Options

The more you move about in your day-to-day life, the more calories you burn. Someone who fidgets a lot, who gets up and down from her desk and paces around throughout the workday, and generally can't sit still for very long, can burn up to several hundred calories more in a day than someone who sits very still. Any physical activity you do — gardening, walking, house cleaning, mowing the lawn — burns calories. The more you perform these activities, the more they count as exercise that can help improve or maintain your fitness level.

The following sections cover other exercises that you may want to include in your routine.

Stretching out

Besides making you feel lighter and looser, a good stretch can help prevent exercise injuries. So even though stretching technically has nothing to do with burning calories, it's not a waste of your time, and it warrants as much attention as any "real" exercise when you're developing a fitness plan.

One of the reasons exercise becomes more difficult as you get older is that physically you become less flexible with age. *Flexibility exercises* (also known as stretches) lengthen and loosen the tendons that hold your muscle to your bone so that you're able to stand straighter, bend easier, and walk with a longer stride. Stretching can also help alleviate the back and leg pain that prevents some people from doing as much exercise as they could.

Never warm up or cool down with stretches. Begin your workout session with warm-up exercises and end with cooling down exercises that are appropriate to the activity. (See "Warming up, cooling down, and other workout essentials," earlier in this chapter for details.) Many types of exercises, such as yoga and balance balls, incorporate stretches, and that may be enough for you if you practice these activities on a regular basis. If you're adding stretches to your routine, however, add them just after you cool down from a rigorous workout, while your muscles are still warm and your heartbeat has fallen back down to the bottom of your target range.

Walking tall

Every fitness expert recommends walking because, if nothing else, it's something that anyone with working feet can do, regardless of individual lifestyle or athletic prowess. Walking is an especially good exercise option for anyone who, right now, can't picture herself at the gym in leotards balanced on an elliptical trainer or spinning herself into a frenzy. Walking is also a good choice for anyone who lives near any types of trails, stretches of beach, or parks.

When you walk, you can actually do it the right way or the wrong way. If you're going to make walking your primary source of physical activity and start walking longer distances, check the tips that follow to ensure you're doing it right. Start by developing a walking routine, just as you would develop any other exercise routine, by picking a time of day that's good for you to walk most days of the week. (See "Easing into an exercise routine," earlier in this chapter for more info.) Consider walking to work, school, or another regular destination, to incorporate exercise into your normal everyday routine. Aim to increase the amount of time you spend walking as well as the distance you go and the speed at which you walk.

To keep your walking routine interesting, walk in different directions than you normally go and walk on different types of terrain. Walking uphill burns more calories and helps you work different muscle groups than walking on a straight path, so seek out opportunities. The following list includes some additional tips for walkers.

- Buy good quality sneakers or walking shoes that fit properly.
- Walk tall; don't slouch!
- Warm up with a slow walk and pick up speed until you get to a brisk walk.
- Keep your arms relaxed and slightly bent at the elbows. Swing them gently as you walk.
- Carry a water bottle and sip from it often.
- Cool down for 5 or 10 minutes by gradually slowing down.

✔ Aim to gradually increase both the amount of time you spend walking and the distance you cover. If walking is your primary physical activity, gradually increase the distance you walk and the pace at which you walk over the course of a couple of months, until you're walking briskly for at least 30 minutes most days.

✔ Invest in a *pedometer,* which measures how far you've walked and gives you a basis for challenging yourself to walk longer and farther. Pedometers are available in all sporting goods stores and in the sporting goods section of most department stores. (See the nearby sidebar "Using exercise gadgets and gizmos" for details on this and other exercise tools.)

Standing burns more calories than sitting, and even very slow walking burns more calories than standing still. Choosing to move at every opportunity can help you burn up to 50 percent more calories than if you simply stand or sit still most of the day. That's why, in addition to formal exercise, fitness experts always recommend nonexercise activities, such as walking instead of driving whenever you can, taking stairs instead of elevators or escalators, and parking your car as far away from the mall as possible when you go shopping, so that you have to walk a few extra steps (and burn a few more calories) to get to the stores.

Finding alternative ways to burn calories

You burn calories all the time, even when you're eating. You burn calories working around the house, but unless you spend the entire day cleaning or repairing homes, housework won't make a huge contribution to your fitness level.

Hard work can be fun if you like what you do. So if you don't like going to a gym, you don't like jogging, and you can't think of anything else to do in the way of formal exercise, then think about what you like to do that involves some level of physical activity. The following are a few examples:

✔ Play basketball or handball with the neighborhood kids or volunteer to coach a little league team on weekends.

✔ If you watch television on a regular basis, invest in fitness equipment that keeps you moving in front of the tube. It may be as simple as a jump rope or a body ball, or as major as a treadmill or stationary bike.

✔ If you like to dance, take dance classes or just get out there and boogie. If you can't get out often, partner up with a dance video and shake it up in your own living room.

Using exercise gadgets and gizmos

Many exercise "accessories" are available to help you measure your fitness level, monitor your progress, and make sure your exercise routine is safe and effective. While many are unnecessary, the following exercise tools can be quite helpful:

✔ A **pedometer,** which is a digital device you attach to your waistband to keep track of the number of steps you take, can help you determine if you're taking enough steps to make a difference in your fitness level. Just remember: When you walk, you take steps, and the more you walk, the more steps you take. The more steps you take, the more calories you burn. So if you're walking to lose weight, it makes sense to count the number of steps you take as a measure of progress. A pedometer can measure the number of steps you take.

The magic number of steps appears to be 10,000, the goal stated in many fitness articles that recommend using a pedometer for step counting. But the truth, according to The American College of Sports Medicine, is that the goal varies from person to person, and 10,000 steps, or 5 miles, a day may not be optimal for everyone. To an exercise walker, building up speed can be as important as walking longer distances. That all translates to this advice: Use your pedometer as a motivating tool and a tracking tool, but not as your only goal-setting tool. As a walker, your best fitness goal isn't to walk 10,000 steps, but to fit in at least 30 minutes of *brisk* walking on most if not all days of the week. If you like to walk for exercise, using a pedometer can help get you 10,000 steps closer to that goal, give or take a few steps. Some studies do show that using a pedometer is a motivator and a challenge for many people to walk more.

✔ During aerobic exercise you may consider wearing a **heart rate monitor** to measure the intensity of your workout and determine whether or not you're working hard enough to reap cardiovascular benefits or too hard and need to slow down. A heart rate monitor eliminates the need for taking your own pulse and figuring out your heart rate as described in the section "Targeting the right heart rate range," earlier in this chapter.

✔ Relatively new to the gizmo scene are **calorie counters** you can attach to your arm, chest, or wrist to find out approximately how many calories you're burning while you exercise. They're only moderately accurate, at best. You may have noticed that some exercise machines have built-in calorie counters that keep track of your burn while you're working out. The new calorie counters may be slightly more accurate than the built-in counters. Some calorie counters measure your heart rate to determine how much oxygen you use and how much heat you produce while exercising. Others measure your skin's temperature and electrical conductivity along with how much heat you're producing and losing while you work out. Extra features include built-in programs to help you keep track of calorie-burning goals and progress.

None of this equipment can claim 100 percent accuracy, but for adults who like their grown-up toys, any and all of these devices can be helpful as motivators and tracking tools. Some gadgets even do double duty, measuring your heart rate and your calorie burn at the same time, for instance. The one thing they can't do is lose weight for you. That's your job!

Exercising for Body and Mind

Some people are as motivated by the mood-elevating and stress-busting effects of exercise as by the promise of improved physical health and weight loss. If stressful, emotional issues are at the core of your overeating (see Chapter 9 for more about this topic), then you stand to gain multiple benefits from adding mind-body exercises such as yoga or t'ai chi to your fitness routine. These ancient, meditative practices are designed to improve both your mental and physical conditions.

The proven physical benefits of mind-body exercises include improved flexibility, balance, and coordination, better breathing and blood circulation, and reduced muscle tension. These benefits can also help prevent injury when you exert yourself during more strenuous exercises. The most often cited psychological benefits include increased self-awareness, mental relaxation, and a general feeling of emotional well-being.

Yoga, pilates, and t'ai chi are three different exercises with a common objective of uniting mind, body, and spirit with the goal of improving your overall health. You don't wear your MP3 player or watch the news while you practice these three arts. The focus is on your inner self, not the outer world. These prac-tices are widely recognized by medical professionals and alternative practitioners as healthful adjuncts to a sound fitness program. Following are brief descriptions of each:

- ✔ Yoga exercises are designed to quiet the mind in order to reduce psychological distress and develop more physical and emotional self-awareness. It's also a stretching, toning, and strengthening exercise. (If you're interested in finding out more about yoga, check out *Yoga For Dummies* by Georg Feuerstein, Larry Payne, and Lilias Folan [Wiley].)

- ✔ Pilates exercises, which are often compared to yoga and grouped with yoga, consist of strengthening movements that work all your body parts, but focus on the abdomen as your core source of strength. Many pilates floor exercises incorporate yoga-like movements. Because the intense movements of pilates require tremendous concentration, the benefits include a self-awareness similar to that developed by practicing yoga and t'ai chi. (If you want more information about incorporating pilates into your exercise program, check out *Pilates For Dummies* by Ellie Herman [Wiley].)

- ✔ T'ai chi exercises promote the development of balance, alignment, and coordination through a series of slow, graceful movements performed in a dance-like fashion. These unique movements also promote relaxation of body and mind. (If t'ai chi interests you, check out *T'ai Chi For Dummies* by Therese Iknoian [Wiley].)

Mind-body exercises were once relegated to private studios, but now they're often the most popular classes at most gyms and fitness clubs, so you can find one just about anywhere. Because these formerly alternative activities are strength building and incorporate plenty of stretching, you can substitute one of these classes for an "abs, buns, and thighs" class or a weight-training session once or twice a week.

Knowing How Much Exercise Is Too Much

Can there be such a thing as too much exercise in this land of couch tomatoes? (I prefer the term couch tomato to couch potato, because it's more realistic. Potatoes can sit around for months and still stay firm, until you cook them. When tomatoes sit around, they quickly get squishy, just like a body that doesn't get enough exercise.) Believe it or not, sometimes you do need to slow down your physical activity rather than keep going. One of those times is when you begin a new exercise program. If you start off too fast or push yourself too far at first, you may burn out, both physically and mentally, before you finish your workout. If that happens, you could quickly lose your motivation, or worse, hurt yourself.

Identifying the warning signs of too much exercise

As good as exercise is for you — and it's very good for most people — too much can take its toll. Exercise puts physical stress on all your body parts and can ultimately lead to permanent damage to muscles, joints, and bones if you work too hard, too soon, or if you don't follow recommended safety precautions.

Even after you've established your workout routine and you're comfortable with the exercises you're doing, sometimes you may need to slow down or call it quits. Keep the following points in mind when exercising:

- ✔ Whenever you're doing aerobic exercise, you should be able to carry on a conversation at the same time. If you're gasping for breath, feeling faint (or dizzy), feeling any pain, or getting nauseous, slow down or take a break.

- ✔ Anytime you're sick, injured, or tired from lack of sleep is a good time to take a day or two off. Just don't let your exercise break last any longer than it has to or you may find it very difficult to get back in the swing of things.

Overexercising to the extreme

Believe it or not, some people become addicted to exercise in the same, obsessive way a food addict becomes addicted to eating certain foods or a gambler becomes addicted to games. It's a psychological addiction, and many experts believe that there's probably a physiological explanation as well. Exercise "addicts" constantly think about exercising, and they work out frantically, every day, to burn off as many calories as they can. If you work out more than an hour a day, seven days a week, and you're not a professional athlete, consider that you may be exercising too much to the detriment of your own health.

Overexercising can be a sign of a true eating disorder. Someone with an eating disorder is obsessed with food, dieting, and, often, exercise. There are several types of eating disorders, but the two that often involve overexercising are anorexia nervosa and bulimia nervosa.

- ✔ People with anorexia are underweight, extremely afraid of being fat, usually eat very little, and spend most of their time trying to purge any and all calories they consume by vomiting, using laxatives, and exercising excessively.

- ✔ People with bulimia are usually normal weight or overweight, often eat excessive amounts of food, and purge or resort to extreme exercising to burn off the extra calories they eat.

Both of these eating disorders have severe nutritional and medical consequences, which in some cases can result in death. Most people who overeat or focus a great deal of attention on their diets don't have eating disorders, but if you or anyone you know shows signs of an eating disorder, immediately seek the help of a professional. You can start by calling any hospital, university medical center, or trusted physician, who can steer you toward the appropriate type of help.

Part III
Overcoming Obstacles and Moving On

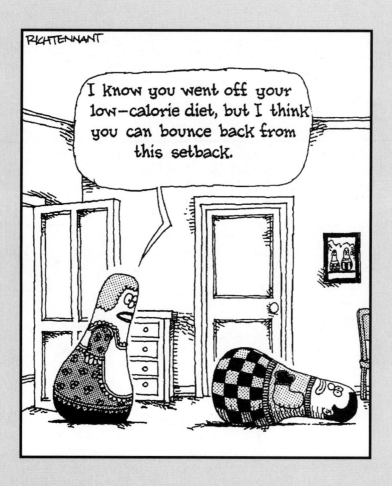

In this part . . .

The chapters in this part deal with everyday frustrations, emotions, and situations that can sabotage even the best thought-out weight-loss plan. Most of these circumstances have nothing to do with your low-calorie diet, but they have everything to do with why and how you gain weight.

Every problem has a solution, and this part offers many. If you're coming up against too many roadblocks in your attempt to lose weight, if you're feeling insecure about your ability to maintain the weight you've lost, or if you feel downright despair over your weight situation, focus on this important part.

Chapter 9

Making Your Way through Trials and Tribulations

- -

In This Chapter

▶ Managing emotional eating dilemmas

▶ Testing your willpower in the long run

▶ Handling special situations away from home

- -

Along the path to weight loss, you're going to run into some inevitable twists and turns. Sometimes you lose your motivation and have to turn around and find it. Maybe you overindulged last night and so now you're thinking of giving up. Perhaps you're bored with your routine, even though it's working for you. You may even get to a point where, no matter what you do, your weight just won't budge, even though you still need to lose 20 pounds. You may feel frustrated and want to give up your goals. Please, don't! You can get your thinking and your behavior back on track. The secret to success is to nip any problems in the bud.

Many people give up (and eventually gain back any weight they lost) when they get thrown off track, lose momentum, or find themselves stuck in a weight-loss rut. But you have to stand strong and renew your commitment to losing weight and keeping it off, especially during these trying times. The type of commitment you need when faced with dieting challenges is to see yourself through every stage of change.

You knew changing your lifestyle wouldn't be easy when you first decided to lose weight, but if you had the motivation to get started on a low-calorie plan, you can find the motivation to keep going. If you cheated on your diet last night, one big meal or one big dessert or even an all-out binge didn't blow everything. If you overeat one day, all you have to do is wake up the next day and get back on track. If you're bored with your diet or exercise routine, remember that you're not stuck with it; it's simply time for a change.

This chapter can help you solve problems common to emotional eaters. You also find ways to cope with everyday dilemmas that are likely to occur in the long run, regardless of the nature of your eating habits, and tips to help you eat sensibly away from home.

Recognizing and Solving Predictable Problems for Emotional Eaters

Food has a way of filling gaps in people's lives. People don't just eat to survive, which can be a big problem. People eat to kill time, to make themselves feel better, and to distract themselves. Many people eat whenever they feel emotional pangs, good or bad, and overeat in response to highly emotional situations. If you're an emotional eater, you eat when you're happy and when you're sad. Eating is the way you deal with your emotions, and what's usually happening is that you're overfeeding yourself to try to "stuff down" feelings that are hard to cope with.

When solving your emotional eating problems, you need to look at the problem in two ways.

✔ **Recognize the emotions that are driving your eating behavior.** For an emotional eater, boredom, loneliness, anger, sadness, anxiety, and everyday frustrations are all potential roadblocks to weight-loss success. Other situations that may cause you to turn to food for relief include

- **Getting rejected.** If you get passed up for a promotion or an intimate relationship goes sour, you may naturally feel insecure or unwanted and turn to food for comfort.

- **Playing the martyr.** When your children talk back to you, your mate ignores you, or you feel taken for granted at work or at home, you may eat instead of expressing your feelings of denigration.

- **Feeling rebellious.** Overeating may help you send out a message that says, "Nobody tells me what to do!"

- **Losing sight of your dreams.** If you're unhappy with the life you live, or you have regrets, you may be overeating to try to make up for not feeling satisfied or complete.

- **Facing challenges.** Success can be as scary as failure; you may overeat to avoid taking that next step.

- **Developing intimacy.** Being overweight may help you cover up your fear of developing an intimate relationship.

✔ **Get to the root of the problem, one way or another.** If you eat to satisfy emotional hunger, as opposed to true physical hunger, you still have to deal with your emotions while you're trying to lose weight. (If you struggle with emotional eating, Chapter 11 has helpful resources.)

In the following sections, I provide tips on how to handle several typical emotional situations while keeping your low-calorie diet on track.

Busting boredom

When you're bored and have nothing to do, what's your first instinct? Do you say "to eat"? Boredom is many a dieter's downfall, but I have an obvious solution: Do something! Find something you enjoy doing, something you can do on a regular basis that has nothing whatsoever to do with eating (unless, of course, you decide to take a class in healthy cooking). Look for something longer lasting and more fruitful, such as taking up a new hobby.

Something like knitting or cabinet making not only keeps you busy, but also provides a reward when you're done — a finished product! If you aren't into hobbies or feel you need to get out of the house, consider volunteering your time at a hospital, museum, or school. If boredom threatens to sabotage your weight-loss goals, check out the list of diversions suggested in Chapter 7.

Dealing with everyday frustrations

For most people, each day brings its share of aggravation, whether you're at work, at school, or at home. Your boss treats you badly, you don't have time to pack a healthy lunch, or you haven't been able to get to the gym in a week. How you handle frustrating situations can make the difference between diet failure and success. Why? Because if you give in to overeating when you feel frustrated, or if you often feel frustrated because circumstances that are seemingly beyond your control are preventing you from eating well, you may feel that you have no choice but to give up on your goals.

In the following sections, I provide tips on handling several common frustrations so that you can stick to your low-calorie plan.

Coping with stress

Anger. Pressure. Change. Any of these stressors can drive bad eating behavior. You may be eating to cope, to give yourself a treat when everything else looks bleak, or to punish yourself. When stress (and eating from stress) gets out of hand, something has to give. You have to find a way to relax and escape the pressure you feel. You may need help. Consider the mind-body exercises in Chapter 8 or some of the counseling options in Chapter 11.

Boosting low confidence

Self-doubt leads to self-criticism, which is known as negative self-talk. Nothing and no one can make you feel all that bad about yourself unless you feel bad about yourself to begin with. Review Chapter 4 for advice about positive self-talk and how it can help you stick to your low-calorie diet plan.

One way to boost your own self-esteem is to force yourself to focus on everything right about your life, rather than on everything wrong with it. At the end of each day, look back and find at least one event that was positive.

- ✔ Look for some accomplishment, big or small. Did you buy a fitness magazine? Did you eat fruit salad for lunch instead of a cheeseburger? If you ate the cheeseburger, did you take a walk after lunch?

- ✔ Look for anything that can make you feel good about yourself and distract from the negative. It doesn't have to have anything to do with your diet or exercise program. Maybe you smiled at a stranger who smiled back. Maybe you cleaned out your kitchen cabinets. Maybe someone thanked you for a job well done. These events are all positive and life affirming, and they deserve recognition.

If you take a few minutes every night to write down your accomplishments in a journal, you'll soon have a good collection of "feel-good" anecdotes to look back on when your confidence needs a boost or when you feel like giving up on yourself.

Handling the pressure of keeping a meal schedule

The pressure of trying to adhere to a "normal" meal schedule may actually be sabotaging your efforts to lose weight. Most people with a history of out-of-control eating, dieting, bingeing, and compulsive overeating benefit from a regular meal routine, but some people just don't fit that mold. You need a plan, but planning three square meals at the usual times of day is fruitless if that plan just doesn't fit into your lifestyle.

You can always make routine eating a long-term goal. (For more about setting goals, see Chapter 4.) For now, have a plan that suits your schedule. The trick is to create your own routine by having the type of food you need available wherever you are, whenever you need it. For instance, if you work late most evenings, stock a shelf in your office or invest in a minifridge to hold foods that can serve as dinner. You can also order an appropriate dinner from local restaurants or delis that deliver your food (see "Dining out at restaurants," later in this chapter to help you eat out the right way).

Feeding your sorrow

Do you overeat because you're unhappy, or are you unhappy because you overeat? That's a chicken-and-egg question if I ever heard one! If you're an emotional overeater, you probably overeat because you're unhappy and then you become even unhappier because you overate. If you find yourself in this state of unhappiness for months on end, with no sign of let-up, you may be clinically depressed. This type of deep unhappiness often leads to self-deprecation and the type of negativity that can really block your best attempts at losing weight and living a healthier lifestyle.

Exercise (which I cover in Chapter 8) helps with sad feelings and mild depression because it raises your levels of *endorphins,* brain chemicals that help improve your general outlook. But if you think you suffer from clinical depression, speak to your physician, who can help you decide if you need further professional help. Chapter 11 provides more information on the type of help that may be available to you.

Meeting Typical Long-Term Challenges and Temptations

For most people, dieting unfortunately is one of those situations where some things get worse before they get better. Early on, you're motivated by hopes and dreams, by the novelty of a new and challenging lifestyle, and I hope, by your initial weight loss. As the weeks and months go by, however, you may have to work harder to prevent old eating habits from sneaking back in, to resist giving in to food cravings, and to stop yourself from all-out bingeing to make up for all the food you haven't been eating. The honeymoon is over and now the real work begins.

The following sections provide tools that can help you face challenges as you continue your low-calorie plan.

Figuring out whether you're truly hungry

What happens when you don't eat? You set yourself up for a binge in the not-so-distant future. Food deprivation never helped anyone lose weight in the long run. The trick is to figure out if you're really hungry, and to eat just enough to satisfy your hunger. One way to know if what you're feeling is true physical hunger, and not emotional hunger, is that when you're truly hungry, you'll feel better by eating just about any type of food. When you're emotionally hungry, you usually crave very specific types of foods that you've used to comfort yourself in the past. (See the following sections for more about cravings and binges.)

The secret to eating without overeating is to eat mindfully, which simply means paying attention to the food you eat and how you eat it. Chapter 4 has info on mindful eating that can help you put this technique into practice.

 One component of mindful eating that dietitians and other weight experts often use is a hunger scale, like the one that follows, that can help you determine just how hungry you are or how full you are. The scale ranges from 0 to 10, with 0 being so hungry you could eat a bucket of beans and 10 being so overstuffed you can't get up out of your chair. You want to avoid these extremes by using this scale to decide when to eat and when to stop. I recommend starting at 2 and stopping at 5; you may have to gradually work your way into that range.

0 Extremely hungry

1 Very hungry

2 Hungry

3 Slightly hungry

4 No longer hungry but not yet full

5 Comfortable

6 Beginning to feel full

7 Beginning to feel too full

8 Uncomfortable

9 Very uncomfortable with a slight stomachache

10 Extremely overstuffed and uncomfortable; possibly nauseous

 Whenever you're following a low-calorie diet and you feel hungry, you need to eat. Period. Don't give it a second thought. Better yet, try not to let yourself get to the point where you actually feel hungry. Eat something.

 If you're an emotional eater — someone who eats when you're excited, angry, distressed — you may turn to food when you're not really hungry. Your challenge (and something to keep in mind the next time you're updating your psychological and behavior goals — see Chapter 4) is to wait until you really feel hungry before you put anything in your mouth. Easier said than done, I know, but try these few tips:

✔ Try to express your feelings with words rather than with food. Write down your feelings if you're not in a position to speak them.

✔ Start walking in the opposite direction of any food source. The walk does you good and the food is less accessible.

✔ Set a timer or watch the clock and wait ten minutes to see if the urge to eat passes.

Satisfying cravings

When you get a craving, you're probably not craving a cucumber salad or a lean slice of chicken. *Cravings* are usually reserved for foods high in sugar, fat, or salt, or some combination of the three. Studies have shown that women are more likely to crave sugar-fat combinations like chocolate cake while men crave protein-fat combos like meat. Surveys have also revealed that, overall, salty foods, breads, and sweet foods top the most-often-craved list.

The hungrier you are, the more you yearn for foods that you may not otherwise be craving. To help control cravings, make sure you eat something every three to five hours.

If you've been depriving yourself of your favorite foods, chances are you're craving them all the time. If that's the case, indulge yourself — with a reasonable amount of food, that is! Deprivation is a way of setting yourself up for a binge, so don't do it. (See the next section for more about binges.) Instead, find a way to enjoy the foods you like in reasonable amounts on a regular basis. Give yourself permission to eat what you want, whenever you want, but not necessarily as much as you want.

Uncovering the clues to your cravings

If you want to know exactly why you get cravings, I can't help you. Scientists aren't sure, but one theory is that cravings are the way your body tells you that you need specific nutrients. I don't buy that one, because nobody *needs* ice cream or chocolate cake or potato chips, although it's quite possible that there's something in ice cream, chocolate cake, and potato chips that fills either an emotional or physical need. According to a small study done at the University of Pennsylvania School of Medicine and the Monell Chemical Senses Center, a physiological change occurs in the brain when you experience a food craving. This research suggests that food cravings activate the same areas of the brain — the hippocampus, insula, and caudate — that are activated when an addict craves drugs, alcohol, or goes on a gambling spree. These areas of the brain are linked to emotion, memory, and reward. That could explain why people crave specific, familiar foods; they're etched into your memory as a reward that soothes the emotions. Other scientific studies have come up with similar findings, but other theories exist as well.

Some experts say people's cravings go back to the beginning of mankind, when cave people filled up on food whenever they came across it. Others say people are simply surrounded by too much food that tastes too good and they just can't resist. Although the jury's still out on this one, most nutrition experts now agree that cravings are somehow linked to brain chemistry and, more often than not, occur when you don't eat enough or you go too long without eating. In other words, your cravings may be a result of real hunger.

Indulging in cravings is good advice for some people, but it isn't for everyone. If you're not satisfied with small amounts of your favorite high-cal foods, or if you know that eating certain foods will set off an episode of binge-eating, then abstinence is your best policy until you have your weight under control.

Avoiding binges

An eating binge means one thing to one person and another thing to the next. Binge eating is relative to individual circumstances and just how much food constitutes a binge for you. Generally, an episode of true *bingeing* is defined as an out-of-control eating episode during which great quantities of food are consumed in a short period of time. The key phrase here is "out of control."

People usually binge in response to an emotional upheaval. Not every emotional overeater binges, but most bingers are emotional overeaters. If you've ever had a bad day at the office or a fight with your mate and then turned around and downed a pint of ice cream along with handfuls of cookies and maybe even more food than that, you went on a binge.

If you binge once in a while but you're able to get back on track the next day without too much residual damage to your physical or mental health, then I don't consider it a big problem. Your solution could be as simple as trying to distract yourself or getting out of the house if you feel a binge coming on, or reviewing your diet strategies to see if maybe you've been too rigid and need to allow in some of the foods you've been denying yourself.

However, if you binge several times a week, for months at a time, you may be showing signs of a clinical eating disorder known, not surprisingly, as *binge-eating disorder*. The signs of binge-eating disorder include

- Quickly eating large amounts of food in one sitting, sometimes when you're not even hungry
- Filling up past the point of satisfaction and to the point of great discomfort
- Planning binges
- Eating alone, or hiding any evidence that you've eaten, to cover up the amount of food you eat
- Feeling ashamed, guilty, disgusted, and depressed about bingeing
- Getting to the point where you avoid loved ones for fear of being discovered

You don't necessarily have an eating disorder just because you binge once in a while. But if you frequently binge and experience guilt, fear, or other behaviors described in this section, then seek treatment from a professional. (Flip to Chapter 11 for more advice.) Dieting isn't a solution for anyone with an eating disorder. Left unchecked, binge eating can put you at a particularly high risk of obesity, which can lead to an assortment of medical problems.

Maintaining your interest and motivation

One reason why I wrote this book is to help you find ways to stay motivated and live a low-calorie lifestyle. I don't want just to help you lose weight right now, but also to help you lay the groundwork for maintaining a healthy weight for the rest of your life. For many people, sticking to a low-calorie lifestyle after the excess weight is gone is harder than losing weight in the first place. That's why keeping your low-cal lifestyle fun and interesting is so important by personalizing your diet plan to suit your own lifestyle and making adjustments and changes whenever your plan starts to stale.

You can use your new diet plan as a tool to prevent boredom and keep your low-cal lifestyle interesting by getting creative with your menus, trying new foods, and discovering new ways to prepare food. The more excited you feel about your food plan, the more motivated you'll be to stick with it. Chapter 7 contains plenty of ideas for "alternative" menu plans and ideas for making your low-cal diet more interesting and more fun. Some of the recipes in Chapters 12 through 15 can also inspire you to try something different once in a while so that your diet doesn't become too routine or too boring.

Breaking through plateaus

Like any mountain you may find yourself climbing, the process of losing weight is tough going uphill. Unlike mountain climbing, however, where reaching a plateau or other flat service is a welcome break for the climber, a weight *plateau,* which is a stable period during which there is little or no change, is no relief to a dieter. A plateau is a source of real frustration because it's a period of time when, for no apparent reason, you stop losing weight before you reach your goal. It happens to just about everyone.

You may be at a plateau stage because you've been slipping on your diet and/or exercise routines. Maybe you've been feeling a bit cocky and thought you could sneak in a little extra food here or there or sneak out of the gym a little sooner than usual. Doing so is okay once in a while, but those added and unburned calories mount up (and usually in places you don't want).

The actual reason you get stuck on a plateau probably has to do with your metabolism slowing down after you've lost a bit of weight. When you lose weight, you inevitably lose some muscle along with excess fat. Along with muscle goes some of your calorie-burning power. As a result, you may need to add weight-bearing exercises to your exercise routine to keep your muscles as strong and healthy as possible. (Chapter 8 can tell you more about that.)

I have good news and bad news about weight plateaus. First, the good news: Eventually, every plateau breaks. The bad news: It can take weeks, or (gulp!) even months. You may get stuck at the same weight for several months, and all the usual calorie counting and burning won't make it budge any quicker. You can only go so low in calories and you can only do so much exercise.

If you're doing all you can do to stay on your low-cal plan, then be patient and hang in there. Whatever you do, don't use a plateau as an excuse to give up. When you reach a plateau, consider the following tips to help you, and maybe, just maybe, you'll break through your plateau stage a little sooner:

- **Remain calm.** Worrying about a weight plateau won't make it go away.

- **Practice positive thinking.** (See Chapter 4 for help.) If you tell yourself, "I can do it," you'll eventually break through your plateau and continue losing weight. If you allow yourself to feel defeated, you may give up and, out of frustration, go back to some of your old overeating habits.

- **Stop weighing yourself for a while.** Instead of weekly weigh-ins, wait two or three weeks. Getting on the scale can be very discouraging when you've reached a plateau. (Chapter 4 has tips on weighing yourself.)

- **Make some changes to your diet.** Now is a good time to try out some of the "alternative" menu plans in Chapter 7 that you can follow for just a day or two. If you're still up around 1,500 calories or more a day, cut back to 1,300 or 1,400 and see what happens after a week or so.

- **Break your exercise routine.** If you haven't been challenging yourself lately, add another 5 or 10 minutes of exercise to what you're already doing on a regular basis. If you're already exercising as much as you can, try something different. For instance, if you normally cycle for 30 minutes, devote 10 of those minutes to an elliptical trainer. (See Chapter 8 for more on exercising.)

- **Attend more meetings or stay more closely in touch with other members if you belong to any type of weight-loss group or program.** Many of your fellow dieters have "been there," and they probably have some encouraging words to say while you wait it out. (See Chapter 11 for more info on joining a group.)

- **Be sure you're drinking at least 8 cups of water every day.** Water aids metabolism and helps you feel full so you're less likely to overeat.

Eating Away from Home with Ease

The best advice anyone can give you if you're eating anywhere outside your own home is to have a plan. You'll always be tempted with restaurant foods, birthday celebrations, holiday feasts, and times when you have to eat on the road. Be prepared! I help you out with great tips in the following sections.

Dining out at restaurants

There are two schools of thought about dieting and eating out at restaurants. The first school says to make low-calorie food choices at the restaurant; the other school says to eat what you want but watch your portion sizes. I know which school I graduated from. Most of the time, when I eat out at a restaurant, I don't want to limit my choices to low-calorie foods. I want to eat food that I don't normally prepare at home. I want to have fun and enjoy my food while I'm out.

In this section you can find helpful tips from both schools, and many of them cross over, depending on where you're eating and how determined you are to stick to your diet when you go out to eat.

These tips may come in handy if you don't want to worry about calories and just want to watch your portion sizes when you eat out:

- ✔ Have an appetizer, side dish salad, or vegetable side dish, and then split an entree with your eating partner.

- ✔ Choose child-size portions when possible.

- ✔ If you order a higher-calorie entree and don't have anyone to share it with, ask for half your dish to be packed in a take-home bag before you even start to eat.

- ✔ Share a dessert.

If you're not ready to tempt the fates, or you're perfectly happy to eat lower calorie foods when you go out to eat, these tips are for you:

- ✔ Stay away from all-you-can-eat buffets unless you're quite confident you'll make wise selections.

- ✔ Order an appetizer as your main course.

- ✔ Scan the menu for dishes that are steamed, poached, grilled, stir-fried without heavy sauces added, boiled, or broiled.

- ✔ Ask for all dressing, gravies, sauces, butter, sour cream, or any other optional toppings on the side.

Whichever approach you take to eating out in restaurants, always ask for a glass of water as soon as you sit down. Also, ask the server to hold the bread that often arrives at the table before you've even ordered. Balance higher-calorie choices with lower-calorie, and always start your meal with a green salad or a bowl of broth-based (clear, not creamy) soup.

No ethnic cuisine is necessarily any healthier or lower in calories than another, although you can probably find more light offerings at, say, Japanese or Southeast Asian restaurants than at Mediterranean or South American restaurants. All cuisines have their fried foods, their starchy foods, and cooking techniques that add too many extra calories to otherwise healthful food. Often, the less "Americanized" the food is at an ethnic restaurant, the lighter the fare. (French food may be one big exception to that rule!) Here's a sampling of the "best of the best" choices for low-calorie dieters at different restaurants:

- **Chinese:** Anything steamed — vegetables, tofu (bean curd), fish or shellfish, chicken, dumplings — with sauce on the side. Use the sauce as a dip instead of pouring it over your food.

- **French:** Meat, poultry, or seafood en brochette or grilled, steamed vegetables; sauces on the side.

- **Greek:** Souvlaki (kabobs) made with chicken, fish, lamb, or pork and vegetables, plain rice, small Greek salad.

- **Indian:** Chicken or seafood Tandoori, lentil dishes, masala (curry) dishes, basmati rice, cucumber raita.

- **Italian:** Mussels marinara, pasta primavera, chicken piccata, spaghetti pomodoro (with tomato-basil sauce), grilled seafood, margherita (or plain) thin-crust pizza.

- **Japanese:** Miso soup, negimaki (scallion wrapped with thin slices of beef), edamame (fresh green soy beans), sushi, sashimi, chirashi, teriyaki, and yakitori (grilled skewer) dishes, noodle soups.

- **Mexican:** Ceviche (fresh seafood marinated in lime juice), fajitas, vegetable chili, burrito, enchilada, or soft taco with chicken, seafood, or vegetables, Tex-Mex salad in a grilled (not fried) tortilla basket, rice and beans (not refried), grilled seafood. Avoid sour cream, cheese, and guacamole toppings; opt instead for diced tomato, onion, and other vegetable toppings.

- **Thai:** Bean thread noodles (glass noodles), green papaya salad, squid salad, grilled or steamed meats.

- **Vietnamese:** Summer rolls, green papaya salad, fish or shellfish wrapped in lettuce with mint and cilantro, fish soups.

Enjoying parties

If the celebration is at your house, you have more control over the type of food that's served. However, if you're partying at someone else's home, you can't assume that the host will serve many low-cal foods. You can take several steps to help prevent yourself from overeating at a party.

- Eat a little bit at home, just before you leave to go to the party. If it's a dinner party, and you don't want to kill your appetite, just be sure to have at least one full glass of water before you leave home and ask for another as soon as you arrive.

✔ Bring your own platter of low-calorie foods, such as cut up vegetables and the Yogurt-Cheese Dip with Spinach and Dill from Chapter 15.

✔ Position yourself away from the buffet table or any place that's a safe distance from temptation.

✔ Always keep a glass of water or seltzer with lemon in your hand.

✔ If you normally drink wine, drink *wine spritzers* — wine diluted with seltzer or club soda — instead, and pack your glass with ice.

✔ Try talking more and eating less.

Celebrating holidays

For many dieters, the problem with holidays is that they're loaded with tradition, and food usually plays a big role in holiday traditions. Traditional foods served at holiday celebrations aren't usually low in calories. What can you do? For one thing, you can bring your favorite lower-calorie vegetable, legume, or rice side dish to the table and introduce a new tradition. I can also think of several other solutions, none of which involve avoiding the big meal. Try out these few ideas:

✔ **Bank some calories.** Don't skip meals throughout the day and then pig out at dinner. However, you can eat very light meals during the day — yogurt with fruit for breakfast, a huge green salad with low-cal dressing for lunch, another piece of fruit for a snack, and plenty of water, all day long — so that you can enjoy normal serving sizes of some of your favorite holiday fare without worrying about your calorie count.

✔ **Drink water or another calorie-free beverage before, during, and after the meal.** You can jazz up a glass of water or seltzer in many calorie-free and near-calorie-free ways. Mint leaves, lemon, lime, or orange slices, a couple of raspberries, or an herbal tea bag can all help a humble glass of water rise to the occasion.

✔ **Remember that it takes 3,500 *extra* calories to gain a pound.** Heavy as Thanksgiving dinner can be, if you've been sticking to a low-calorie plan, you're not likely to blow it with one meal. But if you feel like you blew your diet with a single holiday meal, go to bed, rest easy, wake up the next day, and get back on your plan. You're only one day behind.

Traveling light

Like all "special situations," eating on the road (or in the air or on the tracks) is risky business when you're trying to watch calories and lose weight. You never really know what type of food choices you'll have while you're traveling and when you get to wherever you're going. Your best bet is to have a travel plan.

A travel plan doesn't have to be complicated. Whether you're taking a car trip or traveling on a bus, train, or airplane, you can easily pack a selection of foods that don't require refrigeration so that you're not forced to choose from vending machines, dining car options, or meals you'd just rather not eat or, worse yet, go hungry. Some ideas for easy-to-carry foods that are easy to eat (especially if you've packed your own utensils!) include

- Shelf-stable lowfat milk in 8-ounce containers
- Small bottles of water
- Applesauce and pop-top cans of water-packed or juice-packed fruit in individual serving containers
- Fresh fruit such as apples, cherries, grapes, and pears
- Individual cans or packages of tuna or salmon
- Crackers or pretzels in sealed plastic snack bags
- Individual boxes of cold cereal
- Packets of instant hot cereal (if you have access to boiling water)
- 100-calorie cookie or cracker snack packs

My favorite food and travel anecdote, which is really a bit of advice, is the story of my friend Joyce, who travels to France whenever she gets a chance. She always packs a plastic knife, fork, and spoon in her carry-on bag so that she's prepared to pick up some crusty bread, a small hunk of cheese, and a piece of fruit at a local market and enjoy a picnic meal wherever she goes. That way, she's not limited to hotel or restaurant food. She not only has more control over what she eats, but she also saves money! I followed Joyce's lead several years ago and found it extremely helpful. Everyone laughed when I packed my own chopsticks before I left on a trip to China, but I had the last laugh because I ended up using them every day while I was there. I was on a very hectic schedule and often had no time to sit down for a snack or regular meal. It didn't matter, because I bought packaged or prepared foods to go, and ate in my hotel room or in the vans and buses I was using for transportation. Ever since that time, I've kept a complete set of plastic utensils with me in my handbag (and in my daughter's backpack), at all times. Keeping a set of eating utensils in your bag and your car can open up your options for eating away from home, wherever you go.

Chapter 10

Staying Fit and Stopping Regain in Its Tracks

Maintaining your current weight probably takes just as much patience and open-mindedness as getting to a healthier weight. Maybe even more. Statistically, most people who lose weight aren't able to maintain their weight loss after several years. But you can beat those odds! Plenty of people are able to keep all or most of the weight off and maintain a healthier weight for the rest of their lives. You can be one of them!

This chapter is one of the more serious in this book. I focus on healthy weight maintenance at any age. Sure, losing and maintaining weight gets harder if you wait until you're older to start trying or if you've tried over and over again throughout your life and you've gotten older in the process. But it doesn't matter if you're 20, 40, 60, or older; you lose weight and maintain the loss by following the same rules. You may have to tweak the rules here and there to fit your own circumstances, but they don't change with age.

In addition, this chapter also contains some practical tools to help you maintain your weight loss, such as a formula to help you determine how many calories you can consume now to stay at your current weight and a few menu plans you can use as guides to healthy, calorie-controlled meal planning throughout your lifetime.

Adding Calories and Keeping Up with Your Workouts

The first thing you had to do to start losing weight was accept the notion of change. (What? You haven't started losing weight? Check out Chapter 4 to start your plan.) You had to change something about the way you eat, the way you exercise, and even the way you think. You're probably still changing your ways and adjusting to the many changes you've already made.

Maybe you're noticing that change is a recurring theme when you live a low-calorie lifestyle. Nothing stays the same anywhere, and certainly not in Dietville. You simply move from one stage of weight control to the next. When you get to a healthy weight, or when you decide that cutting calories to lose weight isn't working for you anymore, the next stage is weight maintenance. During this stage, your goal is to stay where you are and prevent weight gain.

Weight maintenance is actually easier than weight loss. First, you're more seasoned in the art of weight control than before you started losing. You've lost weight and you're already a success story! You can now relax some, eat a little more food if you want, put everything you've figured out into practice, and just keep a close eye on yourself. You know that you can lose weight by either reducing calories or exercising, but that a combination of the two is most effective. The same holds true for weight maintenance.

After you enter a weight-maintenance stage, you no longer need a deficit of calories because you're not trying to lose any more weight. On the other hand, you can't celebrate your weight-loss success with random, mindless eating. You still need a plan that includes a calorie-controlled diet and an ongoing exercise routine. In the following sections, I give you tips for adjusting your diet plan and exercise routine so that you can begin maintaining your weight with ease.

Using a formula for the future

To maintain your new weight, you need to figure on taking in at least 25 percent fewer calories than you were when you first started your low-calorie diet. For example, if you were consuming 2,800 calories a day before you started losing and you cut down to an average of, say, 1,400 calories to lose weight, you can raise your calorie limit to about 2,100 for weight mainte-nance. (The difference between 1,400 and 2,100 is 700, which is 25 percent of 2,800.) As it turns out, 700 isn't only 25 percent of 2,800; it's smack dab in the middle of where you started your diet and where you ended it! If you don't know how many calories you were consuming when you started, gradually increase your current calorie allowance by 100 or 200 a day. Evaluate your weight once each week to see if you've lost, gained, or maintained, and then adjust your calorie allowance if necessary.

Like all weight-related formulas and measures, this one is approximate. It can't take into account all your own personal factors that affect how you lose weight and how you gain it, such as your family history and your own personal history of weight loss and weight gain. (See Chapter 2 for more about these topics.) It also can't take into account any changes in your metabolism that may result from losing weight. This formula, like the body measurement and weight-loss formulas in Chapters 2 and 3, is the equivalent of an educated guess. You may have to work with it and adjust your calories up or down a little, in order to make it work perfectly for you.

Planning menus for weight maintenance

A 2,000-calorie menu is a good place for active people to start when developing a weight-maintenance plan. If you're a small-framed woman, or someone who isn't very active, you may need to cut this amount down to somewhere between 1,500 and 2,000 calories. If you're a man, or a very active woman, you may be able to add a couple of hundred calories. Use the following menu plans for at least a week to see how they work for you.

Just as you had to take a basic calorie-controlled menu (see Chapter 6) and adjust it to make it work for you while you were losing weight, you can use the 2,000-calorie weight-maintenance plans that follow as basic guides, and increase or reduce the amount of food slightly until you find your own balance.

As you start increasing the number of calories you consume each day, be sure to remember the following:

✔ You can approach weight maintenance in two ways.

- The first way is to slightly increase the portion sizes of some of the same foods you enjoyed while you were on a low-calorie weight-loss plan.

- Another way is to continue on a nutritionally balanced, lower-calorie plan so you can enjoy more of the favorite foods you may have cut back on or even eliminated while you were losing weight.

The approach you take depends on how confident you are in your ability to stick to reasonable portion sizes of *all* foods.

✔ Now that you're on a maintenance plan, you can relax. If you stick closely to the portion sizes you've discovered are acceptable, and you don't add too many snacks and desserts back into day-to-day meal plans, you can go out to eat at a restaurant or dinner party and enjoy your meal without worrying so much about how your food was prepared or how many calories it contains.

✔ Paying attention to the amount of food you eat, practicing more mindful eating behavior (see Chapter 4 for more about mindful eating), and keeping your goals in mind are all more important at this point than counting every single calorie. By the time you get to a weight-maintenance stage, you know how to eat. You know how important maintaining a positive attitude is and how to incorporate as much physical activity into your life as possible. Following a low-cal lifestyle after you've lost weight is all about putting everything you've discovered into practice on a regular basis.

✔ If you find that your maintenance diet isn't working and you're starting to gain weight, use a lower-calorie menu plan from Chapter 6 to get back on track again and figure out how many calories you can consume, on average, to stay at your maintenance weight.

Now that you're on a maintenance plan, you're eating the same way as anyone else who maintains his or her weight. The only difference between you and a nondieter is that you may still need to follow a strict plan until you're confident that you know exactly how much you can eat and stay at your current weight. You're no longer on a low-calorie diet, but you *are* on a calorie-controlled diet. In fact, anyone and everyone who maintains a healthy weight is on a calorie-controlled diet, whether they know it or not. If they weren't on calorie-controlled diets, they'd be gaining weight!

The following are four menu plans you can use as a guide to just how much food is allowed on a 2,000-calorie maintenance diet plan. Use the basic portion sizes of different foods as guides for substituting similar foods and creating your own menus.

Breakfast No. 1

8 ounces orange juice

1 cup bran flakes or ½ cup cooked oatmeal

1 tablespoon brown sugar

1 banana

1 cup skim milk

Lunch No. 1

Sandwich on 2 slices rye bread made with 3 ounces water-packed tuna and 1 tablespoon light mayonnaise

2 ounces cheese (any variety)

1 pear

Many of the reduced-calorie food products you used while you were on a low-calorie diet plan, such as light bread, reduced-calorie syrups, and light salad dressings, can still be helpful when you're trying to maintain weight at a slightly higher calorie level. For instance, the menus in this chapter use regular bread instead of the light bread you were eating while you were on a low-calorie diet. They also include regular cheese so you can use any variety you like. You now need to decide if you want to make that switch from reduced calorie foods to regular foods. On the other hand, I still base calculations for foods such as mayonnaise, yogurt, salad dressings, and milk, on reduced-calorie and low-fat varieties. As soon as you find your own balance of maintenance calories and exercise, you can decide which foods to hold over from your weight-loss plan.

Dinner No. 1

3-inch square of lasagna (any variety)

1 cup steamed broccoli

1½ cups spinach and orange salad with 1 tablespoon light dressing

2 thin (1-inch) slices Italian bread

2 teaspoons butter

Snacks/Dessert No. 1

½ cup fresh or juice-packed pineapple cubes

½ cup lowfat frozen yogurt or light ice cream

Breakfast No. 2

1 whole-grain or bran English muffin with 2 teaspoons butter and 2 tablespoons fruit spread or jam

2 lean breakfast sausages

1 cup skim milk

When dietitians design weight-loss menus, they often put a lot of milk in the plan to make sure you get enough calcium each day, along with other nutrients in milk that help your body use calcium efficiently. If you don't drink milk, substitute yogurt, cheese, other dairy products, or nondairy products that are fortified with calcium and other vitamins and minerals.

Lunch No. 2

1½ cups vegetarian bean chili topped with 1 ounce shredded cheese

1 small (2-inch) square cornbread

½ cup mango cubes

Dinner No. 2

½ egg roll (any variety)

2 cups beef stir-fry with vegetables

1 cup cooked brown rice

Snacks/Dessert No. 2

2 small almond cookies

1 orange

Breakfast No. 3

6 ounces orange juice

2 scrambled eggs

½ cup hash browns or home-fried potatoes

1 slice whole-grain toast with 1 teaspoon butter and 1 tablespoon fruit spread or jam

½ cup skim milk

Lunch No. 3

1½ cups minestrone soup

Turkey sandwich on 2 slices whole-wheat bread made with 3 ounces turkey and 1 tablespoon light mayonnaise

1 apple

Dinner No. 3

5 ounces broiled fresh tuna or salmon

Rice pilaf made with ½ cup cooked brown rice, 1 tablespoon chopped pistachio nuts, and 1 tablespoon golden raisins

1 cup steamed green beans

Snacks/Dessert No. 3

1 ounce cheese with 2 shredded wheat crackers

1 small (2-inch wide) slice angel food cake with ½ cup raspberries

Breakfast No. 4

¼ cantaloupe

3 small (4-inch) whole-grain pancakes with 2 tablespoons maple syrup and 2 teaspoons butter

½ cup blueberries

½ cup skim milk

Lunch No. 4

Egg salad sandwich on 2 slices whole-grain bread made with ½ cup egg salad and lettuce leaves

8 baby carrots

1 cup fresh lemonade

Dinner No. 4

4 ounces grilled chicken breast or lean boneless pork chop

1 small baked potato topped with ½ cup plain lowfat yogurt

1 cup steamed broccoli

1 tomato, sliced and drizzled with 1 tablespoon light salad dressing

1 small dinner roll with 1 teaspoon butter

Snacks/Dessert No. 4

1 cup mixed fruit salad topped with ¼ cup lowfat vanilla or lemon yogurt

1 frozen fruit bar

Revisiting your exercise routine

After you reach your goal weight or decide to stop losing weight for any reason, your new goal is to maintain a balance of calories and physical activity that can keep you at your current weight. While you were losing weight, you were trying to shift that balance so that you burned more calories than you consumed by eating fewer calories and exercising more. When you reach the maintenance stage, you'll probably want to add more calories to your diet, but you don't necessarily have to increase the amount of exercise you do. However, maintaining the level of physical activity that you reached while you were losing weight is still important.

One of the biggest threats to your exercise routine is boredom. Check out Chapter 8 for suggestions on ways to keep your exercise life interesting.

Age is no excuse for cutting back on physical activity. If you've been active throughout your life or you became more active in your attempt to lose weight, try to maintain the same activity level as you get older to help fight the normal slowing down of your metabolism. If you can't maintain the same level of activity, remember: Any activity is better than no activity at all.

Managing Your Weight for the Long Term

You stop losing weight when the amount of calories you consume routinely equals the number of calories your body uses for energy. At that point, you have to decide whether or not to update your low-calorie plan and continue to try to lose weight or to revise your plan completely and try to maintain your current weight. You don't want to gain back any of the weight you lost.

By losing weight, you've made an investment in your long-term health. The younger you are, the more advantage this decision will have for you *if* you maintain all or most of your weight loss. Typically, if dieters gain back the weight they've lost, they regain even more weight, and their excess weight is higher in fat in proportion to muscle than before they went on a diet. That's one reason why dieting doesn't work for so many people and why weight cycling (*yo-yo dieting*) can be dangerous. If your weight goes up and down and the "up" gets higher and higher with each attempt to lose, you're putting yourself at higher risk of developing weight-related medical problems.

A sure sign of weight-loss success is knowing exactly what works for you and continuing to do it until you reach your goal weight. When you reach a healthier weight, you can't just say, "Now I can stop dieting" and let your old eating habits sneak back in. The point was never to go on a short-term diet or make temporary changes. Instead, you've adopted a low-calorie lifestyle, which means you're committed to eating well and getting physical activity so that you can stay at a healthier weight for the rest of your life.

In the following sections, I tell you how to establish your weight-maintenance plan and explain the special challenges for folks in families with a history of weight problems.

Reviewing what's worked for you

I often hear dieters say, "that diet worked" or "this diet doesn't work." In fact, many weight-loss diets work if people stick to them. Sometimes diets aren't designed for long-term use, however, or they become so monotonous you can't possibly stick to them for more than a month or two.

Dieters who join commercial weight-loss programs are often repeat performers. They've been there before, and they're back again because they feel the program works for them if they just keep working the program. When you're a do-it-yourselfer, you have to create your own program. You have to find the plan, the people, and the activities that work for you and move on from anything (or anyone) that gets in the way of your success.

What works for one dieter may not necessarily work for another. Dieters try all sorts of tricks to lose weight, and they struggle even harder to keep it off. If you're a "career dieter" and you've been on and off different types of diets most of your life, then you're armed with the knowledge of what works and what doesn't work for you. Think back and make a list of all the tips, advice, and new behaviors that felt comfortable to you and contributed to any temporary success you achieved on any type of diet plan. Use that list to remind yourself what you need to do to stay at a healthier weight.

If you're undertaking your first weight-loss diet, then you're lucky. You're not looking back over a lifetime of failed diets and repeated patterns of weight loss followed by weight gain. You're not saddled with the same feelings of hopelessness and defeat that often get in the way of success for more seasoned dieters. You can simply look back over this diet plan, pick out everything that has worked for you, and discard what hasn't. Take the best that this low-calorie weight-loss plan has to offer and move forward with it.

Pushing ahead with new ideas

You may have noticed that the world is overflowing with weight-loss information. You turn on the television and see countless infomercials and sales pitches. You're bombarded with pop-up ads on the Internet. You listen to the radio and hear about every new miracle supplement to help you lose 50 pounds without picking your butt off the couch. You open your e-mail account and you're probably flooded with spam spouting the next best fad. Unfortunately, much of it is *mis*information. But if you can differentiate between advice that comes from a reliable source and advice that comes from someone who is simply trying to sell you a weight-loss plan or fitness product, you can stay well informed.

The following tips can point you toward reliable information:

- **Subscribe to a recognized health, fitness, or healthy cooking magazine.** Use the articles, recipes, and tips you find in these publications to reinforce your commitment to a low-calorie lifestyle.

- **Find helpful Web sites.** Search for sites that can help expand your knowledge of nutrition and weight control. Bookmark the best and visit them often.

✔ **Investigate new ways of eating.** Check out ethnic restaurants, eat vegetarian meals at least once a week, or take a healthy cooking class.

✔ **Check out new exercise classes and programs at your gym.** Do anything you can to keep your exercise life as interesting as your diet life so that you stay motivated to keep up with both.

Coming to terms with your genes

Your genes help determine not only your body shape and type, but also to a certain degree, your propensity to gain, lose, and maintain weight (see Chapter 2 for details). Until such time as scientists find realistic solutions, you really can't fight weight factors that are determined genetically. The power of genetic predisposition became clear in one interesting weight study, wherein adoptees had the same weight patterns as their biological parents, whether they were thin, heavy, or somewhere in between. At the same time, the researchers found no consistent or significant similarities between the weight patterns of adoptive parents and their adopted children.

If you come from a family with a history of being overweight or obesity, losing weight can be more difficult. There's no way around that. But even though losing weight may be more of a struggle for you than someone with a leaner heritage, getting to a healthier weight and staying there is possible. You just may have to work harder at maintaining your weight loss, or perhaps, work a bit harder at developing realistic expectations about your weight.

If you've been dieting most of your life and have never reached your goal weight, your goal weight may no longer be realistic. That's okay; all you have to do is set new goals! You can find help with that in Chapter 4. Just remember, getting real doesn't mean giving up. It just means taking a more rational approach to weight control.

Checking your maintenance plan periodically

When you made a decision to lose weight by living a low-calorie lifestyle, you decided to make permanent changes in your life. Weight maintenance requires an on-going commitment to that lifestyle. From here on in, weight control is all about reinforcing the principals about getting fit that you discovered while you were losing weight.

You'll maintain a healthier weight as long as you continue to live a low-calorie lifestyle that includes well-balanced meals, plenty of physical activity, and a "can-do" attitude. If you feel yourself starting to slip in any of these areas, check out Chapter 4 for tools to help you get back on track.

Recognizing Your Body's Changing Calorie and Nutritional Needs

As you move from a stage of weight loss to the next stage of weight maintenance, at times you may feel as though you've taken on a new identity. Depending on how long it took for you to arrive at this (hopefully) permanent plateau, you may in fact have moved from one stage of life to another. As you revise your diet and exercise plan to accommodate the "new you," you need to pay attention not only to your changing calorie needs but also to your changing nutritional needs. As an adult, you need the same nutrients you needed while you were growing up (for a review of those nutrients, go to Chapter 3), but as your body changes with age, you need some of them in different amounts. The following sections provide info on your body's needs at different ages and various stages of life.

Staying lean and healthy at any age

As you age, the rate at which you burn calories decreases. With every decade, you need 2 percent fewer calories, which isn't a huge decrease. If you maintained your weight at a calorie level of 2,000 when you were 22, you may need to cut that to 1,960 by the time you're 32, and to 1,920 by the time you're 42. In a perfect world, you maintain a healthy weight, stay active, and build up your muscles as you age so that you continue burning calories efficiently, and you don't have to make any huge dietary changes. Life, however, usually gets in the way of everyone's perfect world.

Weight control may be all about counting calories, but *healthful* weight control is all about getting the nutrients you need after you decide to live a low-calorie lifestyle. Getting enough nutrients is easy when you overeat because you're consuming so much food that you're bound to meet your daily requirement for most vitamins and minerals. In fact, instead of feeling guilty next time you sneak in a deluxe cheeseburger, remember that along with all that fat and all those calories, you're getting a good supply of protein, calcium, iron, and B vitamins. Unless you're overeating all the time, such a high-calorie indulgence may even be good for you on occasion.

Whenever your calorie count falls below 1,500, however, getting all the nutrients you need in the amounts you need is difficult. (For a review of necessary nutrients and good food sources, flip to Chapter 3.) It requires careful planning. When I developed the calorie-controlled menu plans in Chapter 6, I did the planning for you and tried to keep those menus as nutritionally balanced as possible within the calorie allowance given.

At different ages and stages of life, it helps to plan calorie-controlled menus, which include specific foods containing specific nutrients that are particularly beneficial during those periods in your life. The recommended calorie intakes for each age group are averages for healthy, moderately active people who aren't trying to lose weight. Depending on your age, height, current weight, and activity level, these figures can vary by several hundred calories.

- 11- to 18-year-olds need plenty of calcium from dairy products or calcium-fortified foods to build healthy bones for later in life because as you age, you stop building bone. The better your bone density at an early age, the less risk you have of developing *osteoporosis,* a disease where you suffer from bone loss, later in life. Girls also need more iron at this stage to offset the loss from menstruation. The average recommended calorie intake for girls in this group is 2,200 calories a day and 2,500 to 3,000 calories for boys.

- 18- to 25-year-olds may need a vitamin C boost from fresh fruits and veggies to move more safely through this experimental stage of life that often includes eating fast foods, smoking cigarettes, drinking alcohol, and getting too little sleep. The average recommended calorie intake for women in this group is 2,200 calories and 2,900 calories for men.

- 25- to 35-year-olds can start thinking about preventing disease as well as preventing weight gain. If you're a woman who plans to become pregnant, be sure to get enough of the B vitamin folic acid (also called *folate*) to prevent the risk of birth defects. Dark green leafy vegetables, legumes, and oranges are naturally high in folic acid. Breads, cereals, pastas, and other grain foods are all fortified with this vitamin. Men and women alike need to be familiar with *antioxidants* — the vitamins, minerals, and phytochemicals described in Chapter 3 that help prevent chronic diseases. The average recommended calorie intake for women in this group is 2,200 calories and 2,900 calories for men.

- 35- to 45-year-olds can start making lower-fat, higher-fiber foods that are rich in lean protein and B vitamins a priority. Soy products, beans, lentils, and other legumes are a great source of low-fat protein and B vitamins. Protein and the B vitamins niacin and riboflavin are essential for keeping your skin, nails, and hair in top condition. The B vitamin folic acid has been shown to protect brain functions, such as memory, in aging adults. The recommended calorie intake for women in this group is 2,200 calories and 2,900 calories for men.

- 45- to 55-year-olds can turn to seafood, soy products, nuts, and wheat germ to provide Omega-3 essential fatty acids that help protect your heart along with foods that are high in fiber and low in saturated fats. During this time, start increasing your calcium intake again to protect against bone loss, and consider introducing more soy foods into your diet. For women, soy foods can help stabilize hormones, and for men, protect against prostate cancer. After age 50, the recommended calorie intake for women in this group drops from 2,200 to 1,900 calories a day; the drop for men is from 2,900 to 2,300 calories.

✔ After you pass age 55, just keep on doing what you're doing (as long as what you're doing is healthful)! Continue to exercise to help offset the slowing down of your metabolism and keep your calories at healthy upper and lower limits. Several of the success stories in Chapter 17 are from people in their 50s and 60s, which just goes to show that it's never too late to start taking care of yourself. The recommended calorie intake for women in this group is 1,900 calories a day and 2,300 calories for men.

Working through normal stages of life

If you're a woman, you have one time in your life when a certain amount of weight gain isn't only inevitable, but it's also encouraged! That's, of course, during pregnancy. Whether you're a woman or a man, midlife is another time when hormonal shifts and a metabolism with a mind of its own can cause weight gain. In the following sections, I offer advice on how to keep both of these types of weight gain under control.

Having a baby

Even if you're overweight, pregnancy *isn't* the time to be on any type of weight-loss diet. Pregnant women need more calories and more nutrients than normal. Reducing calories and losing weight while you're pregnant can be dangerous for the growth and development of the fetus.

If you're overweight before you get pregnant, chances are you'll gain more weight than average during the pregnancy and retain more than a normal-weight woman after delivery. The best solution is to lose weight before you get pregnant. If that's impossible, your doctor may put you on a calorie-controlled diet to help prevent excess weight gain during your pregnancy.

Except under certain conditions, such as when a doctor finds evidence of heart disease, cervical or vaginal complications, or a history of miscarriages, low- to moderate-level exercise is usually encouraged during pregnancy. The type and amount of exercise you do while you're pregnant is a decision that has to be made with your doctor. (Check out *Pregnancy For Dummies,* 2nd Edition, by Joanne Stone, MD, Keith Eddleman, MD, and Mary Duenwald [Wiley] for more information about pregnancy-related issues.)

If you're breastfeeding, you can start eating normally again, but the especially good news is that your metabolism will naturally speed up during this process. If you're breastfeeding exclusively (not supplementing your baby's diet with formula), you may burn up to 600 calories a day. That's the equivalent of two aerobic workouts! So although reducing calories and increasing activity is considered safe for breastfeeding mothers, and normally doesn't affect lactation, you don't have to challenge yourself, because you'll be losing weight naturally. And there's more happy news: At least one study showed that your naturally speedy metabolism during this time helps the weight come off around your hips and butt! (Check out *Breastfeeding For Dummies* by Sharon Perkins, RN, and Carol Vannais, RN [Wiley] for more information about breastfeeding issues.)

Moving into midlife

Staying fit and maintaining a reasonably healthy body weight at an early age can help lower your risk of developing chronic, age-related medical conditions as you get older. (Check out Chapter 16 for an overview of the health problems associated with being overweight and obesity). Still, your body does age and change, and the normal changes associated with aging affect your weight the same way they affect almost every organ in your body.

Menopause and *perimenopause* (the approximately 10-year period of time that precedes actual menopause) are two periods in a woman's life when her hormones are fluctuating wildly and wreaking all types of havoc with her body. Hormonal bouncing can certainly be responsible for shifts in your weight. Even if you've maintained a healthy weight your whole life, you may find yourself starting to gain in your mid-forties to mid-fifties, signaling a time to take action. If you don't already have an exercise routine, develop one. Moving a little more at this point in your life is much easier than starting to eat a whole lot less. And probably healthier for you, too!

The concept of male menopause is controversial, and downright funny to some people, but the fact is that middle-aged men go through their own series of changes. Men who don't get enough exercise lose muscle and get flabby, and those who don't watch what they eat start to gain weight as their metabolism starts to slow down. Depression and mood swings aren't the sole property of menopausal women; men suffer through psychological crises as well and are just as likely to use food as an emotional bandage.

If you're a man or a woman, young or old, who feels excess weight starting to pile on or if you've been dieting for some time and you feel you can't lose any more weight, switch your focus from trying to lose to preventing gain. That still means cutting back on the amount of calories you were eating while you were gaining weight, but you don't have to follow the type of low-calorie diet needed to lose weight. Now you're at a place where your best calorie count falls somewhere between the two extremes. A weight-maintenance diet is your best solution.

Chapter 11

Helping Yourself with Outside Resources

In This Chapter

▶ Requesting help from others

▶ Joining a weight-loss program

▶ Checking out very low-calorie plans

▶ Finding a support meeting

▶ Opening up to the idea of counseling

*I*f you have trouble sticking to a low-calorie weight-loss plan on your own — and many people do — help is available. Maybe all you need is a "diet buddy," someone who holds you accountable and depends on you for his or her own weight-loss success. Maybe you just need to sit down with family and friends and let them know how they can best support you ("Mom, I really love your lasagna, but I can't eat two helpings, so please don't feel bad if I don't ask for more.")

If you don't have a support network of family and friends, if they don't seem to be there when you need them, or if the support of loved ones just isn't enough to keep you motivated and on track, you can turn to one of several different types of programs and groups for support. If you have overeating issues and you feel like no one understands, you may also need the help of a professional counselor.

You really can't know which type of program or counselor will best serve your needs until you compare a few, see what they have to offer, and perhaps even try out several different types of programs until you find the one that works for you. This chapter lays out your options to help you figure out which type of support you actually need.

Asking Other Folks for Help

How do you know when you need help losing weight and sticking to your weight-loss plan? You just know. You can feel your motivation slipping; you find yourself cheating more often on your diet; you start using any old excuse not to exercise.

Losing the weight is up to you. You can't pay someone to lose it for you. You can't swallow a little pill and make it magically disappear forever. You can't dream it away. However, some people know from experience to reach out for help the minute they decide to embark on a program. Maybe you can rely on help and support from your family and friends, especially with any big lifestyle change, such as losing weight. Maybe you need help from outside your circle of family and friends. This chapter is a good start to help you gather together a support group of people who will be with you every step of the way until you've adjusted to all the changes and can live a healthier lifestyle on your own.

When beginning a weight-loss plan, you may just need someone to pay attention to what you're doing, to understand that it can be difficult at times, and to pat yourself on the back when you're doing well. You may need to be in the company of others who are struggling with weight issues or, if the roots of your overeating run deep, you may want to consider private counseling (see "Considering Counseling," later in this chapter). You may need different types of help at different stages of weight loss. Surveys show that people who are successful at losing weight and keeping the weight off are the people who have the most support. Get it wherever you can!

In the following sections, I discuss the pros and cons of involving your loved ones in your weight-loss plans and tell you how to find diet buddies, role models, and even a professional counselor, if you need one.

Talking to friends and family

When you look to others for help and support, your first instinct may be to turn to family members or friends. They know you well, and you know you can trust them. Let your friends and family know what your plans and goals are, and tell them specifically how they can help. No matter how you feel, make your feelings known to the people who are closest to you. They may not know how to help you unless you tell them.

Sometimes, however, the people you count on the most may let you down, especially if they don't understand what you're going through. If losing weight means avoiding Sunday supper at your mother-in-law's house, family members may feel hurt. If losing weight makes you more attractive to other men or women, your mate may surprise you by being less supportive than you expected. And if losing weight means you're going to outshine your best friend, you may not get what you need from her, either. The people who love you love you just the way you are. They may not want you to change. If that's the case, you can't worry about what everyone else wants; you have to be strong enough to take care of yourself.

If ever there was a time to be selfish, this is it. Now is the time to say "No, thanks" to second helpings, no matter who's offering them. You can use the following tips to help you and your friends and family adapt to your new lifestyle:

- ✔ **Set boundaries.** You may have to say no when your partner wants to go out to eat. Explain that it's only for now; after you feel in control of your eating habits, you can eat out all you want. You may or may not want people to comment on your weight as you go along, so let them know. Now is a time to assert yourself; you have to take control without worrying about pleasing everyone else. If you can work up the enormous amount of strength and determination it takes to stick to a low-calorie diet, then you can work up the strength to stand up to anyone who tries to get in your way.

- ✔ **Clearly explain your needs.** Like it or not, you'll probably have some explaining to do when your diet interferes with other people's needs. Help your family and friends understand that this diet is something you have to do right now. Let them know that you're not trying to be antisocial or rude. Tell your loved ones that you don't want it to be just another diet; you're trying to make huge, permanent lifestyle changes. This change is going to take a lot of work, and you need positive reinforcement along the way. Don't apologize for what you're doing, but explain that you won't always have to say "no" to everything that's fun, but for now, you need their understanding.

- ✔ **Be patient and understanding as well.** Your friends and family may not know how to be supportive, and if that's the case, you have to show them. You have to tell them the types of advice and reminders you want to hear and *don't* want to hear. They probably don't realize that they could be hurting your chances of success by keeping food around the house that you find hard to resist or by putting pressure on you to participate in social events that may sabotage your diet.

- ✔ **Thank them for their support.** Let the people you care about know how much you appreciate their attention and support. Don't forget to say thank you.

Reaching out to find diet buddies and role models

When your family and friends can't provide the support you need, you probably need to reach outside your inner circle for help and encouragement. Doing so may just mean looking around the office for someone who may make a good diet buddy or posting a note on a community bulletin board at your church, gym, or school.

Reaching out also means trying to find a role model — someone who has lost a significant amount of weight and kept it off, or someone who never diets but manages to stay in shape. If you know someone like that, try to find out his or her secret! Having the advice of someone who knows what you're going through and who can offer helpful, unbiased advice never hurt anyone.

Wherever you turn for support, look for people who are living happy, healthy lives. Look for people with positive, hopeful attitudes about themselves, their bodies, and their future success. These types of people are your best role models and your best motivators. Model your own behavior after these people. Don't be afraid of their success — or your own!

Sorting through Commercial Weight-Loss Plans

Frustrated dieters founded some of today's most well known commercial weight-loss programs — Weight Watchers, Jenny Craig, and Diet Center. These programs started small and grew into huge businesses that now incorporate their own lines of food products, motivational tools, instructional materials, and Web-based programs. In addition to the biggies, you can find weight-loss programs in YWCAs and YMCAs, community centers, hospitals, and university medical centers. Any of these programs can help you start and stick to a lower-calorie diet and monitor you as you start to lose weight. The secret to success is to stick with the program if it's working for you. Read on in the following sections to find the criteria you can use to evaluate a weight-loss program and decide if it's right for you.

If you plan to lose more than 20 pounds, have any health problems, or take any type of medication on a regular basis, see your doctor for a physical checkup before enrolling in a weight-loss program. Be sure your doctor knows about your weight-loss plans. If you're pregnant, have certain medical conditions, take certain medications, or have a history of eating disorders, you may not be accepted into a commercial weight-loss program without your physician's written consent. Otherwise, most programs accept anyone who has 10 pounds or more to lose.

Figuring out whether a commercial program can help you

Every decade or so, government and consumer groups "crack down" on the diet industry, investigating claims made by weight-loss programs and product manufacturers, and often charging these companies with misleading dieters about the safety, effectiveness, and long-term cost of their programs. The diet industry as a whole has been criticized for not living up to its promises of success for most people, and in most cases, the criticism is warranted.

Evidence shows that no commercial weight-loss program statistically has a very high success rate with respect to long-term weight control. Clients lose weight, but they don't keep it off. That evidence doesn't mean these programs can't help you; they can. Weight-loss programs provide structure, personal attention, and valuable tools to help you stay on track when you're following a low-calorie diet. The better-known programs all have an educational component to help you discover how to eat a nutritionally balanced, lower-calorie diet and develop better eating habits. And the best programs all recommend exercise as part of an overall weight-loss and fitness regime.

So how do you know when you need to turn to a commercial weight-loss program? That's a pretty simple question to answer! If you find that your self-help program isn't working for you or you start to feel that you won't reach your goals on your own, turn to an outside program for guidance, structure, and support. When you choose a good program, that program will complement the low-calorie lifestyle advocated in this book.

You can help ensure your own success by taking on most of the responsibility for your own weight control, rather than turning that responsibility over to any outside plan or program. In other words, use the program and apply any helpful tools they provide to your own low-calorie plan, but don't expect the program to work for you unless you're doing most of the work! At some point, you'll have to become accountable to yourself and no one else. At the same time that you're depending on the advice and expertise of others, you're discovering how to trust yourself to control your own weight in the future.

Asking the right questions

A perfectly good weight-loss program may not be perfect for you. Check around. Before you join any program, ask these questions about each program you check and be sure you feel satisfied with the answers:

- ✔ **How long has the program existed?** Go with the tried and true.

- ✔ **What types of professionals provide services to members? Do doctors, dietitians, nurses, and certified counselors participate in the program?** Unless you participate in a medically supervised weight-loss program (check out "Getting the Scoop on Medically Supervised Programs," later in this chapter), and depending on your individual medical and psychological needs, you may need to seek additional help from professionals such as medical doctors, psychologists, and registered dietitians outside the weight-loss program you choose.

- ✔ **What is the total cost of the program, including special food, supplements, or other products?** Be sure to get the complete cost of participating in the program upfront so you can decide whether or not it's affordable for you. A good program doesn't have to be expensive, and the cost of any individual program isn't an indicator of whether or not it will work for you. You must be able to stick with the program, however, so total cost is one important factor when choosing from among different programs.

- ✔ **How often will you check in or attend educational meetings?** A good commercial program has weekly counseling sessions or group meetings.

- ✔ **How is your weight loss monitored? Is there a weekly weigh-in?** A weight-loss program must include a weekly weigh-in.

- ✔ **Will you get help setting positive lifestyle goals in addition to setting food and weight goals?** Be sure the program includes behavioral counseling (group or individual) to help you break the bad habits that have contributed to your weight gain.

- ✔ **Does the program incorporate or strongly recommend physical activity as a means to weight loss and weight control?** A sound program always includes or recommends some type of exercise program to complement your diet. Avoid any commercial weight-loss plan that focuses on diet alone.

- ✔ **Does the program address the needs of your age group?** A good weight-loss plan takes your age into consideration when making diet adjustments and recommending exercise programs.

- ✔ **If you have a physical or medical condition that requires special attention, does the group address your particular needs?** If you have a chronic medical condition or any dietary restrictions, be sure a physician or dietitian is involved in the program who is qualified to address your particular needs. If the program doesn't have any professionals involved, be aware that you'll have to go outside the program for medical approval of your plan.

✓ **Does the program include a weight-maintenance plan? What are the specifics of this plan?** Every good weight-loss program includes a follow-up plan for members to follow after they reach their goal weight. Don't join any program that ends when you reach your goals.

Picking a suitable plan

Just because someone you know raves about the diet center she goes to doesn't mean it's the right place for you. When picking a diet center, you can start with a recommendation, but you really have to do your own research to find a program that suits your individual needs. Before you make your final decision, check to ensure that the weight-loss plan in question absolutely includes the following if you're to consider it at all:

✓ **The program's diet plan must be safe and sound.** Avoid any plan that recommends fewer than 1,000 to 1,200 calories. At lower calorie levels, getting the nutrients you need from your food is difficult.

✓ **The program's diet plan must ultimately include a wide variety of foods.** If the program requires you to use their own food products in your diet plan, the program needs to have a plan in place to help you return to "normal" eating so you can move on to regular foods that are readily available in the supermarket.

✓ **The program needs to encourage slow, steady weight loss.** You want to lose a pound or two each week.

✓ **The program needs to be goal-oriented.** Avoid any plan that doesn't encourage you to set goals and provide strategies for meeting them.

✓ **The program includes exercise recommendations and behavioral counseling.** In addition to a nutritionally balanced diet plan, exercise recommendations and behavioral counseling are important facets of the program to help you develop better eating habits.

✓ **The program includes a weight-maintenance plan.** Because weight maintenance is much more difficult than weight loss, you don't want to be part of any program that sets you free after you've achieved your goal weight. (See Chapter 10 for more about weight maintenance.)

Just like the health club or gym you decide to join, any diet program that's going to help you succeed at losing weight has to fit your personal lifestyle because it's going to be an important part of your lifestyle for some time to come. Whatever type of program you decide to follow has to be conveniently located, open during hours when you're free to attend, recommend the type of food you're willing to eat, and be generally user-friendly if it's to serve you well in the long run. Before you sign up with any weight-loss program, be sure you're completely comfortable with the cost and methods used and that you also feel satisfied that everyone involved in the program is qualified to do the job they do.

Getting the Scoop on Medically Supervised Programs

You can get help losing weight from a physician in an individual or group medical practice that specializes in weight loss. Physicians who are board-certified in bariatric medicine specialize in obesity, as do endocrinologists and some family doctors. Many physicians also work with registered dietitians to develop individualized diet plans. If you have a chronic medical condition such as diabetes or heart disease, or if you take medication on a regular basis, a medical doctor and/or registered dietitian may be a better choice for you than a commercial weight-loss program.

Medically supervised weight-loss programs that administer very low-calorie diet plans are sometimes appropriate for people who are more than 50 pounds overweight or have a Body Mass Index (BMI) of 30 or more (see Chapter 2 for more about BMI). Medical doctors along with the services of other healthcare professionals, such as nurses and dietitians, supervise these plans.

For very good reason, health professionals monitor very low-calorie diets: The diets are potentially dangerous to your health. Don't ever go on any type of very low-calorie diet or modified fast unless you're under the care of a physician who has given you a preliminary medical exam. While you're following a medically supervised weight-loss plan, you'll be subjected to frequent blood tests, electrocardiograms, and weigh-ins to be sure that you're losing weight at an appropriate rate and that your body can handle the stress of this program.

In the following sections, I explain the basics of medically supervised very low-calorie programs.

Going lower than low

Medically supervised weight-loss programs that administer very low-calorie diets are actually medically supervised fasts. If you join one of these programs, your daily diet will consist of mostly or only a liquid formula that provides 800 calories or less. The average weight loss on this type of modified fast is about 3 to 5 pounds a week, or about 40 pounds in a three-month period, which is the recommended length of time most people spend on this type of diet.

Being on a very low-cal diet does have its benefits, beyond fast weight loss. You're under the constant care of a physician and other healthcare workers. You'll have no food decisions to make because you won't be eating much food, and what you do consume is preformulated. A modified fast can help you break bad eating habits and feel more motivated to continue on a regular weight-loss diet. For some people with urgent medical issues related to their weight, a modified fast is the only way to achieve the type of dramatic weight loss necessary to improve their health.

Any good medically supervised program, like any good weight-loss plan, includes a follow-up maintenance program and will eventually reintroduce you to normal eating.

Exploring your options

You find medically supervised weight-loss programs in hospitals, clinics, medical centers, and sometimes through private physicians. Your primary care physician can probably give you a recommendation for a program. All medically supervised programs are similar in nature, but each plan has its own food products and guidelines. If you're investigating a very low-calorie diet, you'll probably be introduced to one of the following programs:

- ✔ Health Management Resources offers the choice of a very low-calorie diet plan (520 to 800 calories) or a moderately low-calorie diet plan (up to 1,200 calories). HMR plans include liquid meal replacement formulas, prepackaged entrees, soups, and nutrition bars.

   To find out more about what this program offers, check out www. hmrprogram.com for a list of medical centers across the United States that administer HMR weight-loss programs. Or call the customer relations department at 800-418-1367, Monday through Friday from 9 a.m. to 5 p.m.

- ✔ Optifast offers two very low-calorie plans (800 and 950 calories) and a moderately low-calorie plan (1,200 calories). Like all medically supervised programs, Optifast includes liquid meal-replacement formulas plus prepackaged soups and nutrition bars. Weekly education sessions are mandatory. Dieters study new behavior strategies and diet habits while using Optifast products to lose weight, before they're reintroduced to real food.

   Although Optifast products are available to purchase online, anyone who wants to supervise an Optifast program for overweight clients must be a licensed physician. For more information and to find an Optifast provider near you, go to www.optifast.com.

Health Management Resources and Optifast are the big names in medically supervised weight-loss diets, but they aren't the only weight-loss products and programs affiliated with hospitals, medical centers, and physicians who specialize in weight control. Your hospital group or private physician may administer a similar program using products from a different company.

Beware of similar programs and products that are available without medical supervision. Don't ever put yourself on any diet that provides fewer than 800 calories a day. Even 800 calories is too low for most people for more than a day or two, because your body can't get all the nutrients it needs at that calorie level.

Seeking Out Support Groups

Sometimes you just need a friend. After your weight-loss plan is in place, all you have to do is follow it, but doing so is often easier said than done. If you're a compulsive overeater or you have a great deal of weight to lose and you don't have a good support network at home or at work, you may benefit from joining a chapter of a national support group.

All support groups are fundamentally similar, but they each have their own specific set of rules and expectations of their members. Some support groups are more spiritually centered, some are more regimented, and some are more narrowly focused to specific populations than others. You have to shop around to find a group you're comfortable with because even within the same organization, each local chapter group has its own group dynamic.

The two main ones are Overeaters Anonymous (OA) or Taking Off Pounds Sensibly (TOPS). These two nonprofit support groups provide motivation and friendship to anyone who struggles with weight control. Even if you do have a supportive bunch of friends and family (see "Asking Other Folks for Help," earlier in this chapter), you may still need the motivation of others who've "been there."

You can find OA and TOPS support groups all over the country, in almost every city and town, holding meetings in free spaces such as church basements and community centers. They don't endorse or promote any specific weight-loss plan or program. They exist to provide safe places where overweight people can feel free to discuss their ideas and feelings, and seek the help and encouragement of others who fight the same food battles. I discuss these groups and others in the following sections.

Overeaters Anonymous (OA)

OA is a 12-step recovery program for compulsive overeaters that is similar to Alcoholics Anonymous and Narcotics Anonymous. Anyone who is seeking freedom from obsessive overeating is welcome at meetings. The group's foundation is abstinence from overeating, taking it one day at a time, and recovery on physical, emotional, and spiritual levels. Members pay no dues or fees, but usually make voluntary contributions at meetings to help cover expenses.

To find an OA meeting in the United States, Canada, or one of more than 50 countries around the world, start with the OA Web site at www. overeatersanonymous.org. To contact Overeaters Anonymous, call 505-891-2664.

Taking Off Pounds Sensibly (TOPS)

TOPS members provide each other with emotional support, and the organization contributes money for obesity research. Members attend weekly meetings where they weigh in and then attend a group program designed to help them reach their weight-loss goals. The group programs may include handouts, recipes, contests, sharing of personal stories, and lectures by local healthcare professionals.

For more information about TOPS, check out its Web site at www.tops.org. To find a TOPS chapter near you, call 800-932-8677.

Other groups

Although OA and TOPS don't promote any specific types of weight-loss diets, other support groups, such as Compulsive Eaters Anonymous (www.ceahow. org) and Food Addicts Anonymous (www.foodaddictsanonymous.org), do incorporate a strict food plan, known as an abstinence diet, into their programs.

When you join CEA or FAA, you agree to follow a diet that is free of sugar, white flour, and any products made with refined carbohydrates. Although this type of plan is more about abstinence than about losing weight, losing weight and staying healthy is possible by incorporating the rules of abstinence into a well-planned low-calorie diet.

Working the Web for help with losing weight

Many legitimate and well-run support groups have found a home on the Internet. The best sites are affiliated with professional health or weight-loss organizations or include advice from professionals who are affiliated with such organizations. Peer-led groups are sometimes less reliable with respect to accurate weight-loss information, but they can still provide the friendship, support, and advice. Web-based support groups are great if you can't make it to regular meetings, can't find a group meeting in your area, or just want additional access to people with similar issues. Through the message boards and chatrooms you'll find on these sites, you may even find other people who have similar experiences with whom you can start a small support group of your own.

Many helpful Web sites don't include live chats or message boards but do offer helpful, reliable advice for calorie counters, fitness buffs, and anyone concerned with weight control. The best weight-management Web sites include the following:

✔ America on the Move (www.americaon themove.org)

✔ American Council on Exercise (ACE) (www. acefitness.org)

✔ The American Dietetic Association (www. eatright.org)

✔ American Heart Association Fitness Center (www.justmove.org)

✔ The Calorie Control Council (www.calorie control.org)

✔ The National Women's Health Information Center (www.4woman.gov/bodyimage/ index.cfm)

✔ Overcoming Overeating (www.overcoming overeating.com)

✔ The Partnership for Healthy Weight Management (www.consumer.gov/ weightloss)

✔ Shape Up America (www.shapeup.org)

✔ Something Fishy (www.something-fishy. org)

✔ Weight Control Information Network at the National Institutes of Health (http:// win.niddk.nih.gov)

Considering Counseling

If your overeating feels out of control, if you're more than just a little bit overweight and you know that your overeating is tied to emotional issues, if you suffer from a poor or distorted body image, or if all the self-help strategies you've employed just aren't working for you and you don't know why, you may want to consider professional counseling. Depending on your particular problems with food and weight control, you can get that type of counseling from a registered dietitian or state-certified nutritionist, or a certified social worker or psychologist who specializes in eating issues.

These types of professionals offer one-on-one counseling and sometimes work with groups of dieters with related issues who may benefit from each other's experiences and help each other work out the issues that are preventing them from losing weight and keeping the weight off. To figure out whether you would benefit from counseling, which type of counseling would be best for you, and how to find a counselor, read on.

Selecting the best type of counseling for your needs

If you eat to satisfy physical hunger and you overindulge for the fun of it and that's why you've gained weight, all you probably need to get back in shape is a good low-cal diet and exercise plan, along with the advice of a counselor or dietitian and the support of family and friends.

Eating to satisfy emotional hunger is a different story altogether. You may need the help of a mental health professional such as a certified social worker or psychologist who specializes in emotional overeating.

Understanding nutritional therapy

A registered dietitian or state-certified nutritionist can instruct you about eating well and managing your weight. Unlike a psychologist, who concentrates on the underlying reasons for your eating behavior, a dietitian can focus on your diet and eating behavior in the here and now. Unless a dietitian also has a degree in social work or psychology, however, she can't go out of her scope of practice to delve too deeply into the why and how of your eating problems. Likewise, a dietitian can outline exercise programs and explain the role of exercise in a low-calorie lifestyle, but only a qualified trainer or physical therapist can help you develop a safe and productive exercise routine.

Getting psychological counseling

Different types of psychological counseling and different types of people who are qualified to do it are available. The type of therapist who deals with eating behavior is usually a certified social worker or psychologist trained in cognitive-behavioral therapy (CBT). A CBT professional incorporates aspects of

- ✔ **Cognitive therapy,** which helps you to see that your own thinking is getting in the way of your weight-loss success because you're giving yourself a distorted picture of your own life and your ability to take control of your eating and exercise habits
- ✔ **Behavioral therapy,** which can help you change the fact that you react to emotional situations by eating or overeating by substituting other behaviors

By integrating the two disciplines, a CBT professional can help you work through and change the negative thinking patterns, feelings, and behaviors that interfere with your ability to have a normal relationship with food.

All good professionals stay within their scope of practice, giving advice only in their area of expertise. A psychologist or social worker can help you with the behavioral and psychological aspects of weight control, while a registered dietitian can help you with a sound food plan, and a certified trainer or physical therapist can help you with your exercise plan.

Finding a therapist

A referral from a friend or family member is usually a good way to find a therapist, but if no one in your immediate circle has successfully worked with a psychologist, social worker, or dietitian, then the next best place to start is with your primary care physician. If your family doctor is someone you like and respect (and if he or she isn't, maybe you need to find a new doctor), then chances are you'll feel the same way about other healthcare professionals he or she recommends. Hospitals also refer healthcare professionals who are affiliated with them.

If these options don't work for you, try contacting the following groups:

- **American Dietetic Association**

  120 South Riverside Plaza, Suite 2000

  Chicago, IL 60606

  800-877-1600

  To find a registered dietitian in your area, go the ADA Web site at www.eatright.org. Enter your zip code in the box on the left side of the page that says "Find a nutrition professional."

- **American Psychological Association (APA)**

  750 First St. NE

  Washington, DC 20002

  800-964-2000

  The operator will ask for your zip code and use it to connect you to the local referral service. You can also refer to the state association listings at www.apa.org/practice/refer.html.

- **National Association of Social Workers**

  750 First St. NE, Suite 700

  Washington, DC 20002

  www.socialworkers.org

  Click on the box in the left-hand column that says "Find a social worker." Fill in your zip code to search.

Deciding to face your fears

One of the biggest barriers to losing weight is fear. It can be paralyzing. You can't move forward when you're afraid to find out what lies ahead. Some food and fitness fears are common:

- Fearing that you'll be hungry on a low-cal diet
- Fearing that you'll never be able to eat your favorite foods again
- Fearing that any food that contains fat will make you fat
- Fearing that you won't be able to stick to an exercise program after you sign up

You probably don't need intense psychological counseling to deal with these types of fears. You can probably alleviate these fears with the help of a good weight-loss counselor or fitness trainer, or even someone who has been successful at losing weight and keeping it off by watching calories and working out.

But you may have more deeply rooted fears about dealing with overeating and you'll recognize them because they probably affect other areas of your life. If the following fears are interfering with your ability to take care of yourself, you may want to consider psychological counseling to deal with them effectively.

- **Fear of failure.** This fear means that you have thoughts, such as "What if I go through all the trouble of rearranging my life to accommodate a diet and exercise program, and then I give up?", "What if I reach my goal weight but can't keep the weight off?", or "What will other people think if I fail?" Remember that people who are successful at losing weight, or anything else for that matter, have often failed several times before they reached their goals. Those people who keep going gather valuable lessons from their failures and eventually earn success.

- **Fear of your own success.** This fear often means you're getting in your own way with thoughts that include something like, "What if I lose weight and nothing else changes?", "What if I lose weight and people think I'm a different person?", "What if I reach my goals and I don't like the way I look?", or "How will this weight-loss plan change my life, and can I handle it?" If you've been overweight most of your life, your weight is now a familiar part of you and, in some ways, you're comfortable with it. You can't know how you're going to feel when you lose your excess weight, and that can be scary.

- **Fear of change.** If you have long-standing routines in your life — what time you get up, what time you leave work, when and how you eat, what you do before you go to bed — making changes may not be easy.

Remember: What you've been doing about your weight and your fitness level up to this point hasn't been working for you, so you're going to have to make both physical and psychological changes in order to develop a healthier lifestyle.

✔ **Fear of the hidden emotions that trigger your overeating.** You may have an emotional appetite; that is, you eat in response to your emotional state. Anger, frustration, boredom, loneliness, and even happiness are all emotions that can trigger your overeating. Review Chapter 9 for more insight into your emotional appetite.

Part IV
Trying Time-Tested Low-Calorie Recipes

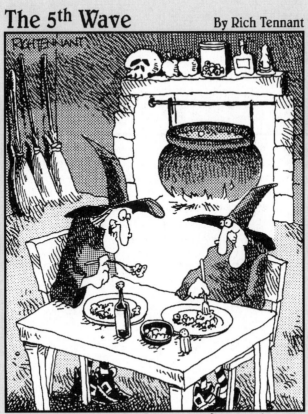

The 5th Wave   By Rich Tennant

"I substitute tofu for eye of newt in all my recipes now. It has half the calories and doesn't wriggle around the cauldron."

In this part . . .

The best way to control the ingredients in your food and become familiar with the amount of calories your food provides is to prepare most of your meals yourself. I realize that making all your meals may not always be possible, but when it is, you want to have tasty, reliable, easy-to-follow recipes on hand. Well, here they are!

You don't need chef training to prepare any of these recipes. Even if you can barely boil your own water, you can find this collection of low-calorie recipes to be as simple as home-cooked food can be. In every category — breakfast, lunch, dinner, snacks, and dessert — you can uncover "made from scratch" recipes that feature plenty of fresh foods but that also make use of some of the most nutritious convenience foods available in the supermarket. And to make everything even easier, you don't have to give a thought to low-calorie "go withs" because I include side dish serving suggestions with recipes that weigh in at less than 300 calories. Bon appetit!

Chapter 12

Benefiting from Breakfast

In This Chapter

▶ Starting the day on a nutritious note

▶ Shaking up your morning meal

▶ Having a berry good day

▶ Waking up to whole grains

▶ Scrambling to get going

*H*ow often have you heard that breakfast is the most important meal of the day? It's true! Your first meal kick-starts your metabolism and provides the initial energy you need for physical and mental activity. When it comes to weight loss, there are more good reasons to eat breakfast than there are to skip it, and this chapter outlines those reasons for you. You can find a variety of recipes here that you can substitute for the suggested breakfasts on the meal plans in Chapter 6.

This chapter contains plenty of tips for eating breakfast on the go, making healthier food choices for breakfast, and preventing breakfast boredom. You can also find ideas that may appeal to you even if you normally skip your morning meal.

Getting Off to a Good Start

Your first diet decisions of the day start with breakfast — when, where, why, and how to have it, along with what to eat. Whether you eat breakfast at 6 a.m. or noon, what follows are some compelling reasons to start the active part of your day with a well-balanced meal, and several ways to make breakfast easier and more appealing, whether you eat it at home, on the job, or, once in a while, on the run.

Recognizing great reasons to eat breakfast

By definition, breakfast is the first meal of the day after a night of fasting. So even though some people "skip" breakfast, everyone actually eats breakfast at some point. Some just eat their first meal a little later in the day! You may not feel hungry when you first wake up in the morning, or you may be afraid that after you start eating, you don't stop, so you put it off as long as possible. Perhaps your day starts later than most people's. These reasons can all be legitimate for delaying breakfast, but for some people, they can also be habits that contribute to weight gain, especially if skipping an early morning breakfast leads to overeating at the end of the day.

Although several medical studies have shown that people who skip breakfast are more likely to consume more calories later in the day, more calories overall, eventually gain weight, and become obese than people who regularly enjoy a morning meal, a small group of people in these studies are successful at losing weight even though they don't eat breakfast. If that is true for you, then it doesn't really matter if you eat breakfast first thing each day. But if you're like most people, routinely eating a balanced breakfast is essential to losing weight and maintaining weight loss.

If you normally don't eat when you first get up, you can try it while you're on this plan and see if eating breakfast stops you from overeating at other meals and also helps you cut back on the overall number of calories you consume each day. And if you normally do eat breakfast, don't stop now. If the act of eating breakfast is contributing to your weight problem, it's because of the amount of food you're eating in the morning. On a low-calorie diet, you eat less, which should help with your weight loss. Losing weight is always about making changes, so either way, you're making some sort of adjustment to your usual breakfast routine that may help you stick to your low-calorie diet.

Sticking to a routine, making healthier breakfast food choices, limiting your breakfast to 300 or 350 calories, and making sure you sit down and eat breakfast before you get too hungry (so that you don't overeat), are all more important to weight control than the time of day you eat your first meal.

When you're down to 1,000 or even 1,500 calories a day, it helps to cut calorie corners wherever you can so that you can fit more food into your diet. Sometimes you may need to cut portion sizes, but other times you can also replace higher calorie foods with lower calorie foods. Table 12-1 has some small, relatively easy breakfast food substitutions that can add up to big calorie savings in the long run if they become permanent new eating habits.

Table 12-1	Calorie-Saving Substitutions	
Replace	*With*	*To Save (calories)*
2 eggs	1 whole egg + 2 egg whites	34
¼ cup half-and-half	¼ cup whole milk	41
1 tablespoon butter	1 tablespoon fruit spread	72
1 tablespoon cream cheese	1 tablespoon light cream cheese	15
1 tablespoon cream cheese	1 tablespoon fat-free cream cheese	25
8 ounces orange juice	1 medium-size orange	40
1 slice regular bread for toast	1 slice light bread	40

If you're not hungry when you wake up in the morning, perhaps you ate late the evening before. The question is: Where does the cycle start? Do you overeat at night because you didn't eat much or at all during the first half of the day, or do you skip meals earlier in the day because you ate so much the night before? If late-night overeating seems to be affecting your weight, the solution may be to start the day with some sort of breakfast and eat a reasonable amount of food at least every three or four hours throughout the day so that you're not famished by late afternoon or early evening. Some people think they're saving calories by not eating in the morning, but that's usually not true. What usually happens is that your body misses those calories and starts screaming for them as the day wears on. Many people who intentionally avoid eating in the early part of the day end up bingeing at night.

Even if skipping breakfast doesn't contribute to your weight problems, the following are several good reasons to eat a balanced meal early in the day:

- ✔ Your first meal of the day wakes up your metabolism and sets your calorie-burning gears in motion for the rest of the day. It makes sense to get your metabolism fired up as soon as possible after you wake up.

- ✔ Breakfast boosts your blood sugar after a night of not eating, providing the energy you need to start your day.

- ✔ Eating a balanced breakfast helps you stay energized and focused throughout the morning.

- ✔ Breakfast is an opportunity to get a lot of the protein, carbohydrate, fiber, vitamin C, calcium, and other vitamins and minerals you need each day to stay healthy and energetic. Skipping this meal may mean you're cutting off a rich source of essential nutrients. (See Chapter 3 for more about the nutrients you need in a low-calorie diet.)

✔ Health experts say that people who eat breakfast have lower cholesterol levels, on average, than people who don't. Over time, eating breakfast can help reduce your risk of developing heart disease.

Keeping your morning meals interesting

Do you avoid eating a balanced, nutritious breakfast because you feel like you're always eating the same foods? How many different ways can you eat bland old bran cereal, right? Whoa! Your morning meal doesn't have to bore you back to sleep.

As with any meal, breakfast can consist of any food you like, as long as you stick to your calorie limit and, ideally, make mostly healthful food choices. You even can mix-and-match your meals. For instance, if you want to eat last night's spaghetti and meatballs again for breakfast today, or a bowl of chicken soup, or even a reheated slice of pizza, go for it! This idea is especially good if you're pressed for time and want to pop something ready-made into the microwave oven for an ultraquick meal. Just remember to stick to your calorie limits and strive for nutritional balance when you're borrowing foods from other meals. Not everyone can eat dinner foods for breakfast, but almost everyone can eat breakfast foods at any meal. Keep that point in mind when you're tweaking your menu plans or can't think of anything you feel like having for dinner.

On days when you want something that resembles an ordinary breakfast, however, you can find that most of the recipes later in this chapter are quick to fix or that you can completely or partially prepare them in advance. You can find plenty of ways to keep your low-calorie breakfasts interesting without spending a lot of early-morning time fiddling around in the kitchen.

Eating on the run

For a low-cal dieter, gobbling down a quick breakfast as you walk out the door may mean consuming the most dangerous calories of all — the forgotten ones! If you're keeping a food diary or any type of record of the calories you consume each day, you may never account for the breakfast you eat on the run. (See Chapter 4 for details on food diaries.) Bringing your breakfast to work with you, where you can sit down and eat it in a more mindful fashion, is another story, however, because you're more likely to keep track of your calories when you're paying attention to what you're eating.

If you find that you often have to pick up and leave home without having breakfast, keep a selection of your favorite packaged foods on hand so you can pack a quick, low-cal breakfast-to-go without a moment's thought. Choose foods that don't require any further preparation or special packing beyond maybe a plastic sandwich bag. Almost any food that comes packaged in individual servings is a good idea. You want to be able to grab and go.

The following list includes some ideas for breakfast foods that are easy to carry and easy to eat after you get where you're going. These are healthy choices that can tide you over until you have time to sit down to a full breakfast. In the portion sizes given, you can easily incorporate these foods into the breakfast and morning snack on your low-calorie diet plan. Pick a few that make sense for you to keep on hand, not only for breakfast but also for light, quick snacks any time of day.

- ✔ One piece of fresh fruit such as apples, oranges, grapes, nectarines, plums, and pears

- ✔ Up to ¼ cup dried fruit

- ✔ ¾ to 1 ounce of string cheese or other single-portion packages of cheese

- ✔ One or two large hard-cooked eggs

- ✔ Cinnamon-raisin bagel (2 ounces; half of a regular bagel or one very small bagel)

- ✔ Cereal in individual boxes with a small container of skim milk

- ✔ Cereal bar (up to 150 calories)

- ✔ Yogurt with granola (up to 200 calories)

- ✔ 6 to 8 ounces of yogurt smoothie

Drinking Up in the Morning

Dieters who normally don't like to eat breakfast are sometimes happy to drink their morning meal from a cup. (And I'm talking about drinking something a little more substantial than a cup of coffee!) If you're that type of dieter, one of the smoothie shakes in this section may put a wake-up smile on your face.

If you don't already own one, check out hand-held immersion blenders in the kitchenware section of your department store (see Figure 12-1). An immersion blender is a rod-shaped appliance with a blade at the end that can be immersed into a tall cup, a pitcher, a bowl, or a saucepan. Basically, you bring the blender to the food, rather than bringing the food to the blender. They're great for mixing up low-cal shakes and smoothies and much quicker and easier to clean than regular blenders. If you cook on a regular basis, you may find many other uses for an immersion blender, such as blending tomato sauces and puréeing vegetable soups directly in the saucepan.

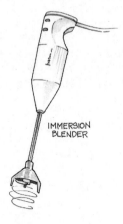

Figure 12-1:
An immersion blender is a handy tool for making shakes and smoothies.

IMMERSION BLENDER

☜ Peanut Butter–Banana Shake

Half of a sliced orange complements this shake and brings your calorie count up to 300. Double, triple, or quadruple the ingredients to make more servings, if you prefer. You can freeze leftover shake mixture in individual freezer-proof containers for up to a month. Transfer frozen shakes from the freezer to the refrigerator to thaw overnight. The shake may discolor, but it will still taste great.

Preparation time: *5 minutes*

Yield: *1 serving*

½ banana, cut up

⅓ cup plain fat-free yogurt

1 tablespoon sugar or honey

1 tablespoon smooth peanut butter

2 ice cubes, cracked

Combine the banana, yogurt, honey, peanut butter, and ice in a blender or food processor. Purée until thick and smooth. If you like thinner shakes, add a tablespoon or two of water or orange juice and purée again until mixed. Serve cold.

Tip: *If your banana is very ripe, you may not need the sugar or honey, thus saving a few calories by leaving it out.*

Per serving: *Calories 244 (From Fat 75); Fat 8g (Saturated 2g); Cholesterol 2mg; Sodium 137mg; Carbohydrate 36g (Dietary Fiber 3g); Protein 9g.*

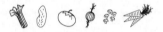

Counting calories at the coffee bar

A cup of Joe just isn't what it used to be. Coffee was once a 15-calorie wake-up call, if you drank it black. A splash of milk and a spoonful or two of sugar may have increased the calorie count to 50, 75, or maybe even 100. Nowadays coffee drinks come in every size and style, and low-cal dieters really have to keep an eye on what they drink at some of the coffee cafes today. A cup of coffee may cost you almost a full day's worth of calories if you don't know what you're ordering. Large-size cups of latte, cappuccino, other drinks with names ending in "appuccino," hot chocolates, white chocolate drinks, or any coffee drink that has "creme" or caramel in its name may contain upwards of 400 calories. Some are as high as 600 or 700 calories.

How do you find out how many calories are in the coffee you're ordering? Ask the server or look around the cafe for the nutrition brochures that many of the larger coffee chains make available in their stores and online.

 Tropical Fruit Smoothie

A bit of dried mint "wakes up" the flavor of this naturally sweet, creamy, eye-opener. To meet your maximum calorie allowance, have your smoothie with a piece of toasted light bread, spread with a teaspoon of butter, peanut butter, or jam.

Preparation time: *10 minutes*

Yield: *2 servings*

1 ripe mango or small papaya, peeled, seeded, and cut up	*½ cup fresh pineapple chunks or pineapple canned in juice, drained*
1 banana, cut up	*½ teaspoon dried mint*
1 cup plain fat-free yogurt	*6 ice cubes, cracked*

Combine the mango, banana, yogurt, pineapple, mint, and ice cubes in a blender or food processor. Whirl until smooth. If you like thinner shakes, add a tablespoon or two of water or orange juice and purée again until mixed. Serve cold.

Per serving: *Calories 210 (From Fat 6); Fat 1g (Saturated 0g); Cholesterol 3mg; Sodium 97mg; Carbohydrate 46g (Dietary Fiber 4g); Protein 8g.*

A wake-up call for caffeine users

Most people who drink coffee or tea in the morning know that the caffeine these drinks contain is a mild stimulant that the body quickly absorbs to provide a "wake up" effect in as little as 15 minutes. A favorite word used by dietitians everywhere is "moderation" and it applies as much to drinking coffee, tea, and other caffeinated beverages as it does to eating. A range of 200 to 300 milligrams (mg) is considered a moderate amount of caffeine. That's the average amount of caffeine in two or three cups of regular brewed coffee, three to five cups of brewed tea, or up to six 12-ounce cans of diet cola or other caffeinated soft drinks.

Caffeine stimulates your central nervous system and, as a result, increases your metabolic rate. That's why many over-the-counter weight-loss supplements contain caffeine as their main active ingredient. If you feel you benefit from the effects of caffeine, however, get it from a drink because caffeine is dehydrating. The caffeine contained in beverages is somewhat offset by the amount of liquid that accompanies it.

Although medical research has dispelled the myth that drinking caffeinated beverages is a potentially dangerous habit for healthy people, you still don't want to overdo it. If caffeine keeps you awake at night or makes you feel nervous, it can interfere with your daily functioning. If caffeine helps cut back on the amount of food you eat in the morning, you're still building up an appetite and may end up eating more calories overall but eating them later in the day. If that's the case, you may also be bingeing on foods that aren't particularly healthful and losing out on essential nutrients you would otherwise be getting from a regular morning meal. Also, if you have any medical problems, such as diabetes, heartburn and reflux, or high blood pressure, speak to your physician on the possible effects of caffeine on your condition.

If you're a heavy user, you probably experience withdrawal symptoms when you cut back on caffeine. Regular use of caffeine creates a physical dependence that can lead to addiction. The withdrawal symptoms of caffeine, which can include headaches, anxiety, irritability, lethargy, and even flu-like symptoms including nausea and muscle pain, can start to kick in within 12 to 24 hours of your last consumption. Psychological studies have shown that some people continue using caffeine simply to avoid the withdrawal symptoms. People who suffer significant withdrawal symptoms have reported missing work and canceling social engagements as a result. That's when some mental health experts say that caffeine can cause as much of a psychological addiction as it can a physical addiction.

Beginning Your Day with Berries

At 30 to 50 calories per ½ cup, strawberries, raspberries, and blueberries are fabulous foods to include on a regular basis in a low-cal diet. They make great snacks and great wake-me-ups whether you eat them out of hand, in a bowl with a low-cal topping, or baked into bars.

In the following recipe, you cook up a delicious custard to serve with berries. If you've never prepared custard, you may prefer to use a double boiler instead of a saucepan to prevent the sauce from burning. If you don't have a double boiler, you can improvise by fitting a larger stainless steel mixing bowl over a smaller saucepan filled with a few inches of simmering water. Make sure the bottom of the bowl sits over, but not in the water, and keep the water at a simmer. Follow the steps in the recipe, but combine the ingredients in the bowl, rather than in the medium saucepan. Using this method, the custard is less likely to stick or burn because it cooks over simmering water rather than over direct heat.

⏱ *Berries with Custard Sauce*

This creamy, cook-ahead custard can help make the idea of fresh fruit more appealing on a low-calorie diet. Have it on hand in the fridge to use as an all-purpose sauce to enhance any fruit you're having for breakfast, a snack, or even dessert. The custard sauce alone provides about 120 calories per ½ cup. Use half that amount when you're serving it with fruit for a low-calorie snack.

Preparation time: *5 minutes*

Cooking time: *10 minutes plus cooling*

Yield: *4 servings*

3 tablespoons sugar	*2 teaspoons vanilla*
1 tablespoon cornstarch	*Pinch ground nutmeg (optional)*
2 egg whites	*4 cups blueberries, raspberries, strawberries,*
1 whole egg	*blackberries, or a combination*
2 cups skim milk	

1 Whisk together the sugar and cornstarch in a medium nonstick saucepan until blended. Whisk in the egg whites, whole egg, and skim milk until smooth.

2 Place the saucepan over low heat and cook, stirring almost constantly, for about 10 minutes or until the custard mixture thickens and coats the spoon. (Don't allow the custard mixture to come to a full boil.) Remove the saucepan from the heat and stir in the vanilla and nutmeg, if using. Cool the custard to room temperature.

3 Divide the berries evenly among four small bowls. Spoon the custard sauce evenly over the berries. Store any leftover custard in a covered container in the refrigerator for up to two days.

Per serving: *Calories 140 (From Fat 12); Fat 1g (Saturated 5g); Cholesterol 28mg; Sodium 62mg; Carbohydrate 29g (Dietary Fiber 4g); Protein 5g.*

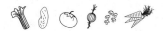

☙ *Blueberry Breakfast Bars*

I'm not encouraging you to eat on the run, but if you don't have time to eat first thing in the morning, or you just don't like to eat the minute you get up, this bar is great to take to work or on the road with you. You'll never miss the butter, which I replace with a healthier and lower-calorie mixture of olive oil and applesauce, and you'll love the taste and texture of fresh berries in this bar. You can have two bars for a 300-calorie breakfast and still have enough calories left over for adding a good splash or two of milk to your coffee.

Preparation time: *10 minutes*

Cooking time: *35 minutes*

Yield: *24 bars*

Nonstick cooking spray	¼ cup light olive oil
1 cup all-purpose flour	1 cup unsweetened applesauce
½ cup whole-wheat flour	1 whole egg
1 teaspoon ground cinnamon	2 egg whites
1 teaspoon baking soda	1 teaspoon vanilla
½ teaspoon salt	3 cups uncooked old-fashioned oats
1 cup packed light brown sugar	1½ cups fresh blueberries
½ cup granulated (white) sugar	

1 Preheat the oven to 350. Line a 13-x-9-x-2-inch baking pan with aluminum foil. Coat the foil with nonstick cooking spray.

2 In a small bowl, whisk together the flours, cinnamon, baking soda, and salt.

3 In a medium bowl with an electric mixer on medium speed, beat the brown sugar, white sugar, oil, and applesauce until blended. Beat in the egg, egg whites, and vanilla. With a wooden spoon, stir in the oats and blueberries. Spread the mixture evenly in a prepared pan.

4 Bake 30 to 35 minutes or until lightly browned around the edges and a wooden pick inserted in the center comes out clean. Cool in the pan on a wire rack for ten minutes. When slightly cooled, lift the foil from the pan and cut into 24 bars.

Per serving: *Calories 150 (From Fat 29); Fat 3g (Saturated 1g); Cholesterol 9mg; Sodium 113mg; Carbohydrate 28g (Dietary Fiber 2g); Protein 3g.*

Bulking Up Your Fiber Intake with Grains

Ask a dietitian how to get more fiber into your diet and the answer will inevitably be: "Eat more whole grains." For breakfast, eating more whole grains means choosing cereals, breads, muffins, pancakes, and other foods made with oats, whole-wheat flour, cornmeal, brans, and other grain products. In this section, you find breakfast recipes that use all these ingredients. Browse through Chapter 3 to find out why you need fiber, how fiber can help you lose weight, and more of the foods that supply it.

◐ Toasted English Muffin with Apple and Cheese

To boost your fiber count, use multigrain, whole-wheat, or oat bran English muffins. Enjoy 6 ounces of your favorite juice or ½ cup orange sections with your muffin.

Preparation time: 5 minutes

Cooking time: 5 minutes

Yield: 2 servings

1 English muffin, split

2 ounces reduced-fat Cheddar or Swiss cheese, grated

1 small apple, quartered, cored, and thinly sliced

Pinch of dried sage, crumbled (optional)

1 Preheat the broiler. Arrange the muffin halves, split side up, on the broiler pan. Broil the muffin 3 to 4 inches from the heat for 30 seconds or until lightly toasted.

2 Sprinkle half of the cheese evenly over the toasted muffin halves. Top with apple slices. Sprinkle with the sage, if using, and then the remaining cheese.

3 Broil the sandwiches for 3 to 4 minutes or until the cheese is melted.

Per serving: Calories 187 (From Fat 65); Fat 7g (Saturated 5g); Cholesterol 22mg; Sodium 131mg; Carbohydrate 23g (Dietary Fiber 2g); Protein 10g.

Toast Topped with Ham, Tomatoes, Asparagus, and Hard-Cooked Egg

You hardly need a recipe because the name says it all. However, I suggest that you follow the recipe because doing so ensures that you stay within your calorie limit. When substituting this dish for a menu-plan breakfast, add a cup of fresh fruit, 6 ounces of fruit juice, or 1 cup of skim milk to bring the calorie count up to approximately 300. If you like, you can omit the eggs in these breakfast sandwiches. You can save 35 or 40 calories if you do.

Preparation time: *15 minutes*

Cooking time: *6 minutes*

Yield: *4 servings*

4 slices light whole-wheat bread	*8 asparagus stalks, trimmed and steamed*
2 tablespoons Dijon mustard	*4 thin slices firm, ripe tomato*
8 thin slices lean deli ham	*2 ounces reduced-fat Swiss cheese, shredded or cut into thin strips*
2 hard-cooked eggs, sliced	

1 Preheat the broiler. Place the bread slices in a single layer on a nonstick baking sheet.

2 Broil the bread 3 to 4 inches from the heat for 30 seconds on each side, or until lightly toasted.

3 Lightly spread each slice of bread with mustard. Top the slices evenly with ham, egg slices, asparagus spears, tomato slices, and cheese.

4 Broil the sandwiches 3 to 4 inches from the heat for 1½ minutes or until the cheese is melted and the sandwich is heated through. Serve hot.

Per serving: *Calories 168 (From Fat 68); Fat 8g (Saturated 3g); Cholesterol 125mg; Sodium 682mg; Carbohydrate 13g (Dietary Fiber 3g); Protein 16g.*

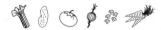

Toast with a topping is a quick and easy way to start the day, and you don't have to limit yourself to a tiny pat of butter or a spoonful of jam. You can top one slice of toasted "light" bread with any of the following and still keep it under 100 calories. ("Light" bread is calculated at 40 calories.)

- ✔ 2 tablespoons cinnamon applesauce
- ✔ 2 tablespoons mashed banana plus ¼ cup strawberry slices
- ✔ 2 tablespoons fruit-flavored cottage cheese
- ✔ 2 tablespoons salsa plus 1 tablespoon light cream cheese
- ✔ 2 tablespoons bean dip
- ✔ 2 tablespoons hummus
- ✔ 1½ tablespoons all-fruit spread
- ✔ 1½ tablespoons low-sugar jam
- ✔ 1½ tablespoons apple butter
- ✔ 1 tablespoon all-fruit spread plus 1 tablespoon light ricotta cheese
- ✔ 1 tablespoon liverwurst
- ✔ 1 tablespoon cheese spread
- ✔ 1 tablespoon guacamole
- ✔ 1 tablespoon low-sugar jam plus 1 tablespoon light cream cheese
- ✔ 2 teaspoons honey
- ✔ 2 teaspoons maple syrup
- ✔ 2 teaspoons lemon curd
- ✔ 2 teaspoons flavored cream cheese
- ✔ 1½ teaspoons peanut butter
- ✔ 1½ teaspoons cashew butter
- ✔ 1½ teaspoons chocolate-hazelnut spread
- ✔ 1½ teaspoons butter
- ✔ 1 teaspoon butter sprinkled with 1 teaspoon cinnamon-sugar
- ✔ 1 teaspoon light cream cheese plus 2 tablespoons crushed pineapple packed in juice
- ✔ 1 slice lean turkey bacon plus 2 slices tomato

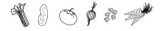 Pumpkin Pancakes

For a 300-calorie breakfast, top two pancakes with ½ cup of cut-up fresh fruit and a tablespoon of light syrup.

Preparation time: *5 minutes*

Cooking time: *20 to 30 minutes*

Yield: *8 servings*

½ cup all-purpose flour	3 eggs
½ cup whole-wheat flour	⅓ cup packed light brown sugar
1½ teaspoons baking powder	1¼ cups lowfat (1%) milk
1 teaspoon pumpkin pie spice	1¼ cups unseasoned canned pumpkin
¼ teaspoon salt	3 tablespoons olive oil

1 Stir together the flours, baking powder, pie spice, and salt in a large bowl. Set aside.

2 In a 2-cup measuring cup or medium bowl, stir together the eggs, brown sugar, milk, pumpkin, and oil. Stir into flour mixture just until smooth.

3 Heat a nonstick griddle or a large nonstick skillet over medium heat. Working in batches, drop ¼ cup of batter at a time onto the hot griddle. Cook until bubbles start to form on the top of the pancakes and the bottoms are golden, about 2 minutes (see Figure 12-2). Turn the pancakes over and cook for 2 minutes longer or until the bottoms are golden brown.

Tip: To partially prepare pancakes in advance and save time in the morning, combine the dry ingredients and the egg-oil mixture and store them separately in the refrigerator overnight. The next morning, take them out of the fridge and let them stand at room temperature for 10 or 15 minutes before mixing the batter and heating up the griddle.

Per serving: Calories 190 (From Fat 70); Fat 8g (Saturated 2g); Cholesterol 81mg; Sodium 193mg; Carbohydrate 25g (Dietary Fiber 3g); Protein 6g.

Figure 12-2:
Turn your pancakes over when you see bubbles on top.

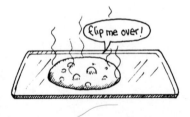

REMEMBER

Health experts recommend that most adults aim for about 25 grams of fiber each day. Breakfast is the one meal that can really help boost your fiber intake and strive to reach that goal, because so many typical American breakfast foods — cereals, fresh fruits, dried fruits, and baked goods — are packed full of the stuff. All whole-grain foods, vegetables, fruits, and legumes (beans, peas, and lentils) are good sources of fiber, providing from 1 to 8 grams per serving. Without having to keep track of yet another set of numbers, you can simply use the following list as a guide to breakfast foods that are comparatively high in fiber. Keep these foods in mind when you're creating your weekly meal plans and incorporate them wherever you can. (I list grains first, followed by fruits.)

- 100 percent bran cereal
- Bran flakes cereal
- Raisin bran cereal
- Shredded wheat
- Granola with raisins
- Whole-grain waffles
- Whole-grain pancakes
- Whole-wheat bread
- Whole-grain bread
- High-fiber breads
- Oatmeal
- Oat bran cereal
- Wheat bran cereal
- Hot wheat cereals
- Bran muffins
- Oat bran English muffins
- Apples
- Dried figs
- Oranges
- Pears
- Prunes
- Strawberries

☙ *Good Morning Cake*

Eat cake for breakfast? When it's a multigrain cake made with yogurt and dried fruit, why not?

Preparation time: *15 minutes*

Cooking time: *30 minutes*

Yield: *8 servings*

Nonstick cooking spray	*1 teaspoon ground cinnamon*
¾ cup chopped mixed dried fruit	*1 teaspoon baking powder*
1 cup boiling water	*½ teaspoon baking soda*
1 cup uncooked old-fashioned oats	*½ teaspoon salt*
1 cup all-purpose flour	*2 eggs*
¼ cup cornmeal	*½ cup plain lowfat yogurt*
½ cup firmly packed light brown sugar	*2 tablespoons olive oil*

1 Preheat the oven to 350. Coat a 9-inch round cake pan with nonstick cooking spray. Line the bottom of the pan with waxed paper. Combine the dried fruits and boiling water in a medium bowl and let stand for 10 minutes. Drain well and set aside.

2 Meanwhile, in a large bowl, stir together the oats, flour, cornmeal, brown sugar, cinnamon, baking powder, baking soda, and salt until well mixed.

3 In another large bowl, stir together the eggs, yogurt, and oil. Make a well in the center of the oat mixture. Pour the egg mixture into the well and stir until the dry ingredients are just moistened. Pour the cake batter into the cake pan. Sprinkle the fruit evenly over the batter, smoothing the top with a rubber spatula.

4 Bake the cake for 30 minutes or until a pick inserted in the center comes out clean. Cool the cake in the pan on a rack for 10 minutes. Turn the cake out onto the rack to cool completely. To serve, cut the cake into 8 wedges.

Per serving: *Calories 259 (From Fat 52); Fat 6g (Saturated 1g); Cholesterol 54mg; Sodium 327mg; Carbohydrate 46g (Dietary Fiber 3g); Protein 6g.*

🍑 Homemade Granola with Pecans and Dried Cherries

Even if you add ½ cup of milk to this cereal, you still have about 100 calories to play with so you can add fresh fruit or fruit juice to the menu or perhaps a couple of strips of lean turkey bacon. One-third cup of this granola also fits into your diet plan as a 100-calorie, snack-size portion.

Preparation time: *10 minutes*

Cooking time: *40 minutes*

Yield: *10 servings (½ cup each)*

3 cups uncooked old-fashioned oats	*⅓ cup honey*
½ cup coarsely chopped pecans	*1 tablespoon vegetable oil*
¼ cup sesame seeds	*1 teaspoon vanilla*
½ teaspoon salt	*1 cup dried cherries, cranberries, blueberries, or golden raisins*

1 Preheat the oven to 300. Combine the oats, pecans, sesame seeds, and salt on a parchment-lined, lipped baking sheet or 13-x-9-inch baking pan.

2 Bake for 30 minutes or until the oats and pecans are toasted. Remove the pan from the oven. Increase the oven temperature to 350.

3 Meanwhile, combine the honey and oil in a small saucepan. Cook this mixture over medium heat for 1 minute. Remove the pan from the heat and stir in the vanilla. Drizzle this syrup evenly over the toasted oat mixture, and then stir to mix well.

4 Bake the granola mixture for 10 minutes or until the oats are crisp, stirring every 2 or 3 minutes.

5 Break up any clumps of granola with a wooden spoon. Stir in the cherries. When the granola is completely cool, store it in a covered, airtight container.

Per serving: Calories 251 (From Fat 83); Fat 9g (Saturated 1g); Cholesterol 0mg; Sodium 121mg; Carbohydrate 37g (Dietary Fiber 4g); Protein 6g.

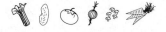

Making Eggs-cellent Breakfasts

In many ways, eggs are the perfect diet food. They're low in calories (about 75 per egg), high in protein, and easy enough for most people to prepare. Eggs are filling, they lend themselves to a variety of food combinations, and they travel well when hard-cooked, so you can take them with you to work, school, or anywhere that you may suffer a hunger attack.

If you're concerned about cholesterol in eggs, you can substitute 2 egg whites for each whole egg called for in most recipes, or follow package directions for using commercial egg substitutes.

Baby Spinach Scramble with Toast

To bring the calorie count for breakfast up to approximately 300, serve these scrambled eggs with a slice of light toast, a teaspoon of butter or a tablespoon of jam, and half a cup of juice or skim milk.

Preparation time: *5 minutes*

Cooking time: *4 minutes*

Yield: *4 servings*

5 eggs	*2 cups baby spinach leaves or finely chopped fresh large-leaf spinach*
5 egg whites	
¼ teaspoon salt	*¼ cup chopped lean ham or 2 lean strips bacon, crumbled*
⅛ teaspoon pepper	
Nonstick cooking spray	*2 green onions, finely chopped*

1 Whisk together the eggs, egg whites, salt, and pepper in a large bowl until well blended.

2 Coat a large nonstick skillet with nonstick cooking spray and place over medium heat. Add the spinach, ham, and onion. Cook, stirring often, for 2 minutes or until the spinach wilts. Transfer the mixture to a small bowl and set aside.

3 Add the egg mixture to the skillet. Cook, gently stirring, for 1 minute or until the eggs start to thicken. Stir in the spinach mixture. Cook, stirring often, for 1 minute longer or until the eggs are cooked through.

Per serving: *Calories 132 (From Fat 60); Fat 7g (Saturated 2g); Cholesterol 270mg; Sodium 433mg; Carbohydrate 3g (Dietary Fiber 1g); Protein 14g.*

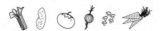

Potato, Bacon, and Cheddar Omelet

When you're on a low-calorie diet, having some recipes that yield just one serving on hand is helpful, especially if it's a recipe for food that doesn't lend itself to reheating or freezing. In this case, you can simply double, triple, or quadruple the recipe if you're serving more than yourself. Serve this omelet with a small piece of fruit or ½ cup orange juice or lowfat milk.

Preparation time: *10 minutes*

Cooking time: *15 minutes*

Yield: *1 serving*

Nonstick cooking spray

½ cup diced peeled potato

¼ cup finely chopped onion

¼ cup fat-free chicken broth or water

Pinch of salt and pepper

1 slice Canadian bacon, chopped

¼ cup finely chopped sweet red pepper

1 egg

2 tablespoons grated reduced-fat Cheddar cheese

2 tablespoons salsa (optional)

1 Lightly coat a small (7-inch) nonstick skillet with nonstick cooking spray. Place over medium-high heat. Add potato and onion. Cook, stirring often, for 2 minutes or until browned.

2 Stir in broth, salt, and pepper. Reduce the heat to medium; cover and cook 5 minutes. Uncover and cook 2 to 3 minutes or until all the liquid evaporates. Stir in the bacon. Transfer the filling mixture to a small bowl and cover to keep warm. Wipe out the skillet with a paper towel.

3 Place the skillet over medium heat. Beat together the egg and cheese until well mixed. Pour the egg mixture into the skillet and cook for 30 seconds.

4 Spoon the filling over half the omelet. Cover and cook for 1 minute or until the egg is set. Fold the egg over the filling, transfer the omelet to a serving plate, sprinkle with red pepper, and top with salsa, if using.

Per serving: *Calories 254 (From Fat 92); Fat 10g (Saturated 4g); Cholesterol 236mg; Sodium 583mg; Carbohydrate 23g (Dietary Fiber 3g); Protein 18g.*

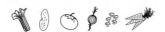

⏰ Huevos Rancheros

Huevos Rancheros is Spanish for "ranch eggs." This traditional breakfast dish of eggs and salsa is served in many restaurants that feature Mexican and Tex-Mex fare.

Preparation time: *15 minutes*

Cooking time: *15 minutes*

Yield: *6 servings*

6 small (6-inch) fat-free flour tortillas

2 teaspoons olive oil

1 sweet green pepper, finely chopped

2 firm-ripe tomatoes, cored, seeded, and finely chopped

1 cup fat-free salsa

1 jalapeno pepper, cored, seeded, and minced

½ teaspoon ground cumin

6 eggs

½ cup shredded reduced-fat Cheddar or Jack cheese

1 avocado, halved, pitted, peeled, and diced

2 tablespoons finely chopped cilantro

1 Preheat the oven to 350. Wrap the tortillas together in one stack in a sheet of aluminum foil. Place the foil pack in the oven for 10 minutes or until the tortillas area heated through. Set the wrapped tortillas aside until ready to serve.

2 Meanwhile, heat the oil in a large nonstick skillet over medium heat. Add the pepper and sauté 2 minutes. Stir in the tomatoes, salsa, jalapeno, and cumin. Reduce the heat to medium-low and simmer for 8 minutes or until the sauce is thickened.

3 Crack the eggs on top of the sauce. Sprinkle the cheese evenly over the eggs. Cover the skillet and cook for 3 to 5 minutes or until the eggs are set.

4 Place one egg and some sauce on top of each warm tortilla. Top with avocado and cilantro and serve hot.

Per serving: Calories 264 (From Fat 116); Fat 13g (Saturated 4g); Cholesterol 219mg; Sodium 487mg; Carbohydrate 26g (Dietary Fiber 5g); Protein 13g.

○ *Spanish Tortilla*

In Spain, this flat, open-face omelet, topped with potatoes, tomatoes, and peppers, is called a tortilla, which confuses some Americans because the recipe doesn't have any tortillas! With a single serving, on a 300-calorie breakfast plan, you have enough calories left over to add a cup of fruit salad.

Preparation time: 10 minutes

Cooking time: 25 minutes

Yield: 4 servings

1 tablespoon olive oil, divided	1 medium Yukon Gold potato, cooked and cut into ½-inch cubes
1 onion, finely chopped	½ teaspoon salt
2 cloves garlic, finely chopped	Nonstick cooking spray
1 sweet red, green, or yellow pepper, finely chopped	5 eggs, lightly beaten
1 firm-ripe tomato, halved, seeded, and finely chopped	¼ cup sliced Spanish olives

1 Heat 2 teaspoons of the oil in a large nonstick skillet over medium heat. Add the onion and garlic and sauté for 5 minutes. Add the pepper and tomato and sauté for 3 minutes longer. Add the potato and salt. Cover the skillet and cook, stirring often and adding a spoonful or two of water if necessary to prevent sticking, for 8 to 10 minutes or until all the vegetables are very tender. Transfer the vegetables to a bowl and cover to keep warm. Wipe out the skillet with a paper towel.

2 Coat the skillet with nonstick cooking spray and place over medium heat. Add the remaining teaspoon of oil, swirling the oil in the pan to evenly coat. Add the eggs. Cook the omelet for 1 minute or until the eggs begin to thicken around the edge of the pan. Run a thin spatula around the inner edge of the skillet to allow the uncooked egg to run underneath the cooked egg. Repeat this for 2 to 3 minutes or until the center of the omelet is set. If necessary, cover the skillet for 1 minute or until the omelet is cooked through.

3 Slide the omelet onto a serving plate. Top the omelet with the vegetable mixture and sprinkle evenly with the olives. Cut the omelet into 4 equal wedges and serve immediately.

Per serving: Calories 194 (From Fat 98); Fat 11g (Saturated 3g); Cholesterol 266mg; Sodium 561mg; Carbohydrate 15g (Dietary Fiber 2g); Protein 10g.

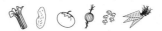

My first favorite thing about the following recipe is the way the strata puffs up and makes a real show of itself in the oven. After it cools down a little, it deflates and looks a little less dramatic, but at that point, all you want to do is eat it, so who cares? My second favorite thing about this recipe is that it looks and tastes *nothing* like diet food! This dish is very satisfying for calorie counters.

Ham and Cheese Breakfast Strata

A *strata* is a casserole that you can prepare the night before and pop into the oven the morning you plan to eat it. In many ways, this combination of bread, cheese, ham, and egg custard is similar to a savory bread pudding. This low-cal version uses mostly egg whites, lowfat milk, light bread, and reduced-fat cheese. You can also try it with hot sauce or a dollop of salsa on the side.

Preparation time: *15 minutes plus standing time*

Cooking time: *25 minutes plus 10 minutes standing time*

Yield: *6 servings*

Nonstick cooking spray	*¼ teaspoon pepper*
8 egg whites	*8 slices light whole-wheat or oat bread*
4 whole eggs	*6 ounces lean ham or Canadian bacon, chopped*
1½ cups skim milk	
2 tablespoons Dijon mustard	*1 cup shredded reduced-fat Cheddar cheese*
¾ teaspoon salt	

1 About 15 minutes before baking, preheat the oven to 425. Coat an 11-x-7-inch baking dish with nonstick cooking spray.

2 Meanwhile, in a medium bowl, beat together the egg whites, whole eggs, milk, mustard, salt, and pepper.

3 Overlap the bread slices in a single layer in the prepared baking dish (see Figure 12-3). Sprinkle evenly with ham. Pour the egg mixture into dish. Sprinkle with cheese. Cover with foil. Let the strata stand for 1 hour before baking or refrigerate for up to 10 hours. (If you refrigerate, let the strata stand at room temperature for 30 minutes before baking.)

4 Bake the strata for 10 minutes. Uncover and bake for 15 minutes longer or until the mixture is set and the top is puffy and golden brown. Remove the strata to a cooling rack and let it stand for10 minutes before slicing and serving.

Per serving: Calories 248 (From Fat 88); Fat 10g (Saturated 5g); Cholesterol 170mg; Sodium 1,098mg; Carbohydrate 18g (Dietary Fiber 2g); Protein 25g.

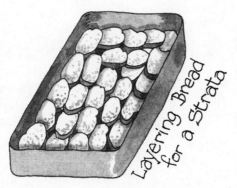

Figure 12-3: Overlap the bread in a strata for even cooking of the egg mixture.

Layering Bread for a Strata

Sausage on the side

You're eating your egg-dominated breakfast, and you're probably craving a bit of sausage. Have you ever tried making your own lean breakfast sausage patties? Doing so is much easier than you may think, just like making turkey burgers but with slightly different seasoning. Two of these patties with a scrambled egg and a slice of light whole-grain toast spread with a spoonful of jam come to just about 300 calories.

In a large bowl, combine 1 pound lean ground turkey or chicken breast, 1 cup cooked rice, ¼ cup unsweetened applesauce, 1 tablespoon Dijon-style mustard, 1 teaspoon salt, ½ teaspoon dried sage, ¼ teaspoon dried marjoram or thyme, and ¼ teaspoon ground black pepper until well mixed. Shape the sausage into twelve 2-inch patties. Cook the patties in a nonstick skillet over medium heat or under a preheated broiler for about 3 minutes on each side.

You can freeze these patties, cooked or uncooked, for up to a couple of months. Stack two patties per package with a sheet of wax paper between to keep them from sticking, and then wrap in freezer-proof paper. Thaw the patties overnight on a plate in the refrigerator before you plan to use them. Add a minute or so to the cooking time if the patties are cooked cold.

Crustless Bacon Quiche

Quiche is a great make-ahead food, something to have on hand in the refrigerator for meals and also for snack attacks. Simply pop a slice in the microwave oven for 20 seconds, and it's ready to eat. When substituting a serving of this quiche for the breakfast listed in any of the 300-calorie menu plans in Chapter 6, add a thin slice of cantaloupe or a couple of fresh strawberries.

Preparation time: *10 minutes*

Cooking time: *35 plus 10 minutes standing*

Yield: *4 main-dish servings or 8 to 12 snack or side-dish servings*

Nonstick cooking spray	1 cup part-skim ricotta cheese
3 slices lean turkey bacon	1 cup plain lowfat yogurt
2 teaspoons olive oil	3 eggs
1 finely chopped onion	½ teaspoon salt
½ cup finely chopped sweet red pepper	¼ teaspoon pepper
1 tablespoon chopped fresh parsley	

1 Preheat the oven to 325. Coat a 9-inch pie plate with nonstick cooking spray.

2 Coat a large nonstick skillet with nonstick cooking spray and place the skillet over medium heat. Add the bacon and cook until crisp. Remove the bacon from the skillet and set aside on paper towels to drain. Wipe out the skillet with a paper towel.

3 In the same skillet, heat the oil over medium heat. Add the onion and sauté for 5 minutes or until tender. Add the peppers and sauté for 2 minutes longer or until just tender. Remove the skillet from the heat and stir in the parsley.

4 Transfer the onion and pepper mixture to a large bowl. Crumble the bacon and add to the bowl. Stir in ricotta cheese, yogurt, eggs, salt, and pepper until well mixed. Turn the quiche mixture into the prepared pie plate.

5 Bake the quiche for 35 to 40 minutes or until just set in the center. Transfer the quiche to a cooling rack for 10 minutes before slicing and serving.

Vary It! *This one basic recipe lends itself to countless low-cal variations. Try substituting 1 cup of cooked, cubed chicken, 2 ounces reduced-fat Cheddar cheese, or 2 ounces finely chopped lean ham for the bacon.*

Per serving: *Calories 236 (From Fat 111); Fat 12g (Saturated 5g); Cholesterol 190mg; Sodium 566mg; Carbohydrate 13g (Dietary Fiber 1g); Protein 18g.*

Chapter 13

Preparing Tasty Lunches

In This Chapter

▶ Brown-bagging your lunch

▶ Dressing up salads

▶ Fixing simple sandwiches

▶ Putting on a pot of soup

*F*inding and eating a low-calorie lunch when you're at work can be a challenge, especially if you don't take a full or regular lunch hour or you wait until you're absolutely famished to take a food break. When you're first starting out on a structured, low-calorie diet, the smartest approach is to bring your lunch from home. You have the most control over how many calories you consume at lunchtime when you prepare your own lunch.

After you have a good sense of how many calories are in the different types of food you eat, and how much food is a reasonable amount of food to eat at one meal, then a trip to the salad bar becomes a great option. You can quickly pick up prepared foods at a salad bar and put together a balanced meal.

In this chapter, you find tips for making healthy, delicious lunches and 15 recipes for portable, 300-calorie lunches, including salads, sandwiches, and a few homemade soups, plus "add-ons" to the menus when calories allow.

Putting Together Midday Meals

Lunch supplies the energy you need to move into your afternoon activities. For a continuous energy flow, have your midday meal no more than 5 hours after breakfast. When you're following a low-calorie diet, a small mid-morning snack can help bridge the energy gap between breakfast and lunch.

Packing a low-cal lunch

If you prepare two or three of the recipes in this chapter over a weekend, you're set with lunch entrees for the entire week. Try pairing some of the recipes and bringing half a serving of a salad and a half-portion of one of the soups one day and a soup-and-half-sandwich combo another day. That way you aren't eating the exact same lunch every day.

Make sure you have a variety of storage containers on hand to use for packing lunches to go. A wide-mouth thermos is best for soups, stews, and other liquid lunches. Invest in a small assortment of lidded containers made for carrying food. (You can find many decent, affordable ones at your local discount store. Look for brands that are microwave-safe if you plan to reheat your lunches.) Keep a set of utensils at work so you don't have to remember to pack plastic forks and spoons.

You always have the option of following the menu plans in Chapter 6 or using them as a guide to preparing lunches that contain just the right number of calories. Remember that the meals on these menu plans are interchangeable so you can eat any one of the meals at any time of day. If you're sticking to 1,200 calories a day right now and you see a breakfast menu on a 1,200-calorie plan that you want for lunch tomorrow, pack it!

Using low-cal leftovers

The easiest lunch you can make is last night's leftover dinner. If you have a microwave oven at work, you can pack pre-portioned leftover food and quickly heat it up at work and eat it before you have time to consider anything else for lunch. Doing so is an especially good idea if you tend to get very hungry by the time you eat lunch so that you're not tempted to run out for higher-calorie fast food just to quickly satisfy that hunger. (See Chapter 14 for delicious dinner ideas that you can use as lunch the next day.)

When you're eating dinner out or ordering in, think about leftovers for your next day's lunch. One of the most common restaurant tips for dieters is to ask for your "doggie bag" in advance so that you're not tempted to eat the entire meal that's served to you. Ask the server to divide your entree in half, serve half now, and bring the leftovers at the end of the meal for you to take home.

Mixing Salads

Main-dish salads are a staple in a low-calorie diet plan because they help fill you up with plenty of nutritious low-cal veggies and still satisfy your hunger because they contain a balance of ingredients that keep you feeling full throughout the afternoon. I give you ideas on salads with chicken, meat, seafood, grains, and fruit in the following sections.

Most foods lack flavor when served ice-cold, so try to remember to take your salad out of the refrigerator at least 30 minutes before you're ready to eat. This step is especially true for pasta and rice salads.

Making salads with meat and poultry

Adding chicken, turkey, or any variety of meat transforms a side-dish salad into an entree. You don't have to add anything else to the dish because you have everything you need for a balanced meal — protein, vegetables, and grains or other starchy carbohydrates such as pasta or rice.

Beefy Romaine Salad with Basil Vinaigrette

This hearty salad is a one-dish lunch that also makes a great light dinner in warm weather months. Use your own leftover meat or use thickly sliced roast beef from your supermarket's deli section.

Preparation time: *10 minutes*

Yield: *4 servings*

1 cup basil leaves

2 tablespoons olive oil

2 tablespoons water

1 tablespoon lemon juice

¼ teaspoon salt

1 clove garlic

8 ounces cooked lean beef, cut into ¼-inch thick strips

1 head Romaine lettuce, trimmed and torn into bite-size pieces

1 large sweet red pepper, halved, seeded, and cut into strips

1 small red onion, halved and thinly sliced

1 Combine the basil, olive oil, water, lemon juice, salt, and garlic in a food processor or blender. Whirl until smooth, about 30 seconds. Pour the vinaigrette into a large serving bowl.

2 Just before serving the salad, add the beef, lettuce, pepper, and onion to the bowl with the vinaigrette. Gently toss.

Per serving: Calories 208 (From Fat 104); Fat 12g (Saturated 3g); Cholesterol 51mg; Sodium 193mg; Carbohydrate 7g (Dietary Fiber 3g); Protein 20g.

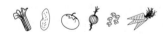

Meaty Potato Salad

This recipe demonstrates an age-old method of cutting fat to cut calories in a creamy salad dressing by replacing half the original amount of mayonnaise with lowfat plain yogurt.

Preparation time: *10 minutes*

Cooking time: *10 minutes*

Yield: *4 servings*

4 cups cubed (1½ inches), unpeeled Yukon gold potatoes

2 tablespoons white wine vinegar or rice wine vinegar

¼ cup light mayonnaise

¼ cup lowfat plain yogurt

1 tablespoon mustard

¼ teaspoon salt

⅛ teaspoon pepper

4 ounces lean ham

½ cup finely chopped red or green onion

¼ cup finely chopped sweet red pepper

¼ cup thinly sliced celery

1 tablespoon finely chopped parsley (optional)

1 Combine the potatoes and enough lightly salted water to cover by 1 inch in a large saucepan. Bring the water to a boil over medium-high heat. Reduce the heat to medium-low and simmer for 10 minutes or until the potatoes are just tender. Drain the potatoes and place in a large bowl. Gently toss the potatoes with the vinegar. Set aside to cool.

2 Meanwhile, in another large bowl, combine the mayonnaise, yogurt, mustard, salt, and pepper until blended. Add the ham, onion, sweet pepper, celery, and parsley. Toss gently to combine. Gently stir in the potatoes. Serve at once or refrigerate to chill before serving.

Vary It! *Substitute an equal amount of any lean meat, poultry, smoked poultry, firm-fleshed fish, or egg white for the ham in this tasty, satisfying lunch entree.*

Per serving: *Calories 253 (From Fat 63); Fat 7g (Saturated 2g); Cholesterol 19mg; Sodium 794mg; Carbohydrate 35g (Dietary Fiber 3g); Protein 11g.*

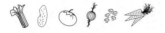

Chicken Salad with Roasted Peppers and Toasted Pine Nuts

Packaged salad greens that include fresh herbs in the mix are a tasty addition to any salad. They also make your cooking life easier by eliminating the need to season your dressing; a simple oil and vinegar mixture works just fine. If you don't have leftover chicken for this recipe and don't feel like cooking, you can use precooked chicken from your supermarket's deli section.

Preparation time: *5 minutes*

Cooking time: *3 minutes*

Yield: *4 servings*

3 ounces pine nuts

2 tablespoons olive oil

1 tablespoon white wine vinegar

1½ cups cubed cooked chicken (8 ounces raw)

6 ounces jarred roasted red peppers, drained and coarsely chopped (about ½ cup)

4 cups mixed salad greens with herbs

1 Place the pine nuts in a small heavy skillet over medium heat. Toast, stirring often, until the nuts just begin to turn golden brown, about 3 minutes. Remove the nuts from the skillet and set aside to cool.

2 Whisk together the olive oil and vinegar in a large salad bowl. Add the chicken, peppers, and pine nuts. Toss to mix. Add salad greens and toss again. Serve at once.

Vary 1t! *Fresh cherry tomatoes work just as well in the place of the red peppers.*

Per serving: *Calories 293 (From Fat 189); Fat 21g (Saturated 4g); Cholesterol 39mg; Sodium 144mg; Carbohydrate 10g (Dietary Fiber 2g); Protein 19g.*

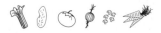

Chinese Chicken Noodle Salad

This recipe is a simple pasta salad with a tasty Asian twist. If you don't have leftover chicken, you can use precooked chicken from your supermarket's deli section. You can use the basic dressing — a soy sauce, sesame oil, and rice wine vinegar combination — on any green salad or side-dish vegetable that you prepare to go with an Asian-style meal. The dressing alone contains 50 calories per tablespoon, which is equivalent to a light dressing. You can serve this dish warm, cool, or at room temperature.

Preparation time: *5 minutes*

Cooking time: *15 minutes*

Yield: *6 servings*

8 ounces angel hair pasta or thin spaghetti

½ head of broccoli, cut into bite-size florets (1½ cups) or 1 box frozen chopped broccoli, thawed

2 tablespoons sesame oil

2 tablespoons rice wine vinegar or white wine vinegar

1 tablespoon soy sauce

3 scallions, trimmed and thinly sliced

1½ cups cubed, cooked chicken (8 ounces)

1 Cook the pasta in a large saucepan of boiling salted water according to the package directions until al dente, or firm to the bite. Add the broccoli to the saucepan for the final 2 minutes of cooking time. Drain thoroughly.

2 Meanwhile, in a large bowl, combine the sesame oil, vinegar, and soy sauce. Stir in scallions and set aside.

3 Add the drained pasta and broccoli to a bowl with the chicken and the reserved sauce and gently toss.

Vary It! *You can substitute an equal amount of leftover pork or cubes of tofu for the chicken in this recipe, if you prefer.*

Per serving: *Calories 245 (From Fat 67); Fat 7g (Saturated 1g); Cholesterol 26mg; Sodium 187mg; Carbohydrate 29g (Dietary Fiber 2g); Protein 15g.*

Diving into seafood salads

Just like meat and poultry, fish and shellfish add the protein necessary to call a low-calorie salad a meal. Compared to other forms of protein, seafood is often lower in calories and fat. And even when you choose slightly fatty seafood such as salmon or albacore tuna, the additional calories aren't usually significant. Furthermore, with these fattier fish you get an added bonus of health-enhancing omega-3 fatty acids that help protect your heart from disease. If these recipes look interesting but you don't eat seafood, you can try them with chicken, turkey, or pork.

Tuna Nicoise Salad

If you bring this salad to work or on a picnic, pack the croutons separately and add them just before eating, or have a small breadstick on the side.

Preparation time: *15 minutes*

Cooking time: *4 minutes*

Yield: *4 servings*

4 cups fresh green beans, trimmed

2 tablespoons olive oil

2 tablespoons white wine vinegar

1 large clove garlic, finely chopped

¼ teaspoon anchovy paste

¼ teaspoon salt

2 cans (6 ounces each) albacore tuna in water, drained

2 large tomatoes, seeded and diced

¼ cup finely chopped red onion

6 imported ripe black olives, pitted and chopped

½ cup croutons

1 Steam the green beans in a steamer basket until tender-crisp, about 4 minutes. Set aside.

2 Meanwhile, stir together the oil, vinegar, garlic, anchovy paste, and salt in a large bowl until well mixed. Add the tuna, tomatoes, onion, and olives. Gently toss. Divide the green beans evenly among four serving plates. Serve the tuna mixture over the green beans and top with the croutons, if using.

Per serving: Calories 244 (From Fat 102); Fat 11g (Saturated 2g); Cholesterol 30mg; Sodium 581mg; Carbohydrate 17g (Dietary Fiber 5g); Protein 20g.

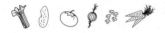

Salmon and Asparagus Salad

You can use fresh, canned, or smoked salmon for this recipe. Serve with four saltine-style crackers or a small breadstick on the side, or top with ⅓ cup croutons.

Preparation time: *5 minutes*

Cooking time: *5 minutes*

Yield: *4 servings*

1½ lbs. fresh asparagus, trimmed	*Salt and pepper*
4 small Yukon gold or new potatoes (8 ounces), peeled if desired, and cut into bite-size pieces	*8 ounces steamed or broiled salmon, boned and flaked*
2 cups watercress, washed and drained	*½ cup light mayonnaise*
1 cup drained, canned or thawed, frozen corn kernels	*¼ cup fresh lemon juice*
	1 tablespoon snipped fresh dill or 1 teaspoon dried dill

1 Place the asparagus spears in a steamer basket over boiling water. Cover and steam for 4 to 5 minutes or until bright green and just tender. Remove steamer basket and rinse asparagus under cold running water. Drain well.

2 Meanwhile, cook the potatoes in lightly salted boiling water to cover for 10 to 12 minutes or until tender. Drain, cool, and cut the potatoes into bite-size chunks.

3 Arrange the watercress, corn, and potatoes on individual salad plates. Place asparagus spears in center of plate. Season with salt and pepper to taste. Top with smoked salmon.

4 Combine mayonnaise, lemon juice, and dill in a bowl. Drizzle over salad.

Per serving: Calories 280 (From Fat 115); Fat 13g (Saturated 3g); Cholesterol 42mg; Sodium 446mg; Carbohydrate 26g (Dietary Fiber 3g); Protein 17g.

Tossing together grain and fruit salads

Salads made with pasta, rice, or even fruit add variety and interest to a low-calorie diet, not to mention numerous nutrients and much-needed fiber. You can fiddle with the three basic recipes in this section by substituting different fruits and vegetables, trying different cheeses, and using different pasta shapes and different types of rice.

☺ Italian Rice Salad

The calories from regular cheese are factored into this recipe so that you're not limited to eating only cheeses that have been modified to reduce fat and calories. If you want to substitute reduced-fat/reduced-calorie cheese such as Swiss or havarti, you can add an extra ounce to the recipe and still come in under 300 calories. If you stick with lower calorie reduced-fat cheese, you can have a ¼ cantaloupe or a slice of honeydew melon on the side.

Preparation time: *5 minutes plus rice cooking time*

Yield: *6 servings (about ¾ cup per serving)*

2 cups cooked white or brown rice

2 cups cherry tomatoes, halved

1 cucumber, peeled, seeded, and diced

1 tablespoon capers, drained and chopped

8 green or black pitted olives, finely chopped

4 ounces fontina or provolone cheese, diced

¼ cup finely chopped fresh basil

¼ cup olive oil

2 tablespoons fresh lemon juice or white wine vinegar (optional)

Salt and pepper

Combine the rice, tomatoes, cucumber, capers, olives, cheese, and basil in a large bowl. Toss the ingredients to mix well. Just before serving, drizzle in the olive oil and lemon juice, if using, and toss again. Season the salad with salt and pepper to taste.

Tip: *Whenever you cook up a pot of rice for dinner, prepare a double batch so that you can use the leftovers to make rice salads such as this one for lunch during the workweek.*

Per serving: *Calories 250 (From Fat 150); Fat 17g (Saturated 5g); Cholesterol 22mg; Sodium 443mg; Carbohydrate 19g (Dietary Fiber 1g); Protein 7g.*

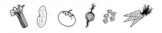

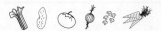 Pasta Salad with Tomato, Mozzarella, and Basil

Whenever you're cooking pasta for dinner, make extra so you'll have it on hand for pasta salads such as this recipe. You can use any stubby-shaped pasta for this recipe. If you like, serve this salad on a bed of fresh spinach leaves without significantly changing the calorie count.

Preparation time: 5 *minutes plus 20 minutes to cook the pasta, if necessary*

Yield: 4 *servings*

1 tablespoon olive oil	2 ounces reduced-fat mozzarella cheese, diced
1 tablespoon lemon juice	¼ cup finely chopped fresh basil
2 cups cooked penne, rotelle, or other stubby shaped pasta	1 large ripe tomato, diced
	Salt and pepper

Whisk together the olive oil and lemon juice in a large bowl. Add the pasta, cheese, and basil. Toss well to combine. Add the tomato and gently toss again. Season the salad with salt and pepper to taste.

Per serving: Calories 176 (From Fat 56); Fat 6g (Saturated 2g); Cholesterol 5mg; Sodium 252mg; Carbohydrate 22g (Dietary Fiber 2g); Protein 8g.

 Whenever you make a rice, pasta, or grain salad in advance, reserve half the dressing to add just before serving. Otherwise, the starchy ingredients soak up all the dressing overnight and dry out the salad. If that happens, you have to add more dressing (and more calories!) to make the salad palatable again. If you're making the salad to take to work, you can still prepare it in advance. Simply carry the leftover dressing in a separate container until you're ready to eat.

The same idea holds true for green salads, mixed vegetable salads, and fruit salads. Add the dressing just before eating so that the ingredients don't soak up the liquids and get soggy.

If your recipe makes more servings than you're going to use in one sitting, dress only the portion you'll be eating at that meal. Pack the leftover salad and dressing separately.

☌ *Pear and Blue Cheese Salad with Walnuts*

This recipe is a little treat for blue cheese lovers. Serve with a small roll or a couple of thin breadsticks to round your calories up to 300.

Preparation time: *10 minutes*

Cooking time: *2 minutes*

Yield: *4 servings*

2 tablespoons finely chopped walnuts	*4 cups torn lettuce leaves*
¼ cup light mayonnaise	*1 small celery rib, thinly sliced*
1 tablespoon fresh lemon juice, divided	*2 green onions, thinly sliced*
2 teaspoons honey	*2 ounces (about ¼ cup) crumbled blue cheese*
2 large firm-ripe red or green pears	

1 Toast the walnuts in a small, heavy, nonstick skillet over medium heat, stirring constantly, for 2 minutes, or until just fragrant. Remove the nuts from the skillet and set aside.

2 Whisk together the mayonnaise, 2 teaspoons of the lemon juice, and the honey in a large serving bowl. If you're not serving or eating the salad right away, refrigerate the dressing until ready to use, up to 5 days.

3 Thinly slice the pears and drizzle them with the remaining lemon juice. Divide the lettuce, pears, celery, and green onions between two serving plates. Drizzle with dressing and sprinkle with blue cheese and toasted nuts.

Per serving: Calories 209 (From Fat 109); Fat 12g (Saturated 4g); Cholesterol 16mg; Sodium 337mg; Carbohydrate 23g (Dietary Fiber 4g); Protein 5g.

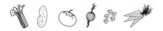

Serving Up Sandwiches

Any type of food that helps you feel full is helpful when you're on a low-calorie diet. Sandwiches certainly fit the bill because, like main dish salads, they often include all the components of a full meal — protein, grain, and vegetables. Any meal or snack that contains several different foods from different food groups can help you feel full longer and provide more sustained energy than if you were to simply grab one type of food for lunch. That's why a sandwich makes more sense for lunch than, say, an all-vegetable salad or a couple of slices of ham on their own.

When you follow the sandwich recipes in this section, you'll know that your lunch contains up to 300 calories. But what about ordering a sandwich at a deli or sandwich shop? When in doubt about the number of calories, eat just half the sandwich and fill up on a green salad with light dressing. You can always have the rest of the sandwich later as a snack or save it for the next day.

⟋ Pita Pizza with Artichokes and Mozzarella Cheese

You can prepare these pita pizzas up through Step 2, and then wrap them tightly in plastic wrap to carry them to work. Unwrap the pizza and microwave each at full power for 1 minute to heat through and melt the cheese. Serve the pizza with a ½ cup serving of soup.

Preparation time: *10 minutes plus thawing time*

Cooking time: *10 minutes*

Yield: *2 servings*

2 small (6 inch) pita breads	*Pinch of dried oregano*	*¼ cup finely chopped tomato*
2 teaspoons olive oil	*3 frozen artichoke hearts, thawed and chopped*	*1 ounce shredded light mozzarella cheese*
1 teaspoon lemon juice		

1 Preheat the oven to 450. Place the pita breads on a nonstick baking sheet.

2 Whisk together the olive oil, lemon juice, and oregano in a medium bowl. Add the artichoke hearts and tomato. Toss gently to coat. Spoon the artichoke mixture evenly over the pita rounds. Sprinkle evenly with the cheese.

3 Bake the pita pizzas for 6 to 8 minutes or until the cheese is melted and the pitas are heated through.

Per serving: Calories 187 (From Fat 66); Fat 7g (Saturated 2g); Cholesterol 7mg; Sodium 302mg; Carbohydrate 24g (Dietary Fiber 4g); Protein 9g.

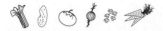

Many sandwich shops pride themselves on the amount of filling they can stuff into a sandwich. They want their customers to feel they're getting a good deal for their money. An overstuffed sandwich is rarely a good deal for a dieter, however, and sometimes even a half sandwich contains too many calories. Remove at least half the meat or other filling in an overstuffed sandwich before you eat it; ask the sandwich maker for a clean piece of foil, if possible, and wrap it to use another time.

☉ Herbed Roast Pepper and Goat Cheese on Crusty Rolls

You can broil these sandwiches at home, cool and wrap them, and then gently reheat them in a toaster oven or microwave oven at work. They're also good cold. To save a little time, you can use jarred roasted red peppers instead of roasting your own.

Preparation time: *5 minutes*

Cooking time: *10 minutes*

Yield: *2 servings*

2 small crusty rolls (2 ounces each), split lengthwise

1 small red onion, thickly sliced

1 sweet red pepper, halved and seeded

2 teaspoons olive oil

1 teaspoon dried rosemary or thyme leaves

Salt and pepper

2 ounces reduced-fat goat cheese, crumbled

1 Preheat the broiler. Place the rolls, cut-side up, on a broiler rack or pan. Broil the rolls for 1 minute or until lightly toasted. Set the bread aside.

2 Place the onion slices and pepper halves, cut-side down, on a clean broiler pan. Sprinkle the rosemary evenly over the vegetables. Drizzle evenly with the olive oil. Salt and pepper to taste.

3 Broil the vegetables 4 to 6 inches from the heat for 5 minutes or until the peppers are charred. Turn the onions over after 2 minutes or when they begin to brown. Remove the charred peppers from oven. Set aside to cool slightly, and then peel off the charred skin and cut the peppers into thick slices.

4 Arrange the peppers and onions over the bottom halves of the toasted bread. Sprinkle the sandwiches evenly with the cheese.

5 Broil the sandwiches side-by-side for 3 minutes or until the cheese is slightly browned. Top the sandwiches with the remaining bread halves, cut in half, and serve.

Tip: If you can't find lower calorie, reduced-fat goat cheese, use regular semisoft goat cheese and reduce the amount to 1 ounce.

Per serving: Calories 289 (From Fat 108); Fat 12g (Saturated 4g); Cholesterol 6mg; Sodium 706mg; Carbohydrate 36g (Dietary Fiber 3g); Protein 8g.

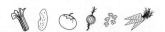

Concerning sandwich condiments and ingredients, mayonnaise may not always be a wise choice because it's so dense in calories. Some diet plans recommend eliminating mayonnaise altogether and choosing lower calorie spreads such as ketchup or mustard, while others recommend using reduced-calorie (light), reduced-fat, or fat-free mayonnaise or a combination of mayonnaise and yogurt.

Because it's a matter of taste as well as a matter of calories, you have to decide what to eat and when. If you're preparing a sandwich made with low-calorie bread and a low-calorie filling, you may well be able to afford the almost 100 calories that come with a tablespoonful of mayonnaise.

Table 13-1 shows a tablespoon-for-tablespoon comparison of the calorie counts of different bread spreads and different combinations that help reduce calories in the creamier condiments.

Table 13-1 Calorie Counts for Common Bread Spreads	
Spread	*Calories per Tablespoon*
Regular mayonnaise	90
Reduced-calorie or "light" mayonnaise	45
Reduced-fat mayonnaise	25
Lowfat plain yogurt	9
½ regular mayo + ½ lowfat yogurt	55
½ reduced-cal mayo + ½ lowfat yogurt	30
Salad dressing (mayonnaise-style)	40
Light salad dressing	25
Mustard	15
Ketchup	15

The following recipe uses light mayonnaise to create a delicious spread for toasted bread.

Toasted Italian Bread with Herbed Tuna-White Bean Spread

This recipe makes 2 cups of topping, which, on its own, provides 25 calories per tablespoon. Plan to make this spread in advance, because it needs at least two hours in the fridge for the flavors to marry. You can also toast the bread in advance and store the slices in an air-proof container until ready to use. This recipe also makes great party fare.

Preparation time: 10 minutes plus 2 hours sitting time for spread

Yield: 8 servings

½ cup parsley leaves	2 tablespoons light ricotta cheese or light cream cheese
¼ cup basil leaves or 2 teaspoons dried basil	1 teaspoon drained capers
¼ cup coarsely chopped red onion	¼ teaspoon salt
1 cup canned cannellini or navy beans, rinsed and drained	1 can (6½ ounces) tuna packed in water, drained
2 tablespoons lemon juice	l loaf Italian bread (12 ounces), cut into 24 slices, toasted
2 tablespoons light mayonnaise	

1 Combine the parsley and basil in a food processor. Process 30 seconds or until finely chopped.

2 Add the onion, beans, lemon juice, mayonnaise, ricotta, capers, and salt. Process with on/off motions for 30 seconds or until the mixture is finely chopped but not smooth, scraping down the side of the processor container with a spatula, as necessary. Add the tuna and process with on/off motion just once or twice to combine.

3 Scrape the mixture into a serving dish or storage container. Cover and refrigerate for at least 2 hours to allow the flavors to blend. Spread the topping on the toast just before serving. Top with pickle slices, if you like.

Tip: For a snack or a lighter lunch, spread this savory topping on cucumber rounds, which are practically calorie-free.

Per serving: Calories 184 (From Fat 32); Fat 4g (Saturated 1g); Cholesterol 10mg; Sodium 474mg; Carbohydrate 27g (Dietary Fiber 3g); Protein 10g.

Savoring Soups

Soup is a great choice on a low-cal diet because broth provides so few calories — it's almost like filling up on flavored water. Each of the recipes in this section comes with side-dish recommendations. Of course you can always skip them and pour yourself another ladleful of soup.

Turkey Noodle Soup

If you've ever wondered what to do with the packaged collection of vegetables in your supermarket called "soup greens" (the package that usually includes an onion, some carrots, some celery, and a turnip or parsnip), this recipe is it. You can pick up that package instead of selecting the individual vegetables used in this soup. Sprinkle a dozen oyster crackers over this soup, if you like, to use up the remaining calories.

Preparation time: *10 minutes*

Cooking time: *50 minutes*

Yield: *4 servings*

1 tablespoon olive oil

1 onion, diced

2 carrots, diced

1 celery stalk, diced

1 clove garlic, minced

1 small turnip, diced

2 cans fat-free chicken broth

1 can (14½ ounces) recipe-ready diced tomatoes

8 ounces turkey tenders

1 teaspoon dried sage or basil

1½ cups broken angel hair pasta or other thin noodles

Salt and pepper

1 Heat the oil in a large nonstick saucepan over medium heat. Add the onion and sauté 5 minutes or until tender. Add the carrot, celery, and garlic, and sauté 5 minutes longer. Add the turnip, chicken broth, tomatoes, turkey tenders, and sage. Simmer 20 to 30 minutes or until turkey is just cooked through. Remove the turkey from the soup to a cutting board.

2 Bring the soup to a boil over medium heat. Add the pasta and cook for 4 minutes or until the noodles are tender.

3 Meanwhile, cut the turkey into bite-size pieces. Stir the turkey back into the soup. Season the soup with salt and pepper to taste.

Per serving: *Calories 266 (From Fat 40); Fat 4g (Saturated 1g); Cholesterol 37mg; Sodium 919mg; Carbohydrate 35g (Dietary Fiber 4g); Protein 22g.*

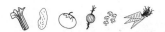

Obviously, different types of soup are going to contribute different amounts of calories, depending on the ingredients, so when you eat soup in a restaurant or order it for take-out at a deli, you're not going to know exactly how many calories it contains. The only thing you can do is think small, especially if it's a creamy or dense soup such as lentil or puréed winter squash soup. In that case, always ask for a cup instead of a bowl and order the small size to go, rather than medium or large.

Spicy Corn Chowder with Ham

Whole milk adds extra creaminess to this hearty classic, but you can stick to skim if you prefer. With a one-cup serving, you can have a small (1-ounce) square of cornbread or half of a corn muffin on the side.

Preparation time: *10 minutes*

Cooking time: *30 minutes*

Yield: *6 servings (scant 1½ cups each)*

1 tablespoon olive oil

1 large onion, diced

2 cans (14½ ounces each) or 4 cups fat-free chicken broth, divided

1 can (15 ounces) corn kernels, drained

2 cups whole milk

1 sweet red or yellow pepper, halved, seeded, and diced

1 jalapeno pepper, halved, seeded, and minced

8 ounces all-purpose potatoes, peeled and cut into ½-inch dice

4 ounces lean ham steak, diced

½ teaspoon salt

1 Heat the oil in a large nonstick saucepan over medium heat. Add the onion and sauté 5 minutes or until tender. Add 1 can (2 cups) of the broth and the corn. Heat the mixture to a boil over high heat. Lower the heat to medium-low and simmer for 5 minutes.

2 Using a slotted spoon or small sieve, transfer 1½ cups of the corn-broth mixture from the saucepan to a food processor or blender. Whirl until almost smooth. Return the pureed mixture back to the saucepan.

3 Stir in the remaining chicken broth, sweet pepper, jalapeno pepper, potatoes, ham, and salt. Bring to a boil over high heat. Lower the heat to medium-low, stir in the milk, and simmer the soup for 15 minutes or until the potatoes are tender.

Vary It! *You can substitute an equal amount of lean turkey bacon or Canadian bacon for the ham in this recipe.*

Per serving: *Calories 188 (From Fat 55); Fat 6g (Saturated 2g); Cholesterol 20mg; Sodium 1,004mg; Carbohydrate 24g (Dietary Fiber 3g); Protein 10g.*

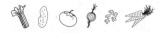

White Bean Soup with Kale and Sausage

This recipe calls for kale, which is a leafy green vegetable that's sweeter than spinach and even more nutritious. You can substitute fresh or frozen spinach, collards, or other leafy greens for the more traditional kale used in this recipe, if you like. To chop fresh kale, be sure to slice across the leaves, as shown in Figure 13-1.

Round out this soup with a slice of light rye bread or sliced tomatoes drizzled with light dressing.

Preparation time: *5 minutes*

Cooking time: *30 minutes*

Yield: *6 servings*

1 tablespoon olive oil, divided

8 ounces hot or sweet lean Italian-style turkey sausages

1 onion, diced

1 carrot, diced

2 large cloves garlic, minced

1 can (19 ounces) white beans, rinsed and drained

1 box (10 ounces) frozen chopped kale, thawed and drained or 4 cups fresh kale, cut up

3 cans (14½ ounces each) or 6 cups fat-free chicken broth

2 tablespoons white or red wine vinegar

Salt and pepper

1 Heat 1 teaspoon of the oil in a large nonstick saucepan over medium heat. Prick the sausages all over with a fork. Add the sausages to the saucepan. Cover and cook for 8 minutes or until well browned and cooked through. Transfer the sausages to paper towels to drain. Carefully wipe out the skillet with a paper towel, if necessary.

2 Heat the remaining 2 teaspoons of oil in the same skillet over medium heat. Add the onion, carrot, and garlic and sauté, stirring often, for 5 minutes or until the vegetables are tender.

3 Meanwhile, thinly slice the sausages. Add the beans, kale, broth, and sausage slices to the soup. Simmer, partially covered, for 15 minutes. Uncover and stir in the vinegar and salt and pepper to taste.

Per serving: Calories 157 (From Fat 43); Fat 5g (Saturated 1g); Cholesterol 24mg; Sodium 957mg; Carbohydrate 16g (Dietary Fiber 4g); Protein 13g.

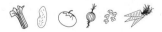

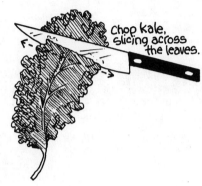

Chop kale, slicing across the leaves.

Figure 13-1:
Use a large chef's knife to chop kale correctly.

Chapter 14

Sitting Down to Delicious Dinners

*T*he one meal of the day that you can, and should, sit down and enjoy is dinner. Unlike breakfast, which is sometimes a hurried affair, and lunch, which is usually part of the workday or nibbled in between household errands, dinner can take place at home in a quiet and relaxed atmosphere. Sitting down and relaxing when you're on a low-calorie diet is important, because it encourages you to sit calmly, be mindful, and enjoy yourself while you eat.

In this chapter, I discuss the benefits of planning your dinners and making time to enjoy them. I also provide you with a variety of delicious low-calorie dinner recipes you can try.

Keeping Supper Simple and Enjoyable

The less you have to worry about what to eat for dinner (and how long you have to eat it) on a day-to-day basis, the easier sticking to your low-calorie diet will be. That's why you need to have a simple system in place that includes some advance meal planning for you and anyone who eats with you and a goal to enjoy your dinner at a reasonable pace.

Planning ahead

The following are some ways you can be sure you have low-calorie dinners on hand when you're ready to eat:

✔ **Be prepared.** Have a stock of low-calorie convenience foods such as canned soups and packaged salad mixes in your cupboards and fridge for those nights when you don't feeling like cooking.

✔ **Keep the basics stocked.** Keep staples such as dry pasta, rice, bottled tomato sauces, light bread, lean meats, eggs, and low-fat dairy products on hand at all times so that you always have the fixings for at least one full meal.

✔ **Plan ahead.** When preparing the specific recipes in this chapter, plan your meal schedule and include the suggested side dishes (or the equivalent) on your shopping list.

✔ **Cook on weekends.** Review your menus for the upcoming week and do as much advance preparation as you can over the weekend when you have more time.

Portioning out

When you prepare a recipe that makes, say, four servings, sticking to that size serving is important. Otherwise you run the risk of adding unwanted calories to your meal. As soon as you prepare the dish, divide it up evenly and put your portion on your plate. If you're eating alone, wrap up the remainders and put them in the refrigerator or freezer as soon as possible after cooking so you're not tempted to go back for more.

Freeze or refrigerate leftovers in single-serving size containers that can go directly into a microwave oven. That way, you have homemade convenience foods on hand that fit right into your low-calorie diet plan for another dinner or a ready-to-go lunch.

Feeding the rest of the family

The recipes and menu ideas in this chapter have been developed to be as balanced, nutritious, and tasty as possible for the amount of calories they provide. Except for the controlled calorie limits, they're no different than anything else you can feed your family. So you don't have to cook separate food for yourself just because you're limiting your calories to 300, unless you want to.

Family members who aren't following this low-calorie plan and who want or need more food for dinner can obviously choose to eat larger portions or expand the meal with other foods.

Preparing Pleasing Poultry Dishes

Poultry has made a name for itself as one of the best low-cal, high-protein food choices for anyone who is trying to lose weight or maintain a healthy weight. Because chicken and turkey are pretty much interchangeable, you can use either one in any of the recipes in this section.

Chicken and turkey parts prepared in a microwave oven cook quickly and turn out moist and tender, just like poultry that has been steamed or stewed. To cook plain poultry, place four even-size pieces (4 to 6 ounces each) in a microwave-safe container. If you prefer, brush the poultry lightly with olive oil or gravy before cooking. Cover the container and cook at full power for 8 minutes. Let it stand for 5 minutes before uncovering. Insert a fork or knife tip into the flesh to be sure juices run clear. Clear juices let you know the poultry is fully cooked.

Fixing quick chicken dinners

When surveyed, home cooks say they serve chicken for dinner more often than any other meat. That makes sense for dieters, too, because chicken is a lean source of high-quality animal protein. Chicken's neutral flavor also makes it easy to incorporate into the tasty, globally-influenced recipes included in this section.

Skillet Chicken Parmesan

This classic dish is prepared in a not-so-classic low-cal style, which simply means measuring ingredients carefully and omitting the initial breading and frying of the chicken breasts.

Preparation time: *5 minutes*

Cooking time: *6 minutes*

Yield: *4 servings*

12 ounces boneless, skinless chicken breasts, cut into four equal pieces

Vegetable cooking spray

½ teaspoon salt

¼ teaspoon pepper

1 cup marinara sauce

½ cup shredded reduced-fat mozzarella cheese

¼ cup grated Parmesan cheese

1 Place the chicken breasts between two sheets of plastic wrap. Pound to ¼-inch thickness with a meat mallet or the bottom of a small heavy saucepan (see Figure 14-1).

2 Coat a large nonstick skillet with vegetable cooking spray and place over medium-high heat.

3 Add the chicken to the skillet. Sprinkle with salt and pepper. Reduce heat to medium. Cook 3 to 5 minutes or until the chicken is lightly browned on the bottom. Turn the chicken over. Add the marinara sauce to the skillet. Cover and cook 2 to 4 minutes longer or until the chicken is just opaque in the center.

4 Sprinkle the mozzarella and Parmesan cheeses evenly over the chicken breasts. Cover and cook 1 to 2 minutes or until the cheese melts. Serve hot.

Tip: You can substitute a serving of chicken and sauce with ½ cup cooked spaghetti and ½ cup steamed broccoli for any 300-calorie meal in the basic menu plans in Chapter 6.

Per serving: *Calories 180 (From Fat 60); Fat 7g (Saturated 3g); Cholesterol 57mg; Sodium 762mg; Carbohydrate 6g (Dietary Fiber 1g); Protein 24g.*

Poached Chicken Breasts with Spinach-Basil Sauce

This dish is an example of true low-calorie fare because it uses both low-calorie ingredients and a low-calorie cooking technique. When you prepare this type of main dish for a 300-calorie meal, you end up with 100 calories to "spend" on the side dish of your choice. This dish is also delicious cold so you can take leftovers for lunch the next day or make it ahead to serve as a cool summer supper.

Preparation time: *10 minutes*

Cooking time: *30 minutes*

Yield: *4 servings*

12 ounces boneless, skinless chicken breast halves, in four equal pieces

1 teaspoon olive oil

1 small onion, diced

2 cups fresh baby spinach leaves, stems removed

¼ cup fresh basil leaves, stems removed

½ cup lowfat plain yogurt

1 teaspoon lemon juice

⅛ teaspoon salt

2 tablespoons shredded basil leaves (optional)

1 Place the chicken breast halves in a large skillet with enough water to cover. Bring the water to a boil. Reduce the heat, cover, and simmer the chicken for 10 minutes or until just cooked through.

2 Meanwhile, heat the oil in a large nonstick skillet over medium heat. Add the onion. Sauté for 5 minutes or until tender. Stir in the spinach and basil and cook until wilted. Turn the mixture into a wire mesh strainer and press lightly with a spoon to drain any excess liquid.

3 Combine the spinach mixture with the yogurt, lemon juice, and salt in a food processor or blender. Whirl for 1 minute or until smoothly puréed, scraping down the side of the container with a rubber spatula, as necessary.

4 Divide the spinach sauce evenly among four serving plates. Cut the chicken breasts into thick slices and arrange on top of the sauce. Sprinkle with shredded basil, if you like.

Per serving: *Calories 130 (From Fat 32); Fat 4g (Saturated 1g); Cholesterol 49mg; Sodium 155mg; Carbohydrate 5g (Dietary Fiber 1g); Protein 19g.*

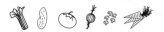

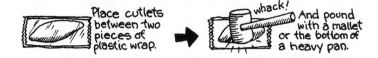

Chicken Cutlets Pounded to an Even Thickness

Place cutlets between two pieces of plastic wrap.

whack! And pound with a mallet or the bottom of a heavy pan.

Indonesian Chicken and Vegetables with Peanut Dipping Sauce

This dish is simple and fun for a casual party, as well as a quick and easy everyday meal. The peanut sauce alone, which is good on just about any meat or vegetable you can think of, contributes 25 calories per tablespoon.

Preparation time: *15 minutes*

Cooking time: *5 minutes*

Yield: *4 servings*

8 ounces boneless, skinless, chicken breast	1 cup water
⅓ cup creamy peanut butter	1 cup mini carrot sticks
⅓ cup cider or rice wine vinegar	2 celery stalks, cut into 2-inch lengths
1 tablespoon soy sauce	1 large sweet red pepper, cut into strips
2 teaspoon sugar	1 cup raw or steamed green beans
2 cloves garlic, finely chopped	1 cup raw or steamed snow peas
¼ teaspoon crushed red pepper flakes	

1 Place the chicken breasts in a medium-size deep skillet and cover with water. Bring the water to a boil over medium heat. Reduce the heat to low and gently simmer for 5 minutes or until the chicken is just cooked through. Drain the chicken and cut into bite-size chunks.

2 Meanwhile, combine the peanut butter, vinegar, soy sauce, sugar, garlic, and red pepper flakes in a small saucepan. Stir until blended. Slowly stir in the 1 cup of water. Bring to a gentle boil over medium heat. Simmer, stirring often, for 2 minutes. Set aside to thicken and cool slightly.

3 Divide the chicken chunks, carrots, celery, pepper, green beans, and snow peas among four serving plates. Divide the sauce among four small cups or bowls and place them in the center of the serving plates. Serve with toothpicks or utensils for dipping the chicken.

Per serving: Calories 247 (From Fat 112); Fat 12g (Saturated 3g); Cholesterol 31mg; Sodium 394mg; Carbohydrate 18g (Dietary Fiber 5g); Protein 19g.

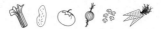

 The following recipe calls for fresh breadcrumbs. You may think that making these crumbs is a difficult task, but it's not! Just place slices of light bread in a food processor and pulse with an on/off motion until fine crumbs are formed. When you're measuring the crumbs, pack them loosely into the measuring cup.

Chicken Breasts with Honey-Mustard Crumb Coating

This recipe is for people who prefer "chicken on the bone" to the boneless cutlets used so often in low-calorie poultry recipes.

Preparation time: *10 minutes*

Cooking time: *20 minutes*

Yield: *4 servings*

Nonstick cooking spray

⅓ cup honey mustard

1 tablespoon lemon juice

4 small chicken breast halves on the bone (6 to 8 ounces each), skin removed

1 cup fresh breadcrumbs (from 2 small slices of light bread)

1 tablespoon olive oil

1 Preheat the oven to 400. Line a baking sheet with aluminum foil and spray the foil with nonstick cooking spray. Combine the honey mustard and lemon juice in a small bowl.

2 Arrange the chicken breasts on the foil-lined sheet. Brush the mustard mixture evenly over each breast. Sprinkle evenly with breadcrumbs, pressing lightly so the crumbs stick. Drizzle with olive oil.

3 Bake the chicken for 20 to 30 minutes or until the crust is crisp and the breasts are just cooked through.

Per serving: Calories 276 (From Fat 96); Fat 11g (Saturated 2g); Cholesterol 76mg; Sodium 176mg; Carbohydrate 15g (Dietary Fiber 0g); Protein 29g.

Jamaican Jerk Chicken Kabobs with Rice

Jerk is a Caribbean style of barbecue that adds unforgettable flavor to a simple chicken dish. In this recipe, the chicken and vegetables are skewered and broiled indoors. You can also cook them on an outdoor grill.

Tools: *16 wooden or metal skewers (6 to 8 inches long)*

Preparation time: *15 minutes plus 15 minutes marinating*

Cooking time: *15 minutes*

Yield: *8 servings (1 kabob per serving)*

¼ cup apple cider vinegar

2 tablespoons light brown sugar

2 tablespoons vegetable oil

2 tablespoons finely chopped garlic

1 tablespoon ground allspice

1 tablespoon finely chopped fresh ginger or ½ teaspoon ground ginger

½ teaspoon salt

¼ teaspoon pepper

Dash or two of hot sauce

1¼ pounds boneless, skinless chicken breasts, cut into 1½-inch cubes

8 green onions, trimmed and cut into 2-inch lengths

2 large sweet green, red, or yellow peppers, cut into 1½-inch pieces

2 cups fresh pineapple chunks or 1 can (20 ounces) pineapple chunks in juice, drained

4 cups hot cooked white or brown rice

1 Soak 16 wooden skewers in a pan of warm water for at least 10 minutes to prevent them from burning. You don't need to prepare metal skewers.

2 Combine the vinegar, sugar, oil, garlic, allspice, ginger, salt, pepper, and hot sauce in a large bowl. Remove 2 tablespoons of the marinade to a small bowl and set aside.

3 Add the chicken cubes to the large bowl of marinade and stir to coat. Set aside at room temperature for 15 minutes.

4 Preheat the broiler or grill.

5 Alternately thread the onion, pepper, and pineapple pieces onto 8 skewers. Thread the marinated chicken cubes onto the remaining 8 skewers. Discard the chicken marinade.

6 Grill or broil skewers 4 to 6 inches from heat for 5 to 10 minutes or until the chicken is cooked through and vegetables are tender-crisp, turning once during cooking time and brushing vegetables with reserved 2 tablespoons of marinade. Serve 1 chicken skewer and 1 vegetable skewer over each ½ cup of hot cooked rice.

Per serving: Calories 232 (From Fat 30); Fat 3g (Saturated 1g); Cholesterol 39mg; Sodium 87mg; Carbohydrate 33g (Dietary Fiber 2g); Protein 17g.

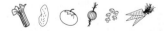

Putting a new twist on turkey

You'd never know that not too long ago, fresh turkey was used mostly for holiday foods and rarely served at regular everyday meals. Now you can buy as many different cuts of turkey in the supermarket as you can chicken, and ground turkey and turkey often substitute for beef or pork in classic dishes such as the stuffed peppers in this section. Even better, you can also buy precooked fresh turkey almost everywhere to use on sandwiches and in recipes that call for cooked or leftover turkey, such as the open-face turkey sandwich recipe in this section.

Hot Turkey Sandwiches

An open-face sandwich on a single slice of bread is one great way to enjoy your favorite flavors by cutting back on the amount of food you eat, rather than eliminating "added" calorie foods like gravy from your diet altogether. Serve this recipe with steamed green beans or a tossed green salad drizzled with 1 or 2 teaspoons of light dressing.

Preparation time: *5 minutes*

Cooking time: *10 minutes*

Yield: *4 servings*

¼ cup chicken broth	*1 teaspoon Dijon-style mustard*
1 cup mushrooms, thinly sliced	*8 ounces sliced cooked turkey breast*
2 cups turkey, chicken, or white gravy	*4 slices light bread, toasted*
¼ teaspoon dried tarragon	

1 Combine the broth and the mushrooms in a heavy nonstick skillet over medium-high heat. Cook for 7 to 10 minutes, or until the mushrooms are tender and the liquid is almost evaporated. Stir in the gravy, tarragon, and mustard. Mix well. Add turkey slices and simmer until hot.

2 Place a slice of toast on each serving plate. Top with turkey and gravy.

Per serving: *Calories 189 (From Fat 33); Fat 4g (Saturated 1g); Cholesterol 50mg; Sodium 912mg; Carbohydrate 16g (Dietary Fiber 2g); Protein 23g.*

Roasted Red Peppers Stuffed with Turkey Sausage and Rice

These are old-fashioned stuffed peppers updated to include lower calorie ingredients such as reduced-fat cheese and lean turkey sausages. Each filled pepper is a 300-calorie meal in itself.

Preparation time: *15 minutes*

Cooking time: *45 minutes*

Yield: *4 servings*

4 large sweet red, yellow, or green peppers, halved lengthwise and seeded

8 ounces lean, sweet Italian-style turkey sausage, removed from casings

1½ cups cooked rice

¾ cup shredded reduced-fat cheddar cheese

1 teaspoon Italian seasoning

1½ cups marinara sauce

1 Preheat the broiler. Arrange the peppers, cut side down, on a broiler pan.

2 Broil the peppers 4 inches from the heat for 3 to 5 minutes, or until they just start to blacken in spots but are still firm. Transfer the peppers, cut side up, to a 9-inch square baking dish. Set aside.

3 Preheat the oven to 375.

4 In a large nonstick skillet, cook the loose sausage over medium heat for 3 to 5 minutes or until just cooked through, breaking up the meat with a wooden spoon. Remove the skillet from the heat and stir in the rice, cheese, and Italian seasoning. Divide the rice mixture evenly among the pepper halves, packing the mixture into the peppers with a spoon. Cover the baking dish with aluminum foil.

5 Bake the peppers for 20 minutes or until tender.

6 Meanwhile, heat the marinara sauce in the same nonstick skillet, scraping up any browned bits of sausage with a wooden spoon. Spoon a little of the sauce over the peppers halfway through baking time. Serve the remaining sauce with the peppers.

Per serving: Calories 304 (From Fat 90); Fat 10g (Saturated 4g); Cholesterol 49mg; Sodium 905mg; Carbohydrate 37g (Dietary Fiber 5g); Protein 19g.

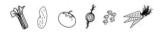

Making the Most of Meat

Meat is great source or protein and hard-to-get minerals such as iron and zinc, but it can also be high in calories, especially when you choose fattier cuts or eat too much of it. That's especially true if a lot of your meat is coming from fast-food restaurants. But the meat you cook at home doesn't have to be a diet-buster or a health hazard. The following are two great ways to enjoy meat without overdoing it:

- **Treat meat more like a condiment than a main dish.** In other words, use very small amounts of meat to flavor foods like soups, stews, rice dishes, pastas, and casseroles dishes, such as lasagna.

- **Cut back on portion sizes.** You probably do the same thing with all your other favorite foods when you're trying to get to or stay at a healthy weight. So if you're a meat-and-potato type, you can continue to enjoy those foods on a low-calorie diet by choosing leaner cuts and eating less meat (and fewer potatoes) overall.

Beefing up your meals

This section includes two easy, beefy recipes that are guaranteed to please dieters and nondieters alike. One is a recipe for kabobs marinated in sweet, teriyaki-style marinade, and the other is a classic steak-and-potatoes combo.

A wonderful, calorie-free way to flavor meats is with dry spice rubs that you simply rub onto the meat with your hands before cooking. A *spice rub* is simply a combination of herbs and/or spices rubbed over the surface of lightly oiled meat before it's cooked. This combination is especially good for beef or lamb. To make a spice rub, combine 1 tablespoon paprika, 2 teaspoons crushed rosemary, 1 teaspoon garlic powder, 1 teaspoon crushed fennel seed, 1 teaspoon dried oregano, 1 teaspoon ground black pepper, ½ teaspoon ground red pepper, and ½ teaspoon salt. Use about 1 tablespoon per pound of meat, and allow the rubbed meat to stand at room temperature for at least 30 minutes or up to 1 hour before cooking so the seasoning mix has a chance to permeate the meat.

Asian Beef Kabobs

A simple soy-sauce–based marinade that you can also use for poultry and fish flavors this recipe. To round the menu out to a 300-calorie meal, serve with ½ cup ramen noodles and a cucumber and radish salad drizzled with rice wine vinegar or another flavored vinegar and a pinch of salt.

Tools: *8 bamboo skewers*

Preparation time: *15 minutes plus 20 minutes marinating*

Cooking time: *5 minutes*

Yield: *4 servings*

2 tablespoons light brown sugar

1½ tablespoons dry sherry

1½ tablespoons soy sauce

1 teaspoon dark sesame oil

1 clove garlic, minced

¼ teaspoon ground ginger

8 ounces boneless beef top sirloin, cut into ¼-inch thick slices

3 green onions, cut into 1½ inch pieces

1 Combine the sugar, sherry, soy sauce, sesame oil, garlic, and ginger in a medium-size bowl. Measure out and reserve 1 tablespoon of the marinade. Add the beef to the bowl with the remaining marinade and stir to coat. Marinate the beef in the refrigerator for at least 20 minutes.

2 Soak 8 bamboo skewers in water for 10 minutes to prevent them from burning under the broiler. (If you're using metal skewers, this step is unnecessary.)

3 Preheat the broiler. Line the broiler pan with foil for easier cleaning. Remove the beef from the marinade and discard the marinade. Alternately thread the beef, weaving back and forth, and green onion pieces onto skewers. Arrange the skewers on the broiler pan.

4 Broil the kabobs about 3 inches from the heat for 3 minutes. Turn the skewers and broil another 2 to 3 minutes or until desired doneness, basting the meat once with the reserved marinade.

Per serving: *Calories 94 (From Fat 29); Fat 3g (Saturated 1g); Cholesterol 32mg; Sodium 199mg; Carbohydrate 4g (Dietary Fiber 0g); Protein 11g.*

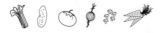

Grilled Steak with Blue Cheese–Mashed Potatoes

Flank steak is a perfect cut for outdoor cooking on a grill. All you need to round out the meal is a tossed green salad drizzled with a teaspoon or two of light dressing.

Preparation time: *5 minutes*

Cooking time: *15 minutes*

Yield: *4 servings*

10 ounces flank steak	*1 tablespoon olive oil or butter*
Salt and pepper to taste	*1½ tablespoons skim milk*
¾ pound all-purpose potatoes, peeled and cut into 1-inch cubes	*2 tablespoons blue cheese, crumbled*

1 Preheat the broiler. Line the broiler pan with aluminum foil for easier cleanup. Place the steak on the broiler pan and sprinkle with salt and pepper.

2 Place the potatoes in a large saucepan with lightly salted water to cover. Heat the water to boiling over medium-high heat. Reduce the heat to low and simmer for 15 minutes or until the potatoes are tender. Drain, reserving some of the water. Add the remaining ingredients and salt and pepper to taste. Mash the potatoes with an electric mixer or potato masher until smooth, adding some reserved cooking liquid if the mixture is too thick.

3 Meanwhile, broil steak 4 inches from the heat for 3 minutes on each side or until desired doneness. Remove the steak from the broiler pan and let stand 5 minutes before slicing on the diagonal (see Figure 14-2).

Per serving: Calories 215 (From Fat 88); Fat 10g (Saturated 4g); Cholesterol 37mg; Sodium 424mg; Carbohydrate 15g (Dietary Fiber 2g); Protein 16g.

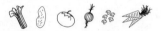

Figure 14-2:
Slice a flank steak across the grain for more tender meat.

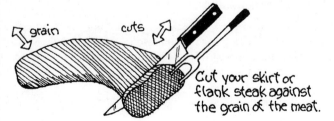

Picking pork and ham

Thanks to changes in agricultural systems and animal feeding, the pork you buy in the supermarket is actually about 30 percent leaner these days than it was 20 or 30 years ago. Those changes mean ounce for ounce, pork is also lower in calories. That's great news for dieters who want to include a variety of meat products in their diets. The recipes in this section make delicious use of lean loin pork chops, today's lower-fat ham, and Canadian-style bacon, which is a precooked, lowfat ham product that's packaged in individual slices just perfect for anyone who's counting calories.

Cranberry Pork Chops

The flavor of pork marries well with almost any fruit. In this recipe, canned cranberry sauce adds fruity flavor and sweetness to a savory sauce. Serve these tasty chops with a cupful of steamed green beans or broccoli on the side.

Preparation time: *15 minutes*

Cooking time: *15 minutes*

Yield: *4 servings*

1½ teaspoons olive oil

4 boneless pork loin chops (3 ounces each)

1 cup diced onion

½ cup finely chopped carrot

1 cup chicken broth

⅓ cup whole-berry or jellied cranberry sauce

1 tablespoon balsamic vinegar or red wine vinegar

1 Heat the oil in a large nonstick skillet over medium-high heat. Add the pork chops and cook for 1 minute on each side. Remove the chops from the skillet and set aside on a warm covered plate.

2 Add the onions and carrots to the skillet and cook over medium heat for 5 minutes or until lightly browned and tender. Return the chops to the skillet and add the broth. Cover, reduce heat to low, and simmer for 5 minutes, until the pork is cooked through-out. (Cooking time depends on the thickness of the chops.) Remove the chops from the skillet to a covered platter to keep warm.

3 Add the cranberry sauce and vinegar to the skillet. Cook over low heat, stirring, for 1 to 2 minutes or until the cranberry sauce is melted and heated through. Return the chops to the skillet and cook just until the pork is heated throughout. Transfer the chops to serving plates. Spoon any remaining sauce over the chops.

Per serving: Calories 214 (From Fat 83); Fat 9g (Saturated 3g); Cholesterol 48mg; Sodium 298mg; Carbohydrate 14g (Dietary Fiber 2g); Protein 18g.

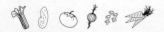

Risotto with Ham and Peas

Creamy, hearty risotto is a slow-cooked Italian rice dish that's especially satisfying to eat when you're on a low-calorie diet. By gradually adding liquid to the rice and stirring constantly as it cooks, you release a starch that creates a very creamy rice mixture. It's best to make risotto with Arborio rice, which you can find in the rice section of most large supermarkets or specialty food shops. Serve with sliced tomatoes, drizzled with just a teaspoon or two of light dressing.

Preparation time: *10 minutes*

Cooking time: *45 minutes*

Yield: *6 servings*

1 tablespoon olive oil	*1 cup frozen green peas or baby green peas*
1 small onion, finely chopped	*6 ounces Canadian-style bacon or lean ham, diced*
1 clove garlic, finely chopped	
1 cup Arborio rice	*½ teaspoon salt*
3½ cups fat-free chicken broth, heated and divided	*¼ teaspoon pepper*
	½ cup grated Parmesan cheese

1 Heat the oil in a medium nonstick saucepan over medium heat. Add onion and sauté 5 minutes. Add garlic and sauté 1 minute longer. Stir in rice.

2 Add ½ cup of the chicken broth and stir often for about 2 minutes or until the broth is absorbed. Add all but ½ cup of the remaining broth, ½ cup at a time, stirring after each addition until the liquid is absorbed.

3 Stir in the peas, ham, salt, pepper, and remaining ½ cup broth. Cook, stirring, for 5 to 8 minutes or until the rice is tender and somewhat creamy. Remove the rice from heat and stir in Parmesan cheese. Serve immediately.

Per serving: *Calories 248 (From Fat 59); Fat 7g (Saturated 3g); Cholesterol 15mg; Sodium 977mg; Carbohydrate 34g (Dietary Fiber 2g); Protein 14g.*

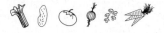

Glazed Ham Steaks

A combination of apple butter and honey mustard elevates the everyday status of humble ham steaks to company-worthy fare. As part of a 300-calorie meal, serve the ham with ½ cup corn kernels, ½ cup creamed spinach, and a small (2-inch) square of cornbread. This menu also makes a great low-calorie holiday meal.

Preparation time: *5 minutes*

Cooking time: *3 minutes*

Yield: *4 servings*

12 ounce lean ham steak	*1 tablespoon honey mustard*
¼ cup apple butter	

1 Preheat the broiler. Lightly score the ham steak with a sharp knife. Cut into four equal pieces and place, scored side-up, on a foil-lined broiler rack.

2 In a small bowl, stir together fruit spread and mustard. Spread evenly over ham steaks.

3 Broil steaks 4 inches from the heat for 3 minutes or until just browned. Be careful not to burn the glaze.

Per serving: *Calories 128 (From Fat 32); Fat 4g (Saturated 1g); Cholesterol 45mg; Sodium 1,134mg; Carbohydrate 10g (Dietary Fiber 0g); Protein 14g.*

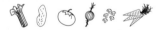

Fishing for Seafood Dinners

Many fish recipes call for cod because it's not only lean and low in calories, but it's also often readily available wherever seafood is sold. Flounder, sole, and snapper are among the fish that are equally low in calories and fat. Because of their mild flavor, you can substitute them in most recipes that call for cod. Shellfish such as shrimp and crab are even lower in calories, but if you're watching your dietary cholesterol, you may want to limit the amount of shrimp you include in your diet. Two of the following recipes use oven-frying and steaming, two low-calorie cooking techniques that work particularly well with seafood.

Cod Stew Provencal

Fennel seed is the "secret" ingredient that gives this soup such a special flavor. If fresh fennel is available, you can use it as a substitute for the celery (see Figure 14-3 to find out what fresh fennel looks like). You can also substitute tilapia if cod is unavailable. To bring this dish up to 300 calories, serve with four saltine crackers or a small breadstick on the side.

Preparation time: *5 minutes*

Cooking time: *20 minutes*

Yield: *4 servings*

1 tablespoon olive oil	*1 bottle (8 ounces) clam juice*
1 onion, finely chopped	*¼ teaspoon fennel seeds, crushed*
1 celery stalk, thinly sliced or 1 fennel bulb, finely chopped	*1 pound cod fillets or other boneless white fish*
1 large Yukon gold potato, cut into ½-inch cubes	*Salt and pepper, to taste*
2 cans (14½ ounces each) diced tomatoes in juice	

1 Heat the olive oil in a large nonstick skillet over medium heat. Add the onion and sauté 5 minutes or until tender. Add celery, and sauté 1 more minute. Add potato and sauté, stirring often, 5 minutes longer.

2 Add the tomatoes with their juice, clam juice, and fennel seeds to the pan. Heat to boiling. Reduce heat to low and simmer for 5 minutes.

3 Add the cod. Partially cover the pan and cook, stirring occasionally to break up the fish, for 5 minutes or until the vegetables are tender and the cod is opaque. Add salt and pepper to taste. Serve hot.

Per serving: Calories 232 (From Fat 38); Fat 4g (Saturated 1g); Cholesterol 48mg; Sodium 923mg; Carbohydrate 23g (Dietary Fiber 2g); Protein 26g.

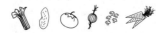

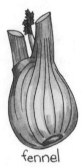

Figure 14-3:
Fresh fennel is a bulb-shaped vegetable that tastes a bit like anise or licorice.

fennel

Oven "Fried" Fish Fillets

When you bite into these fillets with their crispy coating, you'll think you're eating fried fish. To round out a 300-calorie menu, serve the fish with a small ear of corn and a tossed green salad with light dressing.

Preparation time: *10 minutes*

Cooking time: *8 minutes*

Yield: *4 servings*

1 pound flounder or sole fillets, cut into 4 equal pieces

1 tablespoon reduced-fat mayonnaise

⅓ cup dried seasoned breadcrumbs

2 tablespoons fresh parsley, minced

½ teaspoon paprika

1 lemon, cut in wedges

1 Preheat the oven to 450. Lightly coat a baking sheet with nonstick cooking spray.

2 Brush the fish fillets with mayonnaise. Combine the breadcrumbs, parsley, and paprika in a shallow dish. Dredge the coated fillets in the breadcrumb mixture. Arrange the fillets on the prepared baking sheet.

3 Bake the fish for 8 minutes or until the flesh is opaque and flakes easily when a fork is inserted in fillet's center. Serve with lemon wedges.

Per serving: Calories 142 (From Fat 25); Fat 3g (Saturated 1g); Cholesterol 55mg; Sodium 376mg; Carbohydrate 8g (Dietary Fiber 1g); Protein 20g.

Pasta with Tuna, Olives, and Tomatoes

Cherry tomatoes make this a pasta dish that's delicious year-round. A small breadstick on the side brings this dish up to 300 calories.

Preparation time: *15 minutes*

Cooking time: *10 minutes*

Yield: *6 servings*

8 ounces (about 2 cups) uncooked small shaped pasta such as fusilli, rotelle, wheels, or shells

2 cans (6½ ounces each) tuna packed in water

2 cups cherry tomatoes, halved

½ cup pitted imported ripe olives, sliced

¼ cup chopped fresh parsley

1 tablespoon olive oil

1 tablespoon lemon juice or white wine vinegar (optional)

1 Cook the pasta following package directions. Drain well.

2 Meanwhile, combine the tuna, tomatoes, olives, parsley, and oil in a large bowl. Add drained pasta and gently toss. Add lemon juice or vinegar, if you prefer, and toss again. Serve hot.

Vary It! *You can substitute ½ cup chopped sun-dried tomatoes for the fresh tomatoes. If the sun-dried tomatoes come packed in oil, eliminate the olive oil in the recipe.*

Per serving: Calories 242 (From Fat 50); Fat 5g (Saturated 1g); Cholesterol 20mg; Sodium 283mg; Carbohydrate 31g (Dietary Fiber 2g); Protein 17g.

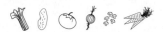

Steamed Ginger Shrimp with Snow Peas

If you don't own a steamer, refer to Chapter 5 for tips on constructing your own from basic pots, pans, and utensils you may already have in your kitchen. In Chapter 5 you can also find basic steaming instructions. Serve this dish with ½ cup hot cooked rice or ramen noodles, flavored with some of the steaming liquid, and sliced tomatoes and cucumbers tossed with light dressing.

Preparation time: *10 minutes plus 30 minutes marinating*

Cooking time: *4 to 8 minutes*

Yield: *4 servings*

¼ cup white wine or chicken broth	24 large shrimp (1 to 1¼ pounds), shelled and deveined
1 tablespoon finely chopped ginger root	
1 tablespoon soy sauce	12 ounces snow peas (about 2 cups)
2 teaspoons finely chopped garlic	1 tablespoon finely chopped cilantro

1 Combine the wine, ginger root, soy sauce, and garlic in a medium bowl. Add the shrimp. Toss gently to coat. Marinate at room temperature for 30 minutes.

2 In a steamer filled with enough boiling water to barely reach the bottom of the steamer tray, arrange the shrimp in the tray in a single layer. Top with snow peas. Pour the remaining marinade over the snow peas. Cover and steam for 4 minutes or until the shrimp are opaque. (This step may be easier to do in two separate batches.)

3 Sprinkle the shrimp with cilantro before serving.

Per serving: Calories 148 (From Fat 12); Fat 1g (Saturated 0g); Cholesterol 210mg; Sodium 475mg; Carbohydrate 7g (Dietary Fiber 2g); Protein 26g.

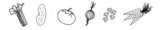

Trying a Variety of Vegetarian Dishes

In books and articles about health and weight control, I often see advice to eat at least one vegetarian dinner a week. I agree with this advice and even suggest that you work at least one vegetarian day into your diet every week, because you can benefit from eating a vegetarian diet in many ways. For one thing, it's a good way to get more fresh vegetables, beans, and grains into your diet, along with the vitamins, minerals, and fiber that come with them. Another reason vegetarian meals are helpful on a low-cal diet is that they add variety to a plan that limits the amount of food you can eat, which can help prevent you from getting bored.

⌕ Simple and Savory Black Bean Chili with Cheese

Hearty foods like chili are a satisfying break from lighter diet fare. To get all 300 of the calories you're entitled to for dinner, stir ¼ cup of rice into your chili bowl or serve with half a dozen baked tortilla chips. Like most tomato-based sauces and stews, chili tastes even better when it's reheated the day after it's made. If you like, substitute a dollop of low-fat plain yogurt or fat-free sour cream for the shredded cheese topping.

Preparation time: *10 minutes*

Cooking time: *30 minutes*

Yield: *6 servings*

1 teaspoon olive oil	*2 cans (14 ounces each) diced tomatoes in juice*
1 large onion, finely chopped	
1 sweet green, red, or yellow pepper, finely chopped	*1 can (8 ounces) corn kernels, drained*
	½ teaspoon chili powder
1 tablespoon finely chopped garlic	*½ teaspoon ground cumin*
2 cans (15 ounces each) black beans, rinsed and drained	*¼ teaspoon ground cinnamon*
	2 ounces (½ cup) shredded reduced-fat cheddar cheese

1 Heat oil in large nonstick skillet over medium heat. Add onion and sauté 5 minutes or until softened. Add sweet pepper and sauté 3 minutes. Add garlic and sauté 1 minute. Stir in the beans, tomatoes with juice, corn, chili powder, cumin, and cinnamon. Cover and simmer gently for 15 minutes, stirring occasionally.

2 Spoon chili into four individual bowls and top with shredded cheese. Serve hot.

Per serving: *Calories 175 (From Fat 36); Fat 4g (Saturated 2g); Cholesterol 7mg; Sodium 715mg; Carbohydrate 27g (Dietary Fiber 7g); Protein 10g.*

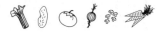

☞ *Tostadas with Avocado, Corn, and Refried Beans*

This easy-to-assemble, one-dish meal quickly satisfies your hunger for classic Tex-Mex food. When you use fat-free beans and reduced-fat cheese, you can pile your tortilla high with flavorful ingredients and still stick to your 300-calorie dinner limit.

Preparation time: *10 minutes*

Cooking time: *7 minutes*

Yield: *4 servings*

4 small (6 inch) corn tortillas

1 can (15 ounces) fat-free refried beans

1 cup prepared salsa, divided

1 can (8 ounces) corn kernels, drained and divided

½ small avocado, diced

½ cup shredded reduced-fat cheese

1 cup shredded crisp lettuce such as iceberg or romaine

½ cup low-fat plain yogurt

2 green onions, thinly sliced

2 tablespoons finely chopped cilantro

1 Preheat the oven to broil. Arrange the tortillas in a single layer on a broiler rack. Broil 4 to 6 inches from the heat for 1 to 2 minutes or until edges start to brown. Set aside.

2 Meanwhile, combine the beans, ½ cup of the salsa, and ½ can of the corn in a medium saucepan. Cook, over medium heat, stirring often, for 5 minutes or until heated through.

3 Combine the remaining salsa, remaining corn, and avocado in a small bowl.

4 Spread the bean mixture evenly over the tortillas. Sprinkle with cheese. Top with lettuce, avocado mixture, yogurt, green onions, and cilantro. Serve warm.

Per serving: *Calories 296 (From Fat 76); Fat 9g (Saturated 3g); Cholesterol 12mg; Sodium 1,012mg; Carbohydrate 44g (Dietary Fiber 10g); Protein 14g.*

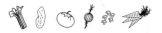

☝ Stuffed Portobello Mushrooms

These giant, meaty mushrooms, packed with hearty white beans, tomatoes, basil, and mozzarella cheese, are practically a meal. Serve them with a small, mixed vegetable salad tossed with a teaspoon or two of light dressing.

Preparation time: *10 minutes*

Cooking time: *15 minutes*

Yield: *4 servings (2 mushrooms per serving)*

8 large portobello mushrooms (2 ounces each), stemmed

1 can (19 ounces) navy beans, rinsed and drained

1 can (14 ounces) diced tomatoes in tomato juice

½ cup chopped fresh basil or 1 tablespoon dried basil

½ cup shredded part-skim mozzarella cheese

¼ teaspoon ground black pepper

2 tablespoons grated Parmesan cheese

1 Preheat the oven to 400. Use a spoon to scrape out the black gills from the mushrooms. Place the mushrooms, stem side down, on a nonstick, rimmed baking sheet. Cover with aluminum foil.

2 Bake the mushrooms for 10 to 15 minutes or until just tender. Remove the mushrooms from the baking sheet and drain on paper towels. Leave the oven on.

3 In a medium bowl, mash the beans slightly with a potato masher or fork. Stir in the tomatoes with their juice, basil, mozzarella cheese, and pepper until mixed. Spoon the mixture evenly into the mushrooms. Sprinkle evenly with Parmesan cheese.

4 Bake for 10 minutes or until heated through.

Per serving: Calories 206 (From Fat 31); Fat 4g (Saturated 2g); Cholesterol 10mg; Sodium 671mg; Carbohydrate 29g (Dietary Fiber 6g); Protein 14g.

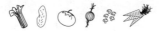

The following recipe for Curried Rice Pilaf features toasted almonds. To toast the almonds, place a small heavy skillet over medium-low heat. Add the almonds and cook, stirring often, until the almonds just begin to turn golden around the edges and become fragrant. Remove the almonds from the skillet immediately and set them aside to cool.

⏂ Curried Rice Pilaf

For maximum flavor in this dish, use basmati, Texmati, jasmine, or another flavorful long-grain rice.

Preparation time: *10 minutes*

Cooking time: *30 minutes*

Yield: *4 servings*

1 tablespoon olive oil	2 tablespoons golden or dark raisins
1 onion, diced	1½ cups chicken broth
¾ cup long-grain white rice	1 small sweet red pepper, finely chopped
1 teaspoon curry powder	1 cup drained garbanzo beans (chick-peas)
¼ teaspoon ground cinnamon	2 tablespoons toasted sliced almonds

1 Heat the oil in a large nonstick skillet over medium heat. Add the onion. Sauté 5 minutes or until tender.

2 Stir in the rice, curry powder, and cinnamon. Add the raisins and broth. Bring to a boil. Lower the heat, cover the skillet, and simmer for 10 minutes.

3 Stir in the pepper and beans. Cover and simmer 5 minutes longer or until the rice is tender. Remove the skillet from the heat and set aside, covered, for 10 minutes.

4 Sprinkle the pilaf with the almonds just before serving.

Per serving: Calories 294 (From Fat 69); Fat 8g (Saturated 1g); Cholesterol 2mg; Sodium 568mg; Carbohydrate 49g (Dietary Fiber 5g); Protein 8g.

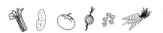

Chapter 15

Fitting In Snacks and Desserts

*W*hen you're counting every calorie in an attempt to lose weight, you may think snacks and desserts are something you'll never see again in this lifetime. Not so! For most dieters, sweet and salty treats are an important part of losing weight and often serve as motivators when you use your snack calories for favorite comfort foods and other special treats. I, myself, live for the moment when I know that I've eaten enough healthy stuff to justify the (heaping) tablespoon or two of chocolate chip cookie dough ice cream I plan into my diet most days.

You don't need to torture yourself about forbidden foods because no foods are forbidden on this diet. True, the foods you may think of as forbidden — cookies, candies, chips, dips, and chocolate chip cookie dough ice cream — are quite limited on a calorie-controlled weight-loss plan. They have to be. But if you can control the amount you eat, then don't feel guilty. This diet doesn't prohibit you from sampling these yummy treats.

The healthiest sweet stuff usually includes some type of fruit, and the healthiest savory snacks are usually made with some type of vegetable matter. If you choose healthier treats most of the time to use for your snack calories, then, as a registered dietitian, I can say without reservation, "Go right ahead and enjoy the cookies, candies, crackers, chips, dips, and chocolate chip cookie dough ice cream you eat (in moderation) from time to time."

In this chapter, I provide some 100-calorie snack and dessert recipes that are healthful, easy to prepare, and fun to eat. I also throw in a list of 50-calorie snacks for those of you who want to break your 100-calorie snack allowance into two extra mini-snacks.

Being Smart about Munching between Meals

If you like to snack but think you have to sneak your snacks or, at the very least, feel guilty about eating them, think again. A well-planned snack can help because it

✔ Provides energy

✔ Keeps your blood sugar steady throughout the day

✔ Fills nutritional gaps in your diet

✔ Facilitates weight loss by preventing you from getting too hungry and overeating at your next meal

For many low-calorie dieters, a snack eaten sometime between lunch and dinner is the most important "meal" of the day because it staves off the hunger and fatigue that often accompanies *afternoon slump,* which is the energy gap that many people suffer toward the end of the workday. An afternoon snack fills that gap and helps tide you over until dinner.

In the following sections, I give you a few tips and tricks for eating snacks and desserts without wrecking your low-calorie plan.

Adding variety to snacks and desserts

To get the most out of your snack calories, think of snacks (and desserts, for that matter) as mini-meals, and balance them the way you would balance a small meal, with a little bit of protein, a little bit of carbohydrate, and maybe a little fat. Balancing snacks and desserts serves the same purpose as balancing the rest of your diet. When you eat different types of foods together, your body metabolizes them at different rates, which means a steadier and longer-lasting supply of energy. Your snacks and desserts will do a better job of tiding you over until your next meal.

For example, instead of eating 100 calories worth of saltine crackers (6 or 7 crackers), have three crackers, half an ounce of reduced-fat cheese, and a few apple or orange slices. This type of snack can compensate for nutrients that may be low or missing in your regular meals. In this example, you're getting calcium, protein, and a little fat from the cheese, different types of carbohydrates, vitamins, and minerals from the fruit and crackers, and sustained energy from the combination of all three foods.

A sweeter way to balance a snack and add some fun is to treat yourself to a chocolate drop or mini-chocolate bar, served with a couple of fresh strawberries and a half cup of skim milk. This snack is loaded with vitamin C and calcium, and provides other nutrients along with a chocolate bonus. Just remember: Don't get carried away. Only one piece of chocolate!

These two examples show how eating between meals can become a healthful, guilt-free habit that doesn't have to affect your weight, or your blood sugar, in a negative way.

Grazing throughout the day

Research over the past few decades has shown that, for some people, *grazing*, or eating small meals and snacks throughout the day instead of three larger meals, can help with weight control and other health issues. More frequent eating may help

- Lower your blood cholesterol
- Control your moods
- Keep your blood sugar steady
- Give you more control over your appetite

Grazing works for low-calorie dieters as long as you aren't random. You still need a low-cal plan (see Chapter 6 to start with a four-week plan), and you need to stick to your calorie limit if you're serious about losing weight. The only difference between grazing and eating three square meals a day is that you're breaking the same number of calories up into smaller meals to be eaten more often.

For many people, however, snacking or grazing is detrimental to their diet. If you're the type of person who isn't satisfied with small portions of your favorite foods or for whom a few bites of food easily leads to a binge, then you probably need to avoid frequent snacking, at least for now. You may even have to forego all snacks and desserts until you feel in better control of your eating habits. If that's the case, take your snack and dessert calories (and the foods that provide those calories) and add them to your regular meals. For instance, rather than having a baked apple at 3 p.m. to hold you over until dinner, add it to your breakfast menu or have it with dinner, rather than later in the evening.

All the low-cal snacks and desserts in the world can't help you lose weight if you overdo it. You have to be able to stop eating when you've used up your calorie allotment. Your body plays a funny trick on you when you eat too much, too often. If you start feeding yourself six or eight times a day, you'll start to feel hungry at those same times every day. That's okay if you're simply dividing an appropriate number of daily calories into that many small meals and snacks. But if you feed that hunger with excess food, then snacking becomes just another bad habit that can lead to weight gain.

Sampling 100-Calorie Snacks

The following sections provide recipes and ideas for quick-to-fix snacks, both savory and sweet. You can eat some of them in the here and now, while you can make others ahead of time for your scheduled snack or if you need to appease a snack attack that comes out of the blue. (Yes, it happens, and yes, give in to it! Better to give in to a craving and allow yourself 100 extra calories worth of satisfaction than to end up bingeing later in the day because you denied yourself a small treat earlier.)

Treating yourself to sweet snacks

The sweet snacks in this section and the desserts later in this chapter are certainly interchangeable. They all contain approximately 100 calories in a single serving. The only difference is that the desserts are just slightly more sophisticated, and perhaps more suitable for serving to company.

If your friends are like mine, they'll welcome the make-it-yourself oozy cookie snack made with marshmallow creme and chocolate syrup (Just a Little S'More) in this section just as readily as the more elegant chilled dessert cup of orange sections in sweet and spicy syrup (Oranges in Spicy Syrup) you can find in the section "Making the most of fruit," later in this chapter.

⊘ Watermelon Freezies

This recipe isn't unlike the semifrozen, slurpable drink snacks you may have enjoyed as a kid at your local convenience store. This one is a little healthier, though, because it contains real fruit, instead of just fruit-flavored sugar syrup, and it fits nicely into your 100-calorie snack slot.

Preparation time: *5 minutes plus freezing time*

Yield: *4 servings*

4 cups cubed seedless watermelon, frozen	*1 tablespoon sugar*
½ can (3 ounces) frozen limeade concentrate, thawed and undiluted	*Pinch of dried mint (optional)*

Combine the frozen watermelon cubes, limeade concentrate, sugar, and mint, if using, in the container of a blender or food processor. Process with on/off motions until smooth. Serve immediately.

Tip: *Put any leftover mixture back in the freezer before it thaws and freeze for up to a month. To serve at another time, take the mixture out of the freezer for 10 minutes before reprocessing.*

Per serving: *Calories 92 (From Fat 1); Fat 0g (Saturated 0g); Cholesterol 0mg; Sodium 5mg; Carbohydrate 27g (Dietary Fiber 1g); Protein 1g.*

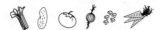

Just a Little S'More

I include this recipe because dieters deserve to have as much fun as everyone else. A take-off on the traditional campfire s'mores, this sweet treat weighs in under 100 calories — if you can eat just one! The recipe is written to yield only one serving. I don't recommend it for anyone who can't keep ingredients like marshmallow creme in the house, for fear of eating the entire jarful during a midnight binge.

Preparation time: *5 minutes*

Yield: *1 cookie*

1 tablespoon marshmallow creme

½ graham cracker (1 square), split into two rectangles

1 teaspoon chocolate syrup

Spread the marshmallow creme onto one of the graham cracker rectangles. Drizzle the creme with the chocolate syrup. Top with the remaining graham cracker rectangle. Enjoy!

Tip: *Sometimes when I make one, I put it on a plate and pop it in the microwave oven for 5 seconds just to warm it slightly.*

Per serving: *Calories 67 (From Fat 7); Fat 1g (Saturated 0g); Cholesterol 0mg; Sodium 51mg; Carbohydrate 14g (Dietary Fiber 0g); Protein 1g.*

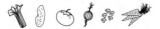

Savoring salty snacks

If you have a salt tooth, rather than a sweet tooth, then you go more for chips, pretzels, and other savory foods when the urge to snack strikes. The recipes in this section are all designed to allow you to eat not just one, but several, and still stick to your 100-calorie snack limit.

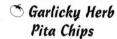
⬆ Garlicky Herb Pita Chips

You can't eat just one, but you don't have to, because they're less than 20 calories apiece. Feel free to eat five or six for a full snack.

Preparation time: *10 minutes*

Cooking time: *15 minutes*

Yield: *64 chips*

8 small (6 inch) pita breads

2 egg whites

¼ cup olive oil

2 large cloves garlic, minced

1 teaspoon dried rosemary, basil, oregano, or Italian seasoning mix, finely crushed

½ teaspoon salt

1 Preheat the oven to 300.

2 Split each pita bread so that you have 16 rounds. Place the rounds, rough side up, on your work surface.

3 Stir together the egg whites, olive oil, garlic, basil, and salt in a small bowl. Brush some of this egg-white mixture over the rough side of each pita round. With a pizza cutter or a knife, cut each pita in 4 equal wedges. Gently cut or pry each wedge apart. You'll have 64 wedges. Place the wedges, coated side up, on baking sheets.

4 Bake the chips, in batches if necessary, for 15 to 20 minutes or until the edges are toasted and the egg-white topping is set. Remove the baking sheets to wire racks. Allow the chips to cool completely before serving.

Per serving: Calories 18 (From Fat 8); Fat 1g (Saturated 0g); Cholesterol 0mg; Sodium 39mg; Carbohydrate 2g (Dietary Fiber 0g); Protein 0g.

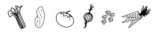

🍎 Salad Scoops

My friend Laurie Mozian, who is also a registered dietitian, shared the basis of this recipe with me years ago. Her version called for spooning the finely chopped vegetable mixture onto rye-crisp crackers or melba toast. You can do that, if you like (keeping it to two or three crackers). But personally, the way I write it is a great way to sneak a few potato chips into your diet.

Preparation time: *10 minutes*

Yield: *4 servings*

1 ripe tomato, halved, seeded, and very finely diced

1 small cucumber or ½ seedless cucumber, peeled, halved lengthwise, seeded and very finely diced

1 tablespoon very finely chopped green onion

2 tablespoons light creamy salad dressing such as blue cheese, creamy Italian, creamy Caesar, or ranch

24 baked potato chips or potato crisps

1 Combine the tomato, cucumber, green onion, and dressing in a small bowl.

2 Spoon a generous tablespoonful of the salad onto each potato chip just before eating.

Per serving: *Calories 86 (From Fat 18); Fat 2g (Saturated 0g); Cholesterol 0mg; Sodium 160mg; Carbohydrate 16g (Dietary Fiber 2g); Protein 2g.*

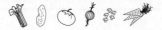

You can serve any of the snacks in this section as party food. If you're invited to someone else's party and you're worried about what you'll eat when you get there, you can offer to bring a tray of low-cal snacks and then position yourself close to that tray so that you're not tempted to reach for any of the higher-calorie foods provided by your host.

☞ Bean and Cheese Nachos

To serve these nachos at a party, simply double, triple, or quadruple the recipe. Even nondieters scarf them up!

Preparation time: *10 minutes*

Cooking time: *8 minutes*

Yield: *8 servings*

2 flour tortillas (8 inches in diameter)

¼ cup fat-free refried beans

¼ cup fat-free salsa

1 tablespoon finely chopped cilantro (optional)

2 ounces shredded reduced-fat cheddar cheese

1 Preheat the oven to 450.

2 Spread the tortillas evenly with the beans. Top with salsa. Sprinkle with cilantro, if desired, then the shredded cheese.

3 Bake the nachos for 8 minutes or until the tortillas are crisp and lightly browned around the edges and the cheese has melted.

4 Use a pizza cutter or sharp knife to cut each tortilla into eight nachos.

Per serving: *Calories 73 (From Fat 23); Fat 3g (Saturated 2g); Cholesterol 6mg; Sodium 136mg; Carbohydrate 9g (Dietary Fiber 1g); Protein 4g.*

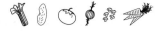

☞ Yogurt-Cheese Dip with Spinach and Dill

This recipe makes about 16 servings if you're planning to use it for a party. For an everyday 100-calorie snack, or as party fare, have 3 tablespoons of dip with a cup of assorted raw vegetable dippers.

Preparation time: *5 minutes*

Yield: *3 cups*

1 package (10 ounces) frozen chopped spinach, thawed and well drained

2 ounces crumbled goat cheese or feta cheese

2 tablespoons chopped fresh dill or 2 teaspoons dried dill

1 clove garlic

1 teaspoon lemon juice

⅛ teaspoon each salt and pepper

2 cups plain lowfat yogurt, divided

1 Combine the spinach, cheese, dill, garlic, lemon juice, salt, and pepper in a food processor. Whirl for 30 seconds, just to combine, scraping down the side of the container with a spatula, as necessary.

2 Add ½ cup of the yogurt to the food processor. Whirl until almost smooth. Stir in the remaining yogurt until well mixed. (Don't process the remaining yogurt, or the mixture will be too thin.)

3 Turn the dip into a serving bowl. Cover and refrigerate until ready to serve.

Per serving: Calories 37 (From Fat 14); Fat 2g (Saturated 1g); Cholesterol 5mg; Sodium 70mg; Carbohydrate 3g (Dietary Fiber 0g); Protein 3g.

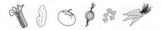

50 snacks worth 50 calories

With 50-calorie snacks, you get to snack more often. You can always double the quantity on any of these snacks to get your full 100 at once, but dividing snacks up into 50-calorie portions can help you bank calories for later on in the day, when you may start feeling desperate for a bite to eat.

- ✔ 25 small thin pretzel sticks
- ✔ 20 tiny fish-shaped crackers
- ✔ 20 mini marshmallows
- ✔ 15 pistachio nuts
- ✔ 15 grapes
- ✔ 10 dry roasted peanuts
- ✔ 8 tiny bear-shaped graham cookies
- ✔ 5 dried apricot halves
- ✔ 5 almonds
- ✔ 5 cashews
- ✔ 5 walnut halves
- ✔ 4 saltine crackers
- ✔ 4 baked tortilla chips with 1 tablespoon salsa
- ✔ 3 dill pickles
- ✔ 3 mini rice cakes
- ✔ 2 brazil nuts
- ✔ 2 small chocolate drops
- ✔ 2 dried dates
- ✔ 2 graham cracker squares
- ✔ 2 saltines with 1 teaspoon peanut butter
- ✔ 2 vanilla wafer cookies
- ✔ 2 cups light microwave popcorn
- ✔ 2 tablespoons dried cranberries
- ✔ 2 tablespoons dried cherries
- ✔ And a partridge in a pear tree (oops, wrong list; keep reading for more great snacks)

- 1 fig bar cookie
- 1 peach
- 1 plum
- 1 flavored rice cake
- 1 mini sesame breadstick
- 1 mini box (½ ounce) raisins
- 1 cup puffed cereal
- 1 cup raw baby carrots
- 1 cup sweet red pepper strips
- 1 cup tomato juice
- 1 cup whole strawberries
- 1 ounce lowfat deli meat
- ½ apple
- ½ grapefruit sprinkled with ½ teaspoon sugar or other sweetener, if you like

- ½ small banana
- ½ cup chicken noodle soup
- ½ cup fresh blueberries
- ½ cup fresh cherries
- ½ cup fresh pineapple
- ½ cup light or juice-packed fruit cocktail
- ½ cup orange sections
- ½ cup cranberry juice
- ½ cup skim milk
- ½ slice light bread toast with 2 teaspoons fruit spread
- ⅓ cup unsweetened applesauce
- ¼ avocado

Dishing Up 100-Calorie Desserts

Dessert eaters will probably want to use their snack calories for an after-dinner sweet. Believing you can find a satisfying dessert for 100 calories or less may sound impossible, but I include six recipes in the following sections.

Making the most of fruit

Nutritionists recommend fresh fruit as the dessert of choice, because it's sweet, easy, packed with nutrients, and comparatively low in calories. What could be bad? Nothing, but if you've ever been on a restricted diet, you know that eating the same foods, the same way, over and over again, no matter how delicious they are, can get boring. And boring spells nothing but trouble for dieters! The following are several recipes that feature fresh fruit in fun and tasty ways.

✆ Cannoli Creme Topping

If you've ever had an Italian cannoli pastry, you can appreciate the flavor of this creamy, sweetened ricotta cheese mixture. This recipe uses it as a topping for fresh fruit that's especially good with a ½ cup of sliced strawberries or a mixture of strawberries, blueberries, and raspberries.

Preparation time: *5 minutes*

Yield: *8 servings (2 generous tablespoons per serving)*

1 cup light ricotta cheese

2 tablespoons superfine sugar

1 teaspoon vanilla

2 tablespoons chocolate chips, chopped, or ½ ounce semisweet chocolate, grated

1 teaspoon grated orange rind (optional)

Combine the cheese, sugar, and vanilla in a blender or food processor. Whirl for a minute or until very smooth, scraping down the side of the container as necessary. Stir in the chocolate chips and orange rind, if using. Refrigerate the topping for up to a week.

Per serving: *Calories 56 (From Fat 18); Fat 2g (Saturated 1g); Cholesterol 8mg; Sodium 28mg; Carbohydrate 6g (Dietary Fiber 0g); Protein 3g.*

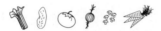

The following recipe features refreshing oranges cut into sections. To cut orange sections, use a small, sharp knife to remove the rind from the orange in a circular fashion, running the knife under the rind and around the fruit (see Figure 15-1). Be sure to cut through the membrane that holds the sections intact. After you have removed the rind, cut down alongside the membrane on both sides of each section to release the sections.

Sectioning an Orange to Eliminate Membranes

Figure 15-1: Use a small, sharp knife to section an orange.

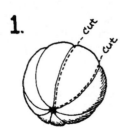

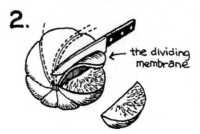

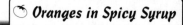 Oranges in Spicy Syrup

This recipe makes four servings as a stand-alone 100-calorie dessert, but you can also use less of this mixture as a topping for a small scoop of light vanilla ice cream or frozen yogurt.

Preparation time: *10 minutes*

Cooking time: *7 minutes plus 15 minutes standing time*

Yield: *4 servings*

¼ cup sugar

¼ cup water

1 tablespoon lemon juice

⅛ teaspoon ground cloves or allspice

2 cups orange sections (about 4 oranges)

1 Combine the sugar, water, lemon juice, and cloves in a small saucepan. Bring to a boil over medium heat. Reduce the heat and simmer for 2 minutes.

2 Add the orange sections to the saucepan. Simmer gently for 5 minutes. Pour the oranges and syrup into a bowl and let the mixture stand for at least 15 minutes or cover and refrigerate overnight.

Vary It! *You can also try this recipe with grapefruit.*

Per serving: *Calories 92 (From Fat 1); Fat 0g (Saturated 0g); Cholesterol 0mg; Sodium 0mg; Carbohydrate 23g (Dietary Fiber 2g); Protein 1g.*

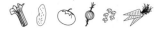

Most low-cal fruit desserts and snacks (including the following recipe for a Raspberry Baked Apple) double as healthful breakfast foods because they're not high in added sugars.

⏱ Raspberry Baked Apple

You can bake this apple the traditional way — in the regular oven — but it will take longer. Substitute any flavor fruit spread you like, and if you're having a light-eating day, and can spare another 25 calories, mix the fruit spread with a tablespoon of fat-free granola or other plain, nugget-shaped cereal or a teaspoon of finely chopped nuts before filling the apple.

Preparation time: 5 minutes

Cooking time: 3 minutes

Yield: 1 serving

1 medium apple, such as Winesap, Stayman, Fuji, or Gala	1 tablespoon natural or low-sugar seedless raspberry fruit spread

1 Peel the apple halfway down from the top. Cut out the core almost to the bottom, leaving a 1-inch opening at the top (see Figure 15-2). Place the apple in a microwave-safe dish. Add 2 tablespoons water to the dish.

2 Cook the apple in the microwave for 3 minutes or until tender. (If you don't have a rotating tray in the oven, turn the apple once halfway through cooking time for more even cooking.)

3 Spoon the fruit spread into the opening in the top of the apple. Microwave for 30 seconds or until the filling is bubbly.

Tip: The best way to eat a baked apple is to halve it first, allow the filling to flow out, and then cut the apple into bite-size pieces.

Per serving: Calories 123 (From Fat 5); Fat 1g (Saturated 0g); Cholesterol 0mg; Sodium 4mg; Carbohydrate 31g (Dietary Fiber 4g); Protein 0g.

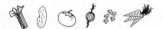

How to Core an Apple

Figure 15-2: Use a sharp paring knife to core an apple safely and easily.

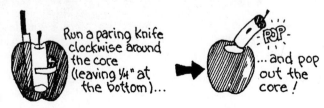

Run a paring knife clockwise around the core (leaving ¼" at the bottom)...

-POP-

...and pop out the core!

☺ Chocolate-Frosted Frozen Banana

This recipe is a great low-cal treat to keep on hand in the freezer for when only something chocolate will satisfy your sweet tooth! (You can find additional chocolate recipes in the next section.) You can use the chocolate to coat strawberries and other fruits too, if you like. That way, you still get a taste of chocolate while having a healthy serving of fruit.

Preparation time: *2 minutes plus freezing time*

Yield: *4 servings*

1 large, firm, ripe banana

1 square (1 ounce) semisweet chocolate

1 teaspoon skim milk

1 Cut the banana in half lengthwise, and then cut each long half in half crosswise to make four equal pieces. Place the banana pieces on a plate and freeze for an hour or two or until just solid.

2 Combine the chocolate square and milk in a ramekin or small cup. Microwave for 45 seconds. Remove the ramekin from the microwave and stir the chocolate mixture with a spoon until it is smooth and spreadable. Spoon or brush the chocolate along the length of the frozen banana pieces. Return the bananas to the freezer for 1 hour or until the chocolate frosting is frozen solid.

3 Wrap each banana separately in freezer paper and keep frozen until ready to eat. To serve, remove the banana pieces from the freezer 15 minutes before serving. Place them on dessert plates and carefully cut them into thin slices. Serve the bananas semifrozen.

Tip: *If you can't wait for the banana to freeze, simply take your share, cut it into thin slices, and spread it with a little of the chocolate frosting while it's still warm.*

Per serving: *Calories 66 (From Fat 27); Fat 3g (Saturated 2g); Cholesterol 0mg; Sodium 1mg; Carbohydrate 11g (Dietary Fiber 1g); Protein 1g.*

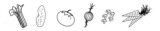

Satisfying your sweet tooth with chocolate

Chocoholics, rejoice! There's room in a low-calorie diet for your favorite food group. In this section you find two recipes that can satisfy your craving without pushing you over your calorie limit.

⏾ Cocoa Meringues

If you can't eat just one of these sweet, crispy drops but you can stop at five or six, then this chocolate cookie is for you! They also make great giveaways for friends who are watching their weight.

Preparation time: *10 minutes*

Cooking time: *90 minutes*

Yield: *50 cookies*

¾ cup superfine sugar

2 tablespoons unsweetened cocoa

6 egg whites, at room temperature

¼ teaspoon cream of tartar

pinch of salt

1½ teaspoons vanilla extract

1 Preheat the oven to 250 degrees. Line a couple of baking sheets with parchment paper or nonstick aluminum foil.

2 In a small bowl, stir together the sugar and cocoa. Set aside.

3 In a large bowl with an electric mixer at medium speed, beat the egg whites until foamy. Beat in the cream of tartar, salt, and vanilla. Add the cocoa and sugar mixture, 1 tablespoon at a time, beating until blended after each addition, until the egg whites are stiff and glossy (see Figure 15-3 to find out what stiff peaks look like). Drop the batter by measuring tablespoonfuls onto the prepared baking sheets.

4 Bake the meringues for 90 minutes. Turn off the oven, open the door slightly, and allow the cookies to cool completely in the oven. (This step takes several hours.) Remove the cookies from the baking sheets with a spatula. Store the meringues in a tightly covered container for up to a few days.

Vary It! *These cookies are even more fabulous if you substitute an equal amount of chocolate extract for the vanilla. If you can't find chocolate extract in your supermarket, check in specialty food shops and baking supply stores.*

Per serving: *Calories 14 (From Fat 0); Fat 0g (Saturated 0g); Cholesterol 0mg; Sodium 9mg; Carbohydrate 3g (Dietary Fiber 0g); Protein 1g.*

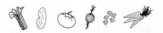

Figure 15-3:
Stiff peaks stand firm and tall while soft peaks fold over slightly on themselves.

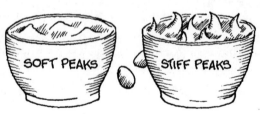

When you need a quick chocolate fix, remember that chocolate syrup has only 13 to 20 calories in a teaspoon. (The calorie range is due to variations among brands. Check the labels on different brands in your supermarket if you want to find the one with the fewest calories.) You can satisfy your need with a drizzle of syrup on fresh strawberries or a couple of banana slices or even a small wedge of angel food cake. Just be aware of how much syrup you're pouring, however, because by the time you're up to 2 tablespoons, you've topped 100 calories, just from the syrup alone.

○ *Chocolate Bread Pudding*

This recipe uses classic calorie-cutting techniques such as using skim milk instead of whole milk and light bread in place of regular bread, and replacing some egg yolks with egg whites to lighten up a traditional dessert.

Preparation time: *10 minutes*

Cooking time: *35 minutes*

Yield: *4 servings*

Nonstick cooking spray	*1 egg yolk*
4 slices light oatmeal bread	*½ cup skim milk*
1 tablespoon sugar	*3 egg whites*
2 teaspoons unsweetened cocoa powder	

1 Preheat the oven to 325.

2 Coat a 1-quart baking dish with nonstick cooking spray. Cut the bread slices into small cubes. Place the cubes in the baking dish.

3 In a large bowl, stir together the sugar and cocoa powder until well mixed. Stir in the egg yolk and milk until blended.

4 In a medium bowl with an electric mixer at medium-high speed, beat the egg whites until stiff peaks form. Carefully fold the whites into the cocoa mixture until almost blended. Be careful not to overmix or you may deflate the beaten whites. Pour this mixture over the bread cubes.

5 Place the baking dish in a larger baking pan. Carefully add enough boiling water to the larger pan to come 1 inch up the side of the baking dish.

6 Bake the bread pudding for 35 minutes or until golden brown and set. Serve warm.

Per serving: Calories 99 (From Fat 16); Fat 2g (Saturated 1g); Cholesterol 54mg; Sodium 162mg; Carbohydrate 14g (Dietary Fiber 2g); Protein 7g.

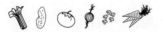

Part V
The Part of Tens

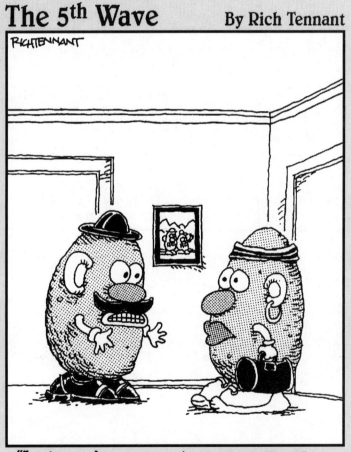

"Look, you're never going to look like Mrs. French Fry, or Mrs. Cheese Stick. Besides, do you have any idea what their calorie intakes are?"

In this part . . .

You find The Part of Tens at the back of every *For Dummies* book you read. In this part, you find almost everything you need to know about successfully losing weight, including ten benefits of following a low-cal diet. And ten people share their own personal weight-loss stories here, to inspire you to follow their lead.

Chapter 16

Ten Benefits of Following a Low-Calorie Diet

In This Chapter

▶ Reaping the physical rewards of a low-calorie lifestyle

▶ Staying healthier and extending your life

*T*he big payback for following a low-calorie diet and losing weight comes from the many ways you'll improve your health and your overall quality of life as you lose weight. These benefits, which I cover in this chapter, can help reduce your risk of developing medical problems now and in the future, and you may even live longer simply because you've chosen to live better.

Looking Good, Feeling Great

I sometimes grow impatient when I read advice suggesting that overweight people need to be comfortable with themselves at any size. I agree with the advice, but it's often militant, not always realistic, and sometimes gives the wrong message. Yes, you must love and care about yourself. Yes, you're a worthwhile person at any size. But if you're not physically and mentally comfortable being overweight, then it doesn't make sense to stay that way. Losing weight may not solve all your problems, but most people I know who have lost weight in the past say they feel better about themselves when they're thinner. Hundreds of people I've spoken with say they want to lose weight to look better and improve the quality of their lifestyles as well as their health. Very few say it's for the sake of their health alone.

You can be "fat and fit," especially if you get plenty of exercise. However, if you're still extremely unhappy when you look in the mirror, then you're carrying around a lot of psychological weight in addition to extra body weight. Wanting to look good is never a negative unless you have unrealistic ideas about how much you want to weigh or what your life is going to be like after you lose weight. If your weight-loss goals are unrealistic, the result could be a painful, lifelong struggle. But if all you want is to get to a comfortable weight so you can feel better about yourself, then make it your goal. (Chapter 4 has more info on setting realistic goals.)

Looking good is a legitimate benefit of weight loss when it comes to improved self-esteem and a positive body image. A trickle-down effect is working here: When you feel good about yourself, you're more likely to take care of your health because you know you're worth it. How do I know this? Well, not many scientific studies have been conducted on the power of positive thinking, but experts do know that poor body image is associated with low self-esteem and low self-esteem is associated with unhealthy behaviors such as abusing alcohol and drugs, avoiding professional help, and overeating.

Boosting Your Energy

The more extra weight you carry on your body, the more energy you use up performing even the simplest tasks. If, for instance, you're 40 pounds out of your healthy weight range, you may as well be wearing a 40-pound backpack. If you can identify with this example, you know that everyday activities, such as walking down the street or doing housework, could be much easier if you took off that backpack.

Although many people assume that energy levels naturally decline as you age, fitness studies have shown that the better you control your body fat, build up your endurance, and develop muscle over the years, the less of a decline you'll see. That's why, even though the mere thought of more exercise might exhaust you, getting active can give you more energy in the long run. I give you the full scoop on working out and getting active in Chapter 8.

Sleeping Better

According to the American Sleep Apnea Association, more than 12 million Americans suffer from *sleep apnea,* a condition that causes people to repeatedly stop breathing for up to a full minute while they sleep. Being overweight is a risk factor for developing sleep apnea and even though the condition is more commonly found in men older than 40, it can affect anyone. (If you want to know all you need to know about sleep apnea and other potential sleeping problems, check out *Sleep Disorders For Dummies* by Max Hirshkowitz, MD, and Patricia Smith [Wiley].)

If you have apnea, your brain wakes you up with each episode to resume breathing, but your sleep quality suffers as a result of these constant awakenings. You may not even know that you have sleep apnea, but you (or your sleeping partner) may recognize some of the symptoms, such as loud snoring and constantly feeling tired throughout the day. Sleep apnea can also cause other medical conditions such as high blood pressure (see "Lowering Your Blood Pressure," later in this chapter), headaches, and impotency.

Saving Your Back

Losing weight can help reduce the load on your lower back and extremities, which in turn can help reduce the symptoms of osteoarthritis and possibly even prevent joint problems. Medical experts also say that being overweight is a cause of osteoarthritis in the hips, knees, and lower back because the extra pressure from excess weight wears away the cartilage that would normally protect these areas. Excess weight in your abdomen puts extra stress on your back muscles. The healthiest solution is to lose weight and work with a physical therapist, or a trainer who is familiar with joint and back problems, to strengthen your abdominal muscles.

Lowering Your Blood Pressure

Blood pressure is the force at which your heart beats to drive blood to your arteries and through your circulatory system. Your blood pressure rises as your heart beats and falls when your heart rests between beats, and that's what's being measured when you get a blood pressure reading. When your pressure reads above the normal range, you have high blood pressure.

Often described as "the silent killer," high blood pressure can cause heart disease, stroke, and kidney failure — all killer diseases. The silent part comes from the fact that you can develop high blood pressure without experiencing any symptoms. So you may have it and not even know it until it leads to a more critical health problem.

As your weight increases, so does your blood pressure. If you're overweight, just losing a few pounds by eating less and moving more can help prevent high blood pressure. If you already have high blood pressure, losing weight can help bring it back into a normal range.

If you're overweight, the way to help prevent and lower high blood pressure is to eat less, exercise more, and lose weight. If you're overweight and take blood pressure–lowering medication, you may be able to reduce your dose or even eliminate the need for medication by losing excess weight.

If you're curious to know more about dealing with high blood pressure, check out *High Blood Pressure For Dummies* by Alan L. Rubin, MD (Wiley).

Maintaining a Healthy Heart

Reducing your weight by a mere 10 percent can lower your risk of developing heart disease. Many factors play into the development of heart disease, including high cholesterol that may be related to your diet, physical inactivity, and being overweight. You can control these factors by eating fewer calories, eating healthier foods, and exercising more. Losing weight can help lower your *LDL cholesterol,* which is the form of cholesterol responsible for clogged arteries, and raise your *HDL cholesterol,* which is the form of cholesterol that is beneficial to your heart because it carries excess dietary fat out of your body. (If you want more information about cholesterol, look for *Controlling Cholesterol For Dummies* by Carol Ann Rinzler and Martin W. Graf, MD [Wiley].)

Even with normal cholesterol levels, you may be at risk of developing heart disease if you're one of 55 million people with *metabolic syndrome,* also known as Syndrome X. This syndrome isn't a disease in and of itself, but rather a collection of risk factors. If you have at least three of the following risk factors, you may be diagnosed with metabolic syndrome:

✔ High blood pressure

✔ High blood glucose (sugar) levels

✔ High blood triglyceride (fat) levels

✔ Low blood levels of protective HDL cholesterol

✔ Insulin resistance

✔ A waist circumference greater than 35 inches in women, 40 in men

The best known treatment for slowing down or reversing the risk factors of metabolic syndrome is to lose weight. Research has shown that a diet providing between 1,100 and 1,950 calories a day can reduce cholesterol levels, blood pressure, and the risk of developing heart disease and diabetes.

Preventing Diabetes

Overweight people are twice as likely to develop non-insulin dependent diabetes than people who are at a healthy weight. Another scary fact: About one-fourth of overweight adults older than 45 are *prediabetic,* a term given to the condition people develop before they get diabetes. Among those people who are prediabetic, almost 95 percent have high cholesterol and more than half have high blood pressure. Scariest fact of all: Approximately 6.5 million people are walking around with undiagnosed diabetes so they're not even included in the statistics. If you're one of them, you're at high risk of developing chronic conditions related to diabetes, such as heart disease and kidney disease.

Cutting calories, balancing your meals, and increasing the amount of exercise you do on a regular basis can reduce your risk of developing diabetes. If you already have diabetes and you're overweight, losing weight can help control your blood sugar levels and decrease your need for medication. Ask your physician if eating less and exercising more can help you.

If you want more information about diabetes, check out *Diabetes For Dummies,* 2nd edition, by Alan L. Rubin, MD (Wiley).

Fighting Cancer

In a study of more than 900,000 adults published in the *New England Journal of Medicine,* being overweight was associated with higher rates of death due to cancer of the esophagus, colon, rectum, liver, gallbladder, pancreas, and kidney, and also higher death rates from non-Hodgkin's lymphoma and multiple myeloma, in both men and women. Heavier men were more likely to die from stomach and prostate cancers; heavier women were more likely to die from cancers of the breast, uterus, cervix, and ovary. From this study, researchers concluded that 14 percent of all deaths from cancer in women and 20 percent of all deaths in men were linked to being overweight and obesity.

Cancer experts list weight loss among their suggestions for preventing cancer because they believe that being overweight and inactive produces changes in the body that encourage cancer cells to thrive and grow. But cancerous conditions also develop in people who aren't overweight, so medical experts don't know if that higher risk is actually due to excess weight or if it's due to eating a high-calorie or high-fat diet.

Some evidence also suggests that if you're overweight, you may get less effective treatment for cancer. Preliminary studies have indicated that heavier women may need more chemotherapy to treat breast cancer than thinner women, but they may not get it because doctors are afraid of administering higher, more toxic levels of the drugs. The side effects of chemotherapy drugs can include damage to the heart and other organs, and the growth of cancer at other sites, so doctors may undertreat their heavier patients.

Simplifying Pregnancy

Being overweight during pregnancy can pose serious problems for both you and your baby. Some studies show that labor takes longer for overweight and obese women. The longer the labor, the increased chance the baby will have to be delivered by Caesarean section.

Overweight pregnant women are at higher risk of developing medical complications, such as high blood pressure, *preeclampsia* (any of several medical conditions associated with high blood pressure during pregnancy), and gestational diabetes. These conditions usually clear up after delivery, but after they occur, they're more likely to develop again later in life. If you require surgery during pregnancy or delivery, your risk of complications increases with increased weight.

Some studies have also shown that women who are obese when they become pregnant have a higher risk of delivering an infant who is stillborn or dies shortly after birth. Women who are simply overweight, however, appear to have the same risk as those of normal weight. (For definitions of "overweight" and "obese," flip to Chapter 2.)

Check out Chapter 10 for more info about pregnancy and weight loss.

Living Longer

Scientific evidence has shown that the maximum lifespan for humans is about 125 years, although few people actually hang around that long. But in the hope of living to their ripest old age, a small but devoted group of people who belong to the Calorie Restriction Society are trying to prove that eating less can help you live longer. Science hasn't been able to prove it in humans yet, but animal studies seem to support the theory that fewer calories can mean a longer life, at least for mice, monkeys, and fruit flies.

Calorie restriction for the purpose of living longer isn't the same as following a low-calorie diet to lose weight, and the concept is too new for most health professions to condone it. My advice to anyone who hopes to live longer by restricting calories is to follow a nutritionally balanced, reduced-calorie diet plan just like the one in this book. If cutting calories turns out to add years to your life, those years will be more enjoyable if you've remained healthy by supplying your body with all the nutrients it needs.

Chapter 17

Ten Low-Calorie Success Stories

In This Chapter

▶ Checking out inspiring stories

▶ Gathering helpful hints

The men and women who contributed the "before and after" stories in this chapter have all battled the bulge. Some have lost weight for the first time in their lives, while others have traveled this road several times finally figuring out that cutting calories and getting more exercise is the key to losing weight. Read their stories as inspirational advice on how you too can begin to control your weight instead of letting your weight control you.

Finally Fitting into My Genes

My unique relationship with food started at a young age. In my family, food was the center of all celebrations, the healing of all wounds, and, before I knew it, one of my best friends. My family was nothing but loving to me, but they never realized that their own food habits might have a negative effect on me in the long run. A good grade got me an ice cream cone; a bad grade got me the same. My mother would bring me bags of potato chips to eat in bed and then at other times scold me for eating snacks that were "meant for my brother." I was confused. Unfortunately, she was too. She could see bad food patterns developing, but she didn't know what to do because she and my father were both struggling with their own weight problems.

I was always a social kid and had a large circle of friends and endless activities to keep me busy. But even then, nothing satisfied me the way food did. It was around the time I turned 8 that I can remember the horror of being called "fatty" or "big butt." I would go home in tears, only to be comforted by cookies. Eating sweets made me feel better. I didn't know any other way.

One vivid memory from adolescence is that of not being able to pull my cheerleading skirt up over my thighs. My mother had one custom-made for me, but the other girls just pointed out that mine was different. I went home in tears. At this point, my mother saw what my weight was doing to me and because she'd struggled with it her entire life, attempted to help me in the only way she knew how, by introducing me to fad diets. We ate grapefruits three times a day. We cut out carbohydrates. We took pills that did unthinkable things to our bowels. We joined a weight-loss program and celebrated the move by going out for ice cream sundaes! None of it taught me anything about my behaviors or how I let my emotions dictate what I would eat.

By the time I got to college, my weight had ballooned to 225 pounds. Although people always tried to tell me I "carried my weight well," 5-feet-7 isn't tall enough to carry 225 pounds. I had let myself go, I knew it, and that's when I became completely introverted. I went to class, went home, and slept as much as I could. I refused to face the outside world. Around the same time, my mother made the decision to undergo gastric bypass surgery. Not only was the surgery a success in helping her lose more than 100 pounds, but it also somehow changed her psychological approach to food. My one-time food buddy had turned into a normal eater! I didn't quite know how to handle it. I felt very alone and that's when I hit rock bottom. I knew that if I didn't put a stop to my overeating, it would be the end of me in more ways than one.

As a result, I joined a weight-loss program. It wasn't the first time I'd joined, but I made a promise to myself it would be the last. It took a lot of patience and it was never easy. It took two years for 60 pounds to come off. Along the way there have been bumps in the road and setbacks I hadn't anticipated. I went off the program at times. Some weeks I skipped meetings. But I never quit. I knew I couldn't turn back. I would never again go back to being the miserable person I was at 225 pounds.

These days, I don't restrict what I eat. If I want a candy bar, I have one. I may choose a smaller one, or one with fewer calories or less fat, but I won't tell myself "I can't have this" because that type of deprivation only leads to trouble. I'm still working to take off another 30 pounds, which will get me to my weight goal, but I've decided not to set a date for that goal. I take my food plan one day at a time, and when I have extra stress in my life, I take it one meal at a time. I draw on all the support I can, including friends, program meetings, published literature, and online research.

At this point, I accept that focusing on weight control will always be part of my life. I know at times I may put on a few pounds, even while I'm still trying to lose. I know I'll work them off because I'm determined never to go back to the person I was before. I just won't let it happen. Being that person wasn't much fun, so I'm determined to stick to the happier "new" me. — Amanda K.

Eating Small Portions All the Time

I never gained the infamous "freshman 15" when I first went to college. It was my junior year that did me in. French was one of my majors, so I decided to take an opportunity to live in France for six months that year. I weighed about 125 pounds before I left, and thanks to a diet that included a few too many freshly baked baguettes and pain au chocolat, came back tipping the scales at 145. Within a few months, I got my weight back down to 125 just by eating less food.

A couple of years later, as a graduation present to myself, I went back to France for another extended stay. I brought those same 20 extra pounds back home to the States with me six months later. Again, I simply started watching how much I ate. I wasn't going to deprive myself of the types of foods I'd come to love, so I simply ate less of them. I lost the weight again and have kept it off for 20 years.

I use the same strategy to maintain weight as I did to lose it. Either I share a high-calorie dish or yummy dessert, or I simply take two or three bites and leave the rest. I don't see it as a loss of money; I see it as a loss of excess calories. I'm spending the same amount of money, regardless of how much I eat.
— Lori T.

Consuming Fewer Calories and Adding More Workouts

For the past 25 years, I've been battling the weight war, always struggling with an extra 10 or 15 pounds. I have tried almost every diet available and purchased every diet "solution" advertised — pills, lotions, teas, fad foods, you name it — in hope of shedding those unwanted pounds. I even tried giving up all forms of chocolate (my favorite food group), but that was an unacceptable and, in the end, unsuccessful strategy. It wasn't until recently that I discovered the only thing that really works and of course it's something I've known deep down for a long time.

After all these years of reading health magazines and newspaper articles about the importance of exercise and good nutrition, it finally sunk in. If you want to lose weight the right and safe way, the only way is by becoming aware of how many calories you consume and, if necessary, cutting back and/or burning off any excess with a good workout. With the help of an article I found in a fitness magazine, I calculated the number of calories I needed to consume each day to maintain my weight. From there I figured out how many calories I should consume to shed a few pounds. I started counting calories every day, factored in how many calories I worked off at the gym, and lost weight.

I still count calories, and if I overindulge one day, I take those calories away from another day during the week. I weigh myself only once a week. Most importantly, I no longer worry or feel guilty when I eat more than I should because I know the formula for getting myself back on track. — Stacey J.

Knowing What Works and Making Time for It

I think I overeat for three reasons: I love food, I'm an anxious person and eating calms me down, and if I don't set a goal or have a strong reason for losing weight, I find it hard to restrain myself. Over the past 30 years, I've lost and regained the same 20 to 40 pounds, and then some. At 6-foot-1, I would be pretty happy if I could maintain my weight around 200 pounds, as long as a lot of that was muscle.

About 15 years ago, just before my wedding, I decided it was time to lose weight again. I went from 251 pounds to 187 pounds in eight months, with the help of a commercial weight-loss program and a rigorous exercise routine. About five years ago, I was back up to 245 pounds, so I rejoined the program, added weight training to my exercise routine, and was down to 210 six months later.

The combination of regular workouts and a structured diet plan works for me every time I stick to them, and stops working when I slack off. These days, I'm back up to 230 pounds, but I finally see the pattern and I know what I have to do. I'm getting back into it and I trust that I'll lose the weight again, but the going is slow because I now have an infant son who needs my attention and takes up all of my spare time. I know that women often have a hard time losing their baby weight, but I'm here to tell you that men gain baby weight too, and have just as much trouble finding the time to work it off!
— Peter S.

Making Four the Magic Number

I don't have a lifetime history of dieting or trying to lose weight; I've been at a healthy weight most of my life. But about ten years ago, I started gaining for no apparent reason. I wasn't doing anything different. I wasn't eating any more than usual or exercising any less. But before I knew it, I was carrying 140 pounds on my 5-foot-2-inch frame and feeling very uncomfortable. Even though I only had 10 pounds to lose, and I lost it within a few weeks by cutting back on the amount of calories I consumed, I had trouble keeping it off. My biggest problem was (and still is) trying to resist the treats and sweets my coworkers bring into the office on a regular basis. At my job, there always seems to be some reason to stop working and have a celebration.

Now I never let my weight creep up by more than 4 pounds. If I let it get that far, I start getting strict again with my diet. I eat half a sandwich for lunch rather than a whole one and I eat plenty of big salads with just a teaspoon of olive oil for dressing. I eat fruit at least three times a day. I also make sure I eat something every two and a half hours so I don't get hungry, even if it's just a cucumber. For lunch, I bring calorie-controlled packaged entrees to the office and heat them up in the microwave oven. And I leave room in my calorie budget for office parties!

As long as I don't let it go any further than 4 pounds, and I stick to a strict plan, I can lose those 4 pounds within a week or two. The secret is to never let it get out of hand. — Sophie M.

Eating Smart While Eating Out and Cruising to a Lower Weight

As a food writer and restaurant reviewer with a weekly newspaper column, I eat lunch and dinner out at least several times a week. To be fair to the restaurant I'm reviewing, I have to go back two or three times to try a good sampling of menu offerings. In addition to the food I eat at restaurants, I attend press events introducing new food products, go on local and international trips sponsored by food associations, and encounter packages of food that routinely arrive on my desk from companies that want me to review their products. A dream job, right? Yes, in many ways, that's true, but it does have its dark side.

I knew when I took this job that I was committing dietary suicide. But I love food and couldn't resist the opportunity. I told myself I would just do it for a year. Six years later, I was 40 pounds heavier, up from a perfect size 8 to a tight size 14, always feeling bloated and miserable, and still writing restaurant reviews. I knew I had to do something, but losing weight isn't easy when you eat for a living. Sure, I could cut back on snacking and eat a little less when I went out, but I knew my only real hope was to start exercising as well.

What actually got me to the gym was an invitation to go on a Mediterranean cruise. You know the joke about cruises: You board as a passenger and disembark as cargo. I knew that if I was going to be sailing and eating for almost two weeks, and starting off at a 40-pound disadvantage, I had to take some preventive measures. Over the course of several weeks, by exercising regularly, canceling my daily midafternoon vending machine visits, foregoing the breadbasket when I went out to eat, and taking "sampling bites" of the food I was reviewing, I managed to lose 12 pounds.

The best part of the story, though, was that I went on that cruise and came home another 8 pounds lighter! When you're hiking steep walkways on a volcanic island, visiting ruins that you can only see by foot, and climbing endless steps to get to a medieval mountaintop town, you don't need an elliptical trainer. Even though, at the end of the day, all roads led back to a cruise ship that offered 1,001 ways to sabotage my diet, I was able to enjoy it because I had done my exercise, and then some. — Cindy K.

Having a Baby, Losing the Weight

By the end of my pregnancy, I had gained nearly 60 pounds. I started at around 130 and ended up close to 190. The baby was two and a half weeks overdue and I was retaining fluid, so with the birth I instantly lost 35 of those pounds. With breastfeeding and a hectic work schedule, I lost another 5 pounds without trying. The remaining 20 stayed right where they were for the next five years.

The first step I took was to add some exercise to my daily routine. I never had a good time to go to a gym, so I started walking, instead of riding, as often as I could. Eventually I added a yoga class every week, and then two or three a week. I started feeling fitter and more flexible, but still had only lost a few of those 20 pounds.

Even though I was very conscientious about my daughter's nutrition, I was just too busy, and too often too tired to prepare healthful meals for myself. I would fill up on high-calorie snacks throughout the day and sweet stuff late at night. I finally joined a weight-loss program, which forced me to look at what I was eating, how much, and when.

The program made me aware of portion control and now I'm less likely to overeat. I never feel deprived because now that I'm paying attention to what I eat, I always seem to have room for a glass of wine or a piece of chocolate at the end of the day. I eat better overall because I've become fussier about the quality of the food I eat. I don't want to waste any calories!

One of the most effective tools the program uses is a weekly weigh-in. Sometimes it reminds me that calories from those cookies I sneak in at midnight when I'm not even hungry start to add up. At other times it's a comfort to know that I'm progressing toward my goal. It has taken me more than a year to lose 15 pounds, and I still have 2 pounds to go to reach my goal weight. It's a slow process but I'm confident that by taking this route, I'll be able to keep those extra pounds off for good. — Juliette K.

Counting Calories as the Years Go By

For years, decades even, I ate whatever I wanted and never gained weight. Even in my late thirties, I was still able to eat large volumes of food — pretty much whatever and whenever I wanted. If I gained a few pounds, I just had to watch it for a week or two and my weight would go back down.

That all seemed to change overnight. I hit my forties and I started feeling thick and heavy. One day I was trying on clothes in a department store that has those 3-way mirrors that show you what you look like from behind. Need I say more? It had been years since I'd seen my backside, and let me tell you, it was a horrifying sight. All I saw when I looked in that mirror was baggy, ripply skin hanging from my thighs, arms that wobbled when I lifted them, and a stomach with accordion folds.

I immediately put myself on a diet and lost about 18 pounds over the course of three months. I didn't go on a lowfat diet, a low-glycemic diet, a high protein diet, a low-carbohydrate diet (bite your tongue!), or any theme diet at all, for that matter. I lost the weight the old-fashioned way, by counting calories. I carried a lined pad with me wherever I went and wrote down everything I ate with the approximate number of calories. When I got to 1,400 calories, I stopped eating for the day. (It only took one day to realize I had to spread those calories out or I wouldn't be able to eat for the rest of the day after lunch!)

A low-calorie diet was the only type of diet I could live with, because it allowed me to eat all types of food. As it turns out, that's the only type of weight-loss diet that really works for anyone, at any age. I should know. I wrote this book! — Susan M.

Buddying Up to Lose Weight

Years ago, I joined a commercial weight-loss program and it helped me lose weight. Recently when I decided to lose 10 pounds more, I figured I could use what I had learned from the program and just do it myself. At the same time, my friend and fellow teacher came into my office and she, too, wanted to shed some pounds. We made it our new year's resolution to lose weight together and support each other along the way.

We first went to the school nurse's office and borrowed her scale for a weigh-in. We decided on a weekly weigh-in in the privacy of our own homes — where we could take our clothes off and weigh a pound less! I dug up some old material from the program and we started our calorie-controlled diets.

We found out that a local sandwich shop would deliver customized lowfat submarine sandwiches to us at school for lunch Monday through Friday. We used our lunch hour to discuss food and to help each other plan ahead when one of us was going to a party or out to eat at a restaurant. We helped each other stay motivated and reminded each other that being thinner was much more appealing than eating an extra couple of meatballs.

One day, months later, my friend came to work and showed me that her pants were very loose. I had lost some weight, too. We knew we couldn't have gotten that far without each other's support. We felt so good about it that we decided to keep going even after we both reached our goal weights. Two and a half years later, I have lost 25 pounds, am down two sizes, bought a whole new wardrobe, and finally threw out my "fat" clothes. My friend lost close to 20 pounds, got pregnant, and gave birth to a healthy baby.

To maintain my weight, I eat pretty much the same thing everyday for breakfast, lunch, and snacks, and always have a light dinner, except on Saturday nights, when I go out to eat. That's when I eat whatever I want, practice a little portion control, and thoroughly enjoy myself. — Nancy B.

Staying Strong with "Want Power"

When I got out of the service, I was extremely fit. In a sense, I had no choice — the Army worked us out and fed us well so that we would be in the best possible shape. I'm a good-size man and, at the time, I weighed 182 pounds.

As I moved up in the business world, I found that along with a fair share of promotions and success came more sedentary office positions, too many social and professional functions, and not enough time to be active. Next thing I knew, I was tipping the scales at 240 pounds.

I was living in New York at the time of the 9/11 terrorist attacks and watched the towers fall from my Brooklyn home. It had a profound affect on me. I was scheduled to have prostate surgery the following day, and of course it was delayed for a month while everyone in the city was trying to figure out how to get their lives back on track again. I didn't realize it at the time, but while I was waiting to have the surgery, I started to become depressed. Before the delay, I had been worried about having the surgery, and now I was worried that I wouldn't be able to have it in time to treat my condition. Although I had my surgery in time and, like most New Yorkers, had started to recover from the events of 9/11, I was still feeling rather morose and apathetic. I began to eat more and more as a way of distracting myself from these feelings and, probably, in an attempt to feel some pleasure.

I may have gotten back on track sooner, but the following summer I fell and broke four ribs. It was a long time before I could move freely again. I kept eating and kept gaining weight. I noticed signs that my weight was starting to affect my health. I found myself gasping for breath one night as I walked from one airport terminal to the next. I went to my doctor, who immediately sent me to a pulmonary specialist. He found I wasn't getting enough air into my lungs and sent me home with a tank of oxygen. I was also diagnosed with sleep apnea. At that point I weighed 343 pounds, and I was scared.

Eight months and many low-cal meals later, I'm down to 272 pounds. I'm still working on my weight, but I know I'll get to my goal of 220 because I'm committed to improving my health. I eat less and at regular times. I've stopped relying on will power; now I rely on "want power." I want this more than anything else right now. I've joined a commercial weight-loss program because I need and believe in the structure of a good diet plan and the help and guidance of counselors who have struggled with weight issues themselves and come out as winners. — Mike C.

Part VI
Appendixes

The 5th Wave   By Rich Tennant

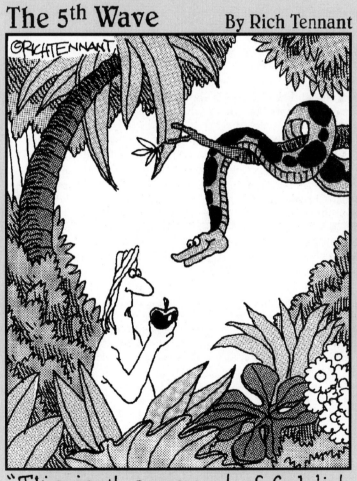

"This isn't some sort of fad diet,
is it?"

In this part . . .

*I*t's pretty obvious what should be included in the appendixes to a book about low-calorie dieting — calorie counts! And that's what you'll find in this part.

Calorie counts are presented in two different ways. In Appendix A, selected individual foods are listed in alphabetical order, along with amount and the number of calories in that amount of food. In Appendix B, foods are categorized into food groups, and one average calorie count is given for all the foods listed in each group. This is a less accurate but quick reference guide that might be a fairly easy way to remember approximate calorie counts when you don't have access to a more complete guide.

And last but not least, Appendix C features a handy metric conversion guide to use when you cook.

Appendix A

Calorie Counts of Select Foods

● ●

*I*n this appendix, you can find the calorie counts of many common foods. Knowing this information can help you make food substitutions when you're adapting the menus in Chapter 6 to your own personal taste or when you're adding foods to increase the number of calories you consume in a day.

I round all figures off to the nearest tenth. Calorie values for similar foods can vary widely, depending on the brand and size you use. Because of space constraints, you won't find every available food in this list. A great Web site that provides more complete information is www.nal.usda.gov/fnic/foodcomp/Data/SR18/nutrlist/sr18list.html. Scroll down to the row marked "Energy (calories)" and click on "A" for an alphabetized list of foods with calorie counts for common portion sizes.

This list can help you fill in calorie counts in your food diary and help you keep track of calories when planning your own menus.

Table A-1	Calorie Counts of Select Foods	
Food	*Amount*	*Calories*
Apple	1 medium	75
Applesauce, unsweetened	½ cup	55
Apricots, raw	1 apricot	15
Apricots, dried	10 halves	85
Artichoke	1 medium	60
Asparagus	4 spears	15
Avocado	1 ounce	45
Bacon	1 slice	35
Bacon, Canadian	1 slice	45

(continued)

Table A-1 (continued)

Food	Amount	Calories
Bagel	4 inch	245
Banana	1 medium	105
Barley, cooked	1/2 cup	95
Beans, baked	½ cup	120
Beans, green, cut-up, cooked	1 cup	45
Beans, kidney, navy, pinto, and so on	½ cup	115
Beef, ribs, cooked	3 ounces	305
Beef, round, cooked	3 ounces	175
Beef, top sirloin, lean only	3 ounces	150
Beets, cooked	½ cup	35
Biscuits, homemade	2 ½ inch	210
Blackberries, raw	1 cup	60
Blueberries	1 cup	85
Bologna	2 slices	175
Bread, banana	1 slice	195
Bread, cornbread	1 piece	180
Bread, cracked wheat	1 slice	65 to 80
Bread, Italian	1 slice	55
Bread, light	1 slice	40
Bread, pita	4 inch	77
Bread, pumpernickel	1 slice	75
Bread, raisin	1 slice	70
Bread, rye	1 slice	80
Bread, white	1 slice	65 to 80
Bread, whole-wheat	1 slice	70
Broccoli, cooked	1 cup	55
Brussels sprouts, cooked	1 cup	55
Butter	1 tablespoon	100

Food	Amount	Calories
Cabbage, cooked	1 cup	25
Cake, angel food	1 piece	70 to 130
Cake, chocolate with frosting	1 piece	235 to 340
Cake, white or yellow with frosting	1 piece	265 to 400
Candy, caramel	1 piece	40
Candy, chocolate covered peanuts	10 pieces	210
Candy, chocolate-covered raisins	10 pieces	40
Candy, jellybeans	10 large	105
Candy, marshmallows	1 cup	160
Candy, milk chocolate	1½ ounces	155
Carbonated beverage, cola	12 ounces	155
Carbonated beverage, ginger ale	12 ounces	125
Carrots, baby, raw	1 small	5
Carrots, cooked	1 cup	55
Carrot, raw	1 medium	30
Catsup	1 tablespoon	15
Cauliflower, cooked	1 cup	30
Celery	1 stalk	5
Cereal, cold	1 cup	110 to 210
Cereal, hot	1 cup	100 to 150
Cereal, rice, puffed	1 cup	50
Cereal, wheat, shredded	2 large biscuits	155
Cheese, American-style	1 ounce	105
Cheese, blue	1 ounce	100
Cheese, cheddar	1 ounce	115
Cheese, cottage, 1 percent fat	1 cup	165
Cheese, cream	1 tablespoon	50
Cheese, cream, fat-free	1 tablespoon	15

(continued)

Table A-1 *(continued)*

Food	Amount	Calories
Cheese, feta	1 ounce	75
Cheese, muenster	1 ounce	105
Cheese, Parmesan, grated	1 tablespoon	22
Cheesecake	1 piece	255
Cherries, fresh	20 cherries	85
Chicken, drumstick, cooked	3 ounces	150
Chicken, thigh, cooked	3 ounces	165
Chicken, white meat, cooked	3 ounces	140
Coconut, meat, raw	1 piece (45 g)	160
Coleslaw	1 cup	85
Collard greens, cooked	1 cup	55
Cookies, butter	1 small cookie	25
Cookies, chocolate chip	1 medium cookie	50 to 130
Cookie, fig bar	1 cookie	55
Cookie, graham cracker	2 squares	60
Cookie, oatmeal	1 medium cookie	65 to 115
Cookie, peanut butter	1 medium cookie	70 to 95
Corn, canned drained	1 cup	165
Crackers, matzo	1 matzo	110
Crackers, melba, plain	4 pieces	80
Crackers, standard	4 crackers	60
Cranberry juice cocktail	8 ounces	145
Cream, half-and-half	1 tablespoon	20
Cream, heavy whipping	1 tablespoon	52
Cream, light whipping	1 tablespoon	45
Croissant	1 croissant	230
Crabmeat	3 ounces	80
Crab, imitation, surimi	3 ounces	85

Food	Amount	Calories
Cucumber	1 large	45
Danish pastry, cheese or fruit	1 danish	265
Doughnut	1 doughnut	200 to 250
Doughnut hole	1 hole	50
Egg, white	1 large	17
Egg, whole	1 large	75
Eggplant, cooked	1 cup	35
Fish, cod	3 ounces	90
Fish, halibut	3 ounces	120 to 225
Fish, orange roughy	3 ounces	75
Fish, salmon, canned	3 ounces	120
Fish, salmon, smoked	3 ounces	100
Fish, salmon, sockeye, cooked	3 ounces	185
Fish, swordfish, cooked	3 ounces	130
Fish, tuna, fresh yellow fin, cooked	3 ounces	120
Fish, tuna, light canned in oil, drained	3 ounces	170
Fish, tuna, light canned in water, drained	3 ounces	99
Frankfurter, beef	1 frankfurter	150
Frankfurter, chicken	1 frankfurter	115
Fruit cocktail, canned in heavy syrup	1 cup	180
Fruit cocktail, canned in juice	1 cup	110
Grape juice	1 cup	130 to 155
Grapes	1 cup	110
Grapefruit juice	1 cup	95 to 115
Grapefruit, pink or white	½ grapefruit	40 to 50
Gravy, beef, canned	¼ cup	30
Gravy, chicken, canned	¼ cup	45
Gravy, mushroom, canned	¼ cup	30

(continued)

Table A-1 *(continued)*

Food	Amount	Calories
Ham, cured, baked	3 ounces	140
Ham, sliced	2 slices	90
Ham, extra-lean, sliced	2 slices	60
Honey	1 tablespoon	65
Hummus, commercial	1 tablespoon	23
Ice cream	½ cup	140 to 250
Jams and preserves	1 tablespoon	55
Kale, cooked	1 cup	35
Kiwi fruit	1 kiwi	45
Lamb, leg, roasted, lean only	3 ounces	160
Lamb, shoulder, braised, lean only	3 ounces	235
Leeks, cooked	1 cup	30
Lemonade, from frozen	1 cup	130
Lentils, cooked	1 cup	230
Lettuce	1 cup	10
Lima beans	½ cup	90
Macaroni, cooked	1 cup	195
Mango	1 mango	135
Margarine	1 tablespoon	100
Mayonnaise, regular	1 tablespoon	100
Melon, cantaloupe	1 cup	55
Melon, honeydew	1 cup	60
Milk, buttermilk	1 cup	100
Milk, chocolate, lowfat, commercial	1 cup	160
Milk, skim	1 cup	80
Milk, whole	1 cup	145
Miso	1 cup	137
Muffin, blueberry	1 standard	160

Food	Amount	Calories
Muffin, corn	1 standard	155
Muffin, English	1 standard	135
Muffin, oat bran	1 standard	155
Mushrooms, raw	1 cup	15
Mustard	1 tablespoon	10
Nectarine	1 medium	60
Noodles, egg, cooked	1 cup	213
Nuts, almonds	1 ounce (24 nuts)	165
Nuts, cashews	1 ounce (18 nuts)	165
Nuts, macadamia	1 ounce (11 nuts)	170
Nuts, pine	1 tablespoon	60
Nuts, pistachio	1 ounce (47 nuts)	161
Nuts, walnuts	1 ounce (14 halves)	185
Oat bran, raw	½ cup	115
Oil, olive or vegetable	1 tablespoon	120
Okra, cooked	1 cup	35
Onion, raw	1 medium onion	45
Onion, green, scallions	1 scallion	5
Onion rings, breaded	10 rings	245
Orange	1 medium	60
Orange juice	1 cup	110
Papaya	1 small	120
Peach	1 medium	40
Peanut butter	1 tablespoon	95
Peanuts, dry roasted or oil roasted	1 ounce (28 nuts)	165 to 170
Pear	1 pear	95
Pear, Asian	1 pear	50 to 115
Peas, green, from frozen	1 cup	125

(continued)

Table A-1 *(continued)*

Food	Amount	Calories
Peas, snow	1 cup	70
Peppers, sweet	1 pepper	25 to 30
Pickle, dill	1 pickle	12
Pie, cherry	1 slice	485
Pie, lemon meringue	1 slice	330
Pie, pecan	1 slice	503
Pineapple, fresh	1 cup	75
Plantain, cooked	1 cup	179
Plum	1 plum	30
Pomegranate	1 pomegranate	150
Pork, loin chop, lean meat	3 ounces	170
Popcorn, light	1 cup	30
Potato salad	1 cup	358
Potato, all-purpose, boiled	1 medium	120
Potato, russet, baked	1 medium	145
Potatoes, mashed with milk and butter	1 cup	235
Prunes, dried, cooked	½ cup	135
Prune juice	1 cup	182
Pudding, chocolate	½ cup	155
Pudding, vanilla	½ cup	145
Radishes	1 radish	1
Raisins	½ cup	215
Raspberries	1 cup	65
Rice, brown, cooked	1 cup	215
Rice, white, cooked	1 cup	205
Salad dressing, regular	1 tablespoon	45 to 75
Sauce, marinara	½ cup	95
Sauce, teriyaki	1 tablespoon	15

Food	Amount	Calories
Shellfish, crab, cooked	1 cup	120
Shellfish, crab, imitation (surimi)	4 ounces	110
Shellfish, scallops, steamed	8 large	45
Sherbet	½ cup	105
Soybeans (edamame)	1 cup	255
Spaghetti, cooked	1 cup	195
Spinach, cooked from frozen	1 cup	60
Squash, summer, cooked, all varieties	1 cup	35
Squash, winter, cooked, all varieties	1 cup	75 to 95
Strawberries	1 strawberry	5
Sugar, white granulated	1 teaspoon	15
Sunflower seeds, dry roasted	¼ cup	185
Sweet potato, baked	1 medium	130
Tangerine	1 medium	45
Tofu	¼ block	60
Tomato	1 tomato	25
Tortilla	1 large	100
Turkey, light and dark	3 ounces	130
Waffle, frozen	1 average	100
Watermelon	1 cup	45
Yogurt, plain, lowfat	8 ounces	145

Source: Adapted from the U.S. Department of Agriculture National Nutrient Database and from information provided by food manufacturers.

Appendix B

Calorie Counts by Food Groups

· ·

*T*his appendix groups foods together and provides approximate calorie counts for specific amounts of foods in each group. Each food, in the amount given, provides approximately the same number of calories. For instance, in the Grains and Starchy Vegetables group, ½ cup pasta has about the same number of calories as half of a 6-inch pita bread or ⅓ cup cooked lentils. Foods listed within the same food group can vary by 10 or 20 calories, which isn't a significant amount or anything you need to worry about when making substitutions within a group. This information is helpful when your focus is on portion control, rather than specific calorie counts of individual foods; it's also a quick and easy tool for low-calorie menu planning.

This quick-count method is less accurate than looking up the exact calories for each and every food (check out Appendix A for more precise counts and for calorie counts of many more individual foods), but it's still a valid way to take control of the amount of calories you consume. For one thing, knowing the approximate number of calories in a few food groups is a lot easier than trying to remember the specific calorie count of every food you eat. This method of calorie counting is similar to the exchange system used by commercial weight-loss groups, medically supervised weight-loss programs, and dietitians who teach portion control. Grouping together foods with similar calorie counts is the first step to understanding standard portion sizes for different types of foods and practicing portion control as a way of limiting your calories. See Chapter 3 for more details about portion control.

Vegetables

Each of these vegetables, measured raw in the amount shown, provides about 25 to 45 calories, depending on form and preparation.

Food	Amount
Artichoke, medium	½
Asparagus	1 cup
Avocado	⅛

(continued)

Food	Amount
Beans, green or wax	1 cup
Beets	1 cup
Broccoli	1 cup
Brussels sprouts	½ cup
Cabbage, raw	2 cups
Carrots	1 cup
Cauliflower	1 cup
Eggplant	1 cup
Greens, cooked: collard, kale, and so on	1 cup
Mushrooms	2 cups
Okra	1 cup
Onion	1 cup
Pea pods	1 cup
Plantain	½ cup
Radish	25 radishes
Spinach	2 cups
Tomato	1 large
Vegetable juice, canned or bottled	½ cup
Zucchini	2 cups

Fruits

Each of these fruits, in the amount shown, provides about 60 to 80 calories.

Food	Amount
Apple	1 small
Applesauce, unsweetened	½ cup
Apricot, fresh	4 medium

Food	Amount
Apricot, dried, and other dried fruit	5 to 7 halves
Banana	½ large
Blackberries	1 cup
Blueberries	¾ cup
Cherries	12
Figs, fresh	2
Fruit juice, canned or bottled	⅓ to ½ cup
Grapefruit	½
Grapes	15
Kiwi fruit	1½
Mandarin oranges, canned	¾ cup
Mango, small	½
Melon, cantaloupe or honeydew, cubes	1 cup
Nectarine	1 medium
Orange	1 medium
Papaya, cubes	1 cup
Peach	1 medium
Pear	1 small
Pineapple, fresh	¾ cup
Plum	2 medium
Pomegranate	½
Raisins	2 tablespoons
Raspberries	1 cup
Strawberries	1¼ cups
Tangerine	2 medium
Watermelon, cubes	1¼ cups

Proteins

These foods, in the amounts shown, provide about 55 to 75 calories.

Food	Amount
Beef, lean: rump roast, chuck steak, ground	1 ounce
Cold cuts and frankfurters (all regular varieties)	1 ounce
Egg	1 large
Fish, lean: Cod, flounder, sole, and so on	2 ounces
Fish, fatty: Salmon, mackerel, swordfish, and so on	1 ounce
Fish, shellfish: Crab, scallop, shrimp	½ cup
Lamb, lean: leg, roast, chop	1 ounce
Legumes, cooked (black beans, red beans, black eye beans, lentils, and so on)	⅓ cup
Peanut butter or other nut butters	1 tablespoon
Pork, lean: Loin, roast, chops	1 ounce
Poultry, chicken, or turkey, dark or light meat, pieces or ground	1 ounce
Shellfish	2 ounces
Tofu	1½ cups
Tuna, canned in oil, drained	1 ounce

Grains and Starchy Vegetables

Each of these foods, in the amount shown, provides approximately 80 calories.

Food	Amount
Bagel	⅓ medium (4-inch)
Bran cereal, concentrated	⅓ cup
Bread, regular	1 slice
Bread, light	1½ to 2 slices

Food	Amount
Breadstick (4 inch)	2
Cold cereal, average	½ to ¾ cup
Cold cereal, puffed	1½ cups
Cooked cereal	½ cup
Corn	½ cup
Corn	6-inch ear
Crackers, saltine	6
Crackers, crisp-bread	2 to 4 slices
English muffin	½
Pita bread (6 inches)	½
Popcorn, air-popped	3 cups
Pasta, cooked	½ cup
Peas, green	½ cup
Potato	1 small
Rice, cooked white or brown	⅓ cup
Roll, dinner	1 ounce
Squash, winter, mashed	1 cup
Sweet potato, mashed	⅓ cup
Tortilla, 6-inch	1
Waffle, 4½-inch square	1

Dairy Products

Each of these foods, in the amounts shown, provide about 100 calories.

Food	Amount
Cheese, hard or semi-soft	1 ounce
Milk, lowfat (1 percent)	¾ cup
Milk, skim	1 cup

(continued)

Food	Amount
Milk, whole	⅔ cup
Reduced-fat cheese, hard or semi-soft	1½ to 2 ounces
Yogurt, lowfat flavored	½ cup
Yogurt, lowfat plain	1 cup

Fats and High-Fat Foods

Each of these foods, in the amount shown, provides about 45 calories.

Food	Amount
Butter or margarine	1 teaspoon
Butter or margarine, reduced calorie	1 tablespoon
Cream, heavy whipping	1 tablespoon
Cream, light whipping	1 tablespoon
Cream cheese, fat-free	3 tablespoons
Cream cheese, regular	1 tablespoon
Mayonnaise	1 teaspoon
Mayonnaise, reduced-calorie	1 tablespoon
Oil, olive, peanut, or vegetable	1 teaspoon
Olives	5 large
Salad dressing, mayonnaise-type	2 teaspoons
Salad dressing, mayonnaise-type, reduced calorie	1 tablespoon

Appendix C

Metric Conversion Guide

∙ ∙

*N**ote:* The recipes in this book were not developed or tested using metric measures. There may be some variation in quality when converting to metric units.

Common Abbreviations

Abbreviation(s)	What It Stands For
C, c	cup
g	gram
kg	kilogram
L, l	liter
lb	pound
mL, ml	milliliter
oz	ounce
pt	pint
t, tsp	teaspoon
T, TB, Tbl, Tbsp	tablespoon

Volume

U.S. Units	Canadian Metric	Australian Metric
¼ teaspoon	1 milliliter	1 milliliter
½ teaspoon	2 milliliters	2 milliliters
1 teaspoon	5 milliliters	5 milliliters
1 tablespoon	15 milliliters	20 milliliters

(continued)

Volume *(continued)*

U.S. Units	Canadian Metric	Australian Metric
¼ cup	50 milliliters	60 milliliters
⅓ cup	75 milliliters	80 milliliters
½ cup	125 milliliters	125 milliliters
⅔ cup	150 milliliters	170 milliliters
¾ cup	175 milliliters	190 milliliters
1 cup	250 milliliters	250 milliliters
1 quart	1 liter	1 liter
1½ quarts	1.5 liters	1.5 liters
2 quarts	2 liters	2 liters
2½ quarts	2.5 liters	2.5 liters
3 quarts	3 liters	3 liters
4 quarts	4 liters	4 liters

Weight

U.S. Units	Canadian Metric	Australian Metric
1 ounce	30 grams	30 grams
2 ounces	55 grams	60 grams
3 ounces	85 grams	90 grams
4 ounces (¼ pound)	115 grams	125 grams
8 ounces (½ pound)	225 grams	225 grams
16 ounces (1 pound)	455 grams	500 grams
1 pound	455 grams	½ kilogram

Measurements

Inches	Centimeters
½	1.5
1	2.5

Inches	Centimeters
2	5.0
3	7.5
4	10.0
5	12.5
6	15.0
7	17.5
8	20.5
9	23.0
10	25.5
11	28.0
12	30.5
13	33.0

Temperature (Degrees)

Fahrenheit	Celsius
32	0
212	100
250	120
275	140
300	150
325	160
350	180
375	190
400	200
425	220
450	230
475	240
500	260

Index

USINESS, CAREERS & PERSONAL FINANCE

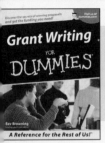

0-7645-5307-0   0-7645-5331-3 *†

Also available:
- Accounting For Dummies †
  0-7645-5314-3
- Business Plans Kit For Dummies †
  0-7645-5365-8
- Cover Letters For Dummies
  0-7645-5224-4
- Frugal Living For Dummies
  0-7645-5403-4
- Leadership For Dummies
  0-7645-5176-0
- Managing For Dummies
  0-7645-1771-6

- Marketing For Dummies
  0-7645-5600-2
- Personal Finance For Dummies *
  0-7645-2590-5
- Project Management For Dummies
  0-7645-5283-X
- Resumes For Dummies †
  0-7645-5471-9
- Selling For Dummies
  0-7645-5363-1
- Small Business Kit For Dummies *†
  0-7645-5093-4

OME & BUSINESS COMPUTER BASICS

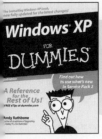 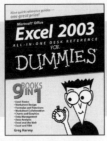

0-7645-4074-2   0-7645-3758-X

Also available:
- ACT! 6 For Dummies
  0-7645-2645-6
- iLife '04 All-in-One Desk Reference
  For Dummies
  0-7645-7347-0
- iPAQ For Dummies
  0-7645-6769-1
- Mac OS X Panther Timesaving
  Techniques For Dummies
  0-7645-5812-9
- Macs For Dummies
  0-7645-5656-8

- Microsoft Money 2004 For Dummies
  0-7645-4195-1
- Office 2003 All-in-One Desk Reference
  For Dummies
  0-7645-3883-7
- Outlook 2003 For Dummies
  0-7645-3759-8
- PCs For Dummies
  0-7645-4074-2
- TiVo For Dummies
  0-7645-6923-6
- Upgrading and Fixing PCs For Dummies
  0-7645-1665-5
- Windows XP Timesaving Techniques
  For Dummies
  0-7645-3748-2

OD, HOME, GARDEN, HOBBIES, MUSIC & PETS

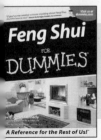 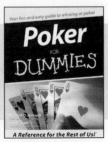

0-7645-5295-3   0-7645-5232-5

Also available:
- Bass Guitar For Dummies
  0-7645-2487-9
- Diabetes Cookbook For Dummies
  0-7645-5230-9
- Gardening For Dummies *
  0-7645-5130-2
- Guitar For Dummies
  0-7645-5106-X
- Holiday Decorating For Dummies
  0-7645-2570-0
- Home Improvement All-in-One
  For Dummies
  0-7645-5680-0

- Knitting For Dummies
  0-7645-5395-X
- Piano For Dummies
  0-7645-5105-1
- Puppies For Dummies
  0-7645-5255-4
- Scrapbooking For Dummies
  0-7645-7208-3
- Senior Dogs For Dummies
  0-7645-5818-8
- Singing For Dummies
  0-7645-2475-5
- 30-Minute Meals For Dummies
  0-7645-2589-1

TERNET & DIGITAL MEDIA

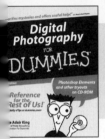 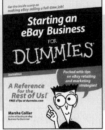

0-7645-1664-7   0-7645-6924-4

Also available:
- 2005 Online Shopping Directory
  For Dummies
  0-7645-7495-7
- CD & DVD Recording For Dummies
  0-7645-5956-7
- eBay For Dummies
  0-7645-5654-1
- Fighting Spam For Dummies
  0-7645-5965-6
- Genealogy Online For Dummies
  0-7645-5964-8
- Google For Dummies
  0-7645-4420-9

- Home Recording For Musicians
  For Dummies
  0-7645-1634-5
- The Internet For Dummies
  0-7645-4173-0
- iPod & iTunes For Dummies
  0-7645-7772-7
- Preventing Identity Theft For Dummies
  0-7645-7336-5
- Pro Tools All-in-One Desk Reference
  For Dummies
  0-7645-5714-9
- Roxio Easy Media Creator For Dummies
  0-7645-7131-1

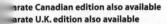

arate Canadian edition also available
arate U.K. edition also available

ble wherever books are sold. For more information or to order direct: U.S. customers visit www.dummies.com or call 1-877-762-2974.
stomers visit www.wileyeurope.com or call 0800 243407. Canadian customers visit www.wiley.ca or call 1-800-567-4797.

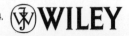

SPORTS, FITNESS, PARENTING, RELIGION & SPIRITUALITY

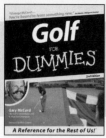
0-7645-5146-9

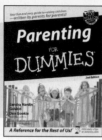
0-7645-5418-2

Also available:

- Adoption For Dummies
  0-7645-5488-3
- Basketball For Dummies
  0-7645-5248-1
- The Bible For Dummies
  0-7645-5296-1
- Buddhism For Dummies
  0-7645-5359-3
- Catholicism For Dummies
  0-7645-5391-7
- Hockey For Dummies
  0-7645-5228-7

- Judaism For Dummies
  0-7645-5299-6
- Martial Arts For Dummies
  0-7645-5358-5
- Pilates For Dummies
  0-7645-5397-6
- Religion For Dummies
  0-7645-5264-3
- Teaching Kids to Read For Dummies
  0-7645-4043-2
- Weight Training For Dummies
  0-7645-5168-X
- Yoga For Dummies
  0-7645-5117-5

TRAVEL

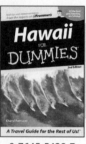
0-7645-5438-7

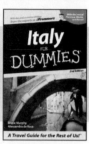
0-7645-5453-0

Also available:

- Alaska For Dummies
  0-7645-1761-9
- Arizona For Dummies
  0-7645-6938-4
- Cancún and the Yucatán For Dummies
  0-7645-2437-2
- Cruise Vacations For Dummies
  0-7645-6941-4
- Europe For Dummies
  0-7645-5456-5
- Ireland For Dummies
  0-7645-5455-7

- Las Vegas For Dummies
  0-7645-5448-4
- London For Dummies
  0-7645-4277-X
- New York City For Dummies
  0-7645-6945-7
- Paris For Dummies
  0-7645-5494-8
- RV Vacations For Dummies
  0-7645-5443-3
- Walt Disney World & Orlando For Dumm
  0-7645-6943-0

GRAPHICS, DESIGN & WEB DEVELOPMENT

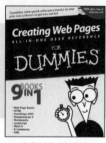
0-7645-4345-8

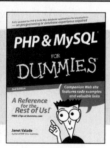
0-7645-5589-8

Also available:

- Adobe Acrobat 6 PDF For Dummies
  0-7645-3760-1
- Building a Web Site For Dummies
  0-7645-7144-3
- Dreamweaver MX 2004 For Dummies
  0-7645-4342-3
- FrontPage 2003 For Dummies
  0-7645-3882-9
- HTML 4 For Dummies
  0-7645-1995-6
- Illustrator CS For Dummies
  0-7645-4084-X

- Macromedia Flash MX 2004 For Dumm
  0-7645-4358-X
- Photoshop 7 All-in-One Desk
  Reference For Dummies
  0-7645-1667-1
- Photoshop CS Timesaving Technique
  For Dummies
  0-7645-6782-9
- PHP 5 For Dummies
  0-7645-4166-8
- PowerPoint 2003 For Dummies
  0-7645-3908-6
- QuarkXPress 6 For Dummies
  0-7645-2593-X

NETWORKING, SECURITY, PROGRAMMING & DATABASES

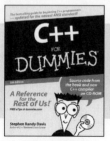
0-7645-6852-3

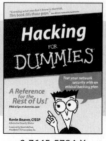
0-7645-5784-X

Also available:

- A+ Certification For Dummies
  0-7645-4187-0
- Access 2003 All-in-One Desk
  Reference For Dummies
  0-7645-3988-4
- Beginning Programming For Dummies
  0-7645-4997-9
- C For Dummies
  0-7645-7068-4
- Firewalls For Dummies
  0-7645-4048-3
- Home Networking For Dummies
  0-7645-42796

- Network Security For Dummies
  0-7645-1679-5
- Networking For Dummies
  0-7645-1677-9
- TCP/IP For Dummies
  0-7645-1760-0
- VBA For Dummies
  0-7645-3989-2
- Wireless All In-One Desk Reference
  For Dummies
  0-7645-7496-5
- Wireless Home Networking For Dumm
  0-7645-3910-8